General Practice at a Glance

Dedication

We dedicate this book to Dr Grant Blair, gifted GP teacher and inspirational colleague and friend, who died during the production of this book.

This title is also available as an e-book.
For more details, please see www.wiley.com/buy/9780470655511
or scan this QR code:

General Practice at a Glance

Paul Booton

Professor of General Practice and Primary Care
St George's, University of London
Formerly Director of Primary Care Education, Imperial College
London
General Practitioner, London

Carol Cooper

Honorary Teaching Fellow
Department of Primary Care and Public Health
Imperial College Medical School, London
General Practitioner, London

Graham Easton

Deputy Director of Primary Care Education
Department of Primary Care and Public Health
Imperial College Medical School, London
General Practitioner, London

Margaret Harper

Honorary Teaching Fellow
Department of Primary Care and Public Health
Imperial College Medical School, London
General Practitioner, London

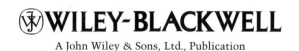
WILEY-BLACKWELL

A John Wiley & Sons, Ltd., Publication

This edition first published 2013 © 2013 by Paul Booton, Carol Cooper, Graham Easton, and Margaret Harper

Wiley-Blackwell is an imprint of John Wiley & Sons, formed by the merger of Wiley's global Scientific, Technical and Medical business with Blackwell Publishing.

Registered office: John Wiley & Sons, Ltd, The Atrium, Southern Gate, Chichester, West Sussex, PO19 8SQ, UK

Editorial offices: 9600 Garsington Road, Oxford, OX4 2DQ, UK
The Atrium, Southern Gate, Chichester, West Sussex, PO19 8SQ, UK
350 Main Street, Malden, MA 02148-5020, USA
2121 State Avenue, Ames, Iowa 50014-8300, USA
111 River Street, Hoboken, NJ 07030-5774, USA

For details of our global editorial offices, for customer services and for information about how to apply for permission to reuse the copyright material in this book please see our website at www.wiley.com/wiley-blackwell.

Library of Congress Cataloging-in-Publication Data is available

A catalogue record for this book is available from the British Library.

Wiley also publishes its books in a variety of electronic formats. Some content that appears in print may not be available in electronic books.

Cover design: Meaden Creative
Illustrations: Graeme Chambers

Set in 9/11.5 pt Times by Toppan Best-set Premedia Limited
Printed and bound in Malaysia by Vivar Printing Sdn Bhd

2   2014

Contents

Contributors

Cressida Amiel
Academic Trainee in Primary Care
Imperial College London
General Practitioner, London

Joanne Athos
Senior Clinical Teaching Fellow
Imperial College London
General Practitioner, London

Catherine Baudains
Academic Trainee in Primary Care
Imperial College London
General Practitioner, London

Grant Blair
Honorary Senior Clinical Lecturer
Imperial College London
General Practitioner, London

Sipra Guha
Honorary Senior Clinical Lecturer
Imperial College London
General Practitioner, London

Oliver Hart
General Practitioner, Sheffield

Rosalind Herbert
Senior Clinical Teaching Fellow
Imperial College London
General Practitioner, London

Richard Hooker
Honorary Senior Clinical Lecturer
Imperial College London
General Practitioner, London

Stella Major
Associate Professor of Family Medicine
United Arab Emirates University
Honorary Senior Clinical Lecturer
Imperial College London

Jan Maniera
Honorary Senior Clinical Lecturer
Imperial College London
General Practitioner, London

Emma Metters
Academic Trainee in Primary Care
Imperial College London
General Practitioner, London

Aisha Newth
Senior Clinical Teaching Fellow
Imperial College London
General Practitioner, London

Sian Powell
Senior Clinical Teaching Fellow
Imperial College London
General Practitioner, London

Adrian Raby
Clinical Lecturer in Medical Ethics and Law
Imperial College London
General Practitioner, London

Sarvesh Saini
Senior Clinical Teaching Fellow
Imperial College London
General Practitioner, London

Sonia Saxena
Senior Lecturer in Primary Care
Imperial College London
General Practitioner, London

Edward Shaoul
Honorary Senior Clinical Lecturer
Imperial College London
General Practitioner, London

James Stratford-Martin
Senior Clinical Teaching Fellow
Imperial College London
General Practitioner, London

Vineet Thapar
Associate Director
Postgraduate GP Specialty Training
London Deanery
General Practitioner, London

Anju Verma
Clinical Teaching Fellow
Imperial College London
General Practitioner, London

Anna Whiteford
Undergraduate GP Teacher
Imperial College London
General Practitioner, Hertfordshire

Bronwen Williams
Academic Trainee in Primary Care
Imperial College London
General Practitioner, London

Preface

General practice has seen huge changes in recent years as more medical care moves into the community. As a result, medical students and junior doctors are spending much more time in general practice – not just to find out about the specialty but to give them the clinical experience they need.

This book attempts to meet those challenges in a relevant, clear and concise 'at-a-glance' way. The book is not a dumbed-down version of hospital management. It's about the unique approach of general practice, where unsorted problems are the staple diet. Here GPs rely on clinical skills rather than huge scanners, and you as the student can understand what is being done and why.

The book focuses on key topics that commonly arise in general practice. It uses a symptom-based approach: patients don't complain of COPD or heart failure, they say they are breathless. Most of the ailments are common everyday conditions, but importantly our book includes rare conditions that must not be missed. 'Red flags' are a key feature. The book makes use of the relevant guidelines to ensure students are kept abreast of current thinking in clinical management. The chapters are written by working GPs, the majority of whom are linked to the academic department of primary care at London's Imperial College Medical School. We believe this combination gives students hands-on practical advice informed by the best available evidence for practice. There are resources and further reading at the back of the book, which is not simply a dry list of references but a wide range of resources including websites to enhance your learning and broaden your horizons.

For medical students, time spent in primary care is a golden opportunity to meet and assess patients with a huge range of medical problems who present a real diagnostic challenge. It's also a chance to see how structured medical care can provide excellent management of chronic diseases and how the primary care team link together to deliver care across the practice patch. General practice is also the ideal place to acquire skills such as focused history-taking and thinking on your feet, skills that will serve you well in any field of practice. If you become a specialist, you'll also find it helpful to be familiar with what happens to your patients before they are referred to you and after you discharge them. This is your guide book to those opportunities. When it comes to your exams, you will find it a useful revision tool. Furthermore, we hope it opens the 'art and mystery' of general practice to foundation and specialty trainees in general practice and to practice nurses and other clinical staff who need a concise summary of clinical primary care.

Paul Booton
Carol Cooper
Graham Easton
Margaret Harper

Acknowledgements

In addition to sources shown in individual figures, there are some figures from Wiley-Blackwell texts.

Chapter 17 Childhood rashes
Pictures of ammoniacal dermatitis, *Candida* nappy rash, seborrhoeic nappy rash, measles, fifth disease, scarlet fever, Henoch–Schönlein purpura, herpes simplex (cold sores), impetigo and molluscum contagiosum from *Paediatrics at a Glance*, 3rd edition. Lawrence Miall, Mary Rudolf and Dominic Smith. © 2012 John Wiley & Sons, Ltd. Published 2012 by John Wiley & Sons, Ltd.

Pictures of strawberry naevus (haemangioma), portwine stain, meningococcal septicaemia and ITP from *Paediatrics at a Glance*, 2nd edition. Lawrence Miall, Mary Rudolf and Malcolm Levene. © 2007 Lawrence Miall, Mary Rudolf and Malcolm Levene. Published 2007 by Blackwell Publishing Ltd.

Picture of chickenpox from *Textbook of Pediatric Dermatology*, 2nd edition. J. Harper, A. Oranje and N.S. Prose. Published 2006 by Blackwell Publishing Ltd., Oxford.

Chapter 19 Musculoskeletal problems in children
pGALS figure used by kind permission of Arthritis Research UK (www.arthritisresearchuk.org) from: pGALS – A screening examination of the musculoskeletal system in school-aged children. Reports on the Rheumatic Diseases (Series 5), Hands On 15. H. Foster and S. Jandial. Arthritis Research Campaign; 2008 June.

Chapter 20 Common sexual problems
Picture of vacuum device or pump from *ABC of Sexual Health*, 2nd edition. John Tomlinson (Editor). © 2005 Blackwell Publishing Ltd. BMJ Books.

Chapter 21 Sexually transmitted infections and HIV
Pictures of common STIs from *ABC of Sexually Transmitted Infections*, 6th edition. Edited by Karen E. Rogstad. © 2011 Blackwell Publishing Ltd. Published 2011 by Blackwell Publishing Ltd.

Chapter 36 Peripheral vascular disease and leg ulcers
Pictures 36b–d from *ABC of Arterial and Venous Disease*, 2nd edition. Richard Donnelly and Nick J.M. London (Editors). © 2009 Blackwell Publishing Ltd. BMJ Books.

Chapter 52 Ear symptoms
Picture of normal ear, nasal polyposis, skin prick test from *ABC of Ear, Nose and Throat*, 5th edition. Harold S. Ludman and Patrick Bradley (Editors). © 2007 Blackwell Publishing Ltd. BMJ Books.

Chapter 55 Eczema, psoriasis
Pictures of eczema, psoriasis, basal cell carcinoma and keratoses from *Lecture Notes: Dermatology*, 10th edition. © R.A.C. Graham-Brown and D.A. Burns. Published 2011 by Blackwell Publishing Ltd.

Picture of malignant melanoma and squamous cell carcinoma from *ABC of Skin Cancer*. S. Rapjar and J. Marsden. © 2008 by Blackwell Publishing Ltd. BMJ Books.

Chapter 56 Other skin problems
Pictures of acne, acne rosacea, seborrhoeic dermatitis, pityriasis rosea, fungal infection, tinea corporis, warts, molluscum and shingles from *Lecture Notes: Dermatology*, 10th edition. © R.A.C. Graham-Brown and D.A. Burns. Published 2011 by Blackwell Publishing Ltd.

Pictures of pityriasis versicolor and scabies from *ABC of Dermatology*, 5th edition. Paul K. Buxton and Rachael Morris-Jones (Editors). © 2009 Blackwell Publishing Ltd. BMJ Books.

Picture of herpes simplex (cold sores) from *Paediatrics at a Glance*, 3rd edition. Lawrence Miall, Mary Rudolf and Dominic Smith. © 2012 John Wiley & Sons, Ltd. Published 2012 by John Wiley & Sons, Ltd.

Chapter 65 Allergy and hay fever
From *ABC of Ear, Nose and Throat*, 5th edition. Harold S. Ludman and Patrick Bradley (Editors). © 2007 Blackwell Publishing Ltd. BMJ Books.

Key to symbol used in the text

► A red flag indicates symptoms, signs or investigations which point to serious conditions that must not be missed.

Abbreviations

AAG	acute angle glaucoma
A&E	accident and emergency department
ABCD2	age, blood pressure, clinical features, duration and diabetes risk scoring system
ABPI	Ankle–Brachial Pressure Index
ACE	angiotensin-converting enzyme
ADHD	attention deficit hyperactivity disorder
AOM	acute otitis media
APH	antepartum haemorrhage
APS	antiphospholipid syndrome
ARB	angiotensin-receptor blocker
ARMD	age-related macular degeneration
AST	aspartate aminotransferase
BASHH	British Association for Sexual Health and HIV
BCC	basal cell carcinoma
b.d.	twice daily
BMI	body mass index
BNF	British National Formulary
BP	blood pressure
BPH	benign prostatic hyperplasia
BRAO	branch retinal artery occlusion
BTS	British Thoracic Society
CAMHS	Child and Adolescent Mental Health Service
CBT	cognitive behavioural therapy
CBT-BN	cognitive behavioural therapy for bulimia nervosa
CCDC	Consultant in Communicable Disease Control
CCP	cyclic citrullinated peptide
CHPP	Child Health Promotion Programme
CMHT	community mental health team
CNS	central nervous system
COCP	combined oral contraceptive pill
COPD	chronic obstructive pulmonary disease
CPA	care programme approach
CPAP	continuous positive airways pressure
CPN	community psychiatric nurse
CRAO	central retinal artery occlusion
CRP	C-reactive protein
CSF	cerebrospinal fluid
CT	computerised tomography
CTS	carpal tunnel syndrome
CVA	cerebrovascular accident
CVD	cardiovascular disease
DCIS	ductal carcinoma *in situ*
DDH	developmental dysplasia of the hip
DEXA	dual energy X-ray absorptiometry
DJD	degenerative joint disease
DMARD	disease-modifying anti-rheumatic drug
DRE	digital rectal examination
DVLA	Driver and Vehicle Licensing Agency
DVT	deep vein thrombosis
ECG	electrocardiography/electrocardiogram
ED	erectile dysfunction
EDD	expected date of delivery
EEG	electroencephalography/electroencephalogram
eGFR	estimated glomerular filtration rate
EMS	early morning stiffness
ENT	ear, nose and throat
EPU	Early Pregnancy Unit
ESR	erythrocyte sedimentation rate
FAST	Face, Arm, Speech Test
FB	foreign body
FBC	full blood count
FSH	follicle-stimulating hormone
GAD	generalised anxiety disorder
GC	gonococcus
GCA	giant-cell arteritis
GDM	gestational diabetes
GGT	gamma-glutamyl transpepstdase
GLP	glucagon-like peptide
GOR	gastro-oesophageal reflux
GORD	gastro-oesophageal reflux disease
GPSI	GP with a special interest
GUM	genito-urinary medicine
Hb	haemoglobin
hCG	human chorionic gonadotrophin
HDL	high density lipoprotein
HELLP	(syndrome characterised by) haemolysis, elevated liver enzyme levels and low platelet count
HiB	*Haemophilus influenzae* type B
HIV	human immunodeficiency virus
HPV	human papilloma virus
HRT	hormone replacement therapy
HSV	herpes simplex virus
HVS	high vaginal swab
IBD	inflammatory bowel disease
IBS	irritable bowel syndrome
IgE	immunoglobulin E
IPSS	International Prostate Symptom Score
ITP	idiopathic thrombocytopenic purpura
IUD	intrauterine device
IUS	intrauterine system
JIA	juvenile idiopathic arthritis
JVP	jugular venous pressure
LCIS	lobular carcinoma *in situ*
LDL	low density lipoprotein
LFT	liver function test
LH	luteinising hormone
LMP	last menstrual period
MCA	Mental Capacity Act 2007
MCV	mean cell volume
MI	myocardial infarction
MMR	measles, mumps and rubella
MMSE	Mini Mental State Examination
MRI	magnetic resonance imaging
MSU	mid stream urine (test)
NICE	National Institute for Clinical Excellence
NSAID	non-steroidal anti-inflammatory drug
NSU	non-specific urethritis
OCP	oral contraceptive pill
o.d.	once daily

OSA	obstructive sleep apnoea (syndrome)	**SIDS**	sudden infant death syndrome
OTC	over-the-counter	**SMR**	standardised mortality ratio
PCOS	polycystic ovary syndrome	**SPF**	sun protection factor
PD	panic disorder	**SSRI**	selective serotonin reuptake inhibitor
PEFR	peak expiratory flow rate	**STI**	sexually transmitted infection
PID	pelvic inflammatory disease	**SVT**	supraventricular tachycardia
pMDI	metered dose inhaler	**T1D**	type 1 diabetes
PMH	past medical history	**T2D**	type 2 diabetes
PMR	polymyalgia rheumatica	**TB**	tuberculosis
PMS	premenstrual syndrome	**TENS**	transcutaneous electrical nerve stimulation
POAG	primary/chronic open angle glaucoma	**TFT**	thyroid function test
POP	progestogen-only pill	**TG**	triglycerides
PPI	proton pump inhibitor	**TIA**	transient ischaemic attack
PSA	prostate specific antigen	**TSH**	thyroid stimulating hormone
PUVA	psoralen with ultraviolet A (treatment)	**U&E**	urea and electrolytes
QOF	Quality and Outcomes Framework	**URTI**	upper respiratory tract infection
RA	rheumatoid arthritis	**UTI**	urinary tract infection
RBC	red blood cell	**VA**	visual acuity
ROM	range of movement	**VDU**	visual display unit
RR	respiratory rate	**VEGF**	vascular endothelial growth factor
RSI	repetitive strain injury	**VUR**	vesico-ureteric reflux
RSV	respiratory syncytial virus	**WCC**	white cell count
SCC	squamous cell carcinoma	**WHO**	World Health Organization
SEA	significant event analysis		

Introduction: how to make the most of your GP attachment

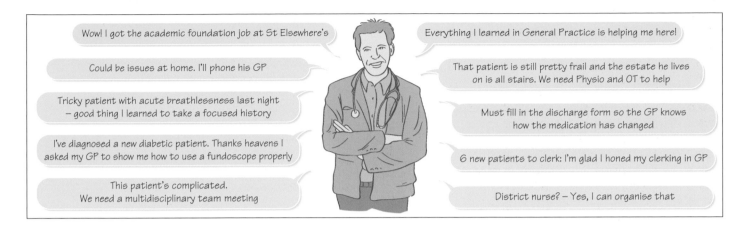

'What you do in general practice is refer patients with serious problems and get rid of the trivia' (medical student about to start a GP attachment). If only life were so simple . . .

General practice gives you opportunities to work with patients, doctors and the primary care team in ways which it may be difficult or impossible to find elsewhere in your undergraduate training.

Opportunities with patients

• **Unsorted problems.** Most patients come with a problem, not a diagnosis. This is a prime opportunity to talk to patients who do not yet have a diagnosis and hone your diagnostic acumen.
• **Learn to take a focused history.** There is probably no better place to practise taking a focused history than primary care.
• **Management.** Planning management with patients with relatively simple problems is an ideal place to start thinking through management issues, gets you into the habit of integrating management thinking into your clerkings and gives you practice negotiating your plan with the patient.
• **Patients at home.** Visiting patients at home gives a much broader insight into their lives and what makes them and their families tick. It provides a chance to see how people live with their illness, in their home with their family and in their own community.

Opportunities with doctors

• **One-to-one.** Generally, you will be attached to a practice individually or in pairs, usually with one tutor taking main responsibility for you. There will be few other opportunities in your career for such a close learning relationship.
• **Looking after your learning needs.** This is a great time to think about your personal learning needs and to set yourself some goals. Am I confident using an ophthalmoscope? Can I examine the cranial nerves? One-to-one sessions with your GP tutor are a great opportunity to look at your personal learning needs and find ways to address them. The tutor may be able to find you a patient with the problem you want to explore – diabetic eye changes, aortic stenosis.
• **Get feedback.** Such a close working relationship is ideal for gaining worthwhile feedback on your performance. Ask for feedback if it is not offered.

Opportunities with the primary care team

• **Multidisciplinary learning.** You'll probably work with different members of the primary care team during your attachment. It is an opportunity to see the different skills that different disciplines bring and how the team relate to each other and work together.
• **Being where healthcare happens.** Most patients' problems are dealt with in primary care, by the doctor, by the practice team or by the wider community team. Whichever branch of medicine you go into it is crucial to understand how care is delivered in the community. This is even more important if you end up as a hospital doctor as your GP attachment is often your only opportunity to see life beyond hospital (although if you are lucky you may get a 4-month foundation post in general practice).

What can you do

Be organised. Turn up when you are meant to and be on time (this may mean leaving home too early the first day, just to be sure).

Be enthusiastic. Get stuck in to the different opportunities offered (even if you don't see the relevance initially) – people are far more keen to help someone who shows enthusiasm.

Be realistic. Set goals for yourself that are realistic and that you can meet in this setting.

Be an ambassador. Create a good impression at the practice and they will not only be keen to help you, but keen to take future students.

Ask questions. Always ask questions. Don't be intimidated when those questions seem very basic or if everyone else seems to know the answers.

Deal with problems. If you find a problem getting to work or are going to be late let the practice know straight away. Clinics will often have been arranged specially for your benefit. If there is a problem with the practice (your tutor makes a pass at you, the practice is being run by locums and no-one knows why you are there) get in touch with the GP team at the medical school straight away. If the practice problem can't be quickly fixed they will move you to a new practice. If you wait till the attachment has finished there is little anyone can do to help.

1 The 10-minute consultation: taking a history

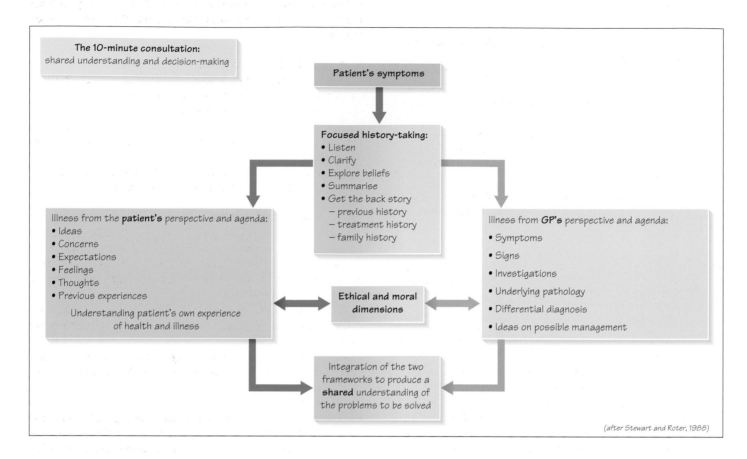

The 10-minute consultation:
shared understanding and decision-making

Patient's symptoms

Focused history-taking:
- Listen
- Clarify
- Explore beliefs
- Summarise
- Get the back story
  - previous history
  - treatment history
  - family history

Illness from the patient's perspective and agenda:
- Ideas
- Concerns
- Expectations
- Feelings
- Thoughts
- Previous experiences

Understanding patient's own experience
of health and illness

Ethical and moral dimensions

Illness from GP's perspective and agenda:
- Symptoms
- Signs
- Investigations
- Underlying pathology
- Differential diagnosis
- Ideas on possible management

Integration of the two
frameworks to produce a
shared understanding of
the problems to be solved

(after Stewart and Roter, 1988)

At finals you could spend 20–40 minutes clerking your patient. So how can a 10-minute consultation in general practice produce an adequate assessment?

- Continuity of care means the patient and their history are often familiar.
- The 10-minute consultation is an average. A quick consultation, like a repeat medication request, saves time which can be spent on trickier problems.
- You don't need to do everything in one consultation. It can help to watch a problem develop over several visits.
- Making diagnoses is honed through practice, enabling GPs to recognise patterns of illness quickly. This is not 'taking short-cuts': it's about the expertise to focus on key areas.

As a student, don't rush to assess a patient in 10 minutes. Take the time you need to understand your patient's problem fully. Speed comes with experience.

What's the difference between a focused history and a traditional one?

- Traditional history-taking is useful when you first learn to interview patients as it teaches you a structure and a list of questions to ask.
- You'll notice senior doctors often ask surprisingly few questions, yet get a better view of the problem.

- This 'focused history' requires judgement about what to explore and what to set aside. Judgement is based on many things including knowledge and experience.
- Learning focused history-taking is an important transition between student and doctor. General practice is the ideal setting to practise this because you will see many undiagnosed patients on whom to hone your skills.

Focused history-taking in a nutshell
Listen

- *'What can I do for you today?'* Students often hope to save time by getting straight to the point with direct questions. The opposite happens. You get a better foundation for exploring the problem if you give the patient the time to tell their story from their perspective: start with an open question and then listen.
- The *'golden minute'* (give the patient a minute to speak without interruption) gives your patient time to frame their problem in their own way.
- *'Go on . . . tell me more . . .'* If the patient falters, encourage them to carry on. Use non-verbal encouragement through head nodding and eye contact.
- *'You were saying the pain is worse at night . . .'* Reflection can get help your patient going again.

General Practice at a Glance, First Edition. Paul Booton, Carol Cooper, Graham Easton, and Margaret Harper.

• Don't fear *silence,* particularly in emotionally charged situations. Give the patient space to formulate their thoughts.

Clarify

• *'When were you last completely well?'* Establish the timetable of the patient's symptoms.
• *'Can you describe the pain?'* Analyse each symptom. Mnemonics can help, such as SOCRATES: Site, Onset, Character, Radiation, Associated factors, Timescale, Exacerbating/relieving factors, Severity.
• *'What do you mean by indigestion?'* Understand what the patient means, especially if they use medical terms. 'Migraine' often means 'bad headache', 'blood pressure' may mean dizziness, headaches or almost anything else.
• Ask *red flag* questions to detect serious underlying conditions. In back pain, ask about incontinence and urinary problems, history of cancer and TB.

Explore beliefs

• *'What are your thoughts about this?'* The patient may have a very good idea of their diagnosis, 'It's just the same as my aunt had.' Equally, they may have a very misleading idea, 'This website said it's typical of *Candida* infection.' Knowing your patients' **ideas** may help you diagnostically, or help your patients away from incorrect formulations.
• *'In your darkest moments what do you think this might be?'* Look for hidden agendas and explore your patients' **concerns**. Patients with headaches often worry about brain tumours or meningitis. They rarely volunteer this for fear of looking foolish, maybe because they're afraid they may be right. Your diagnosis and treatment may be spot on, but if you haven't uncovered these concerns and put your patient's mind at rest, you send away a worried patient.
• *'What are you hoping we can do?'* What are your patient's **expectations** for treatment. When you come to plan management, taking your patient's expectations on board will help you achieve **concordance** with your patient (see Chapter 2).
• Above all, don't try to guess what your patient is thinking. There's no point reassuring your patient about something that never worried them. Their real concerns (which might seem bizarre to you or to the next patient) may be life and death to them.

Summarise

'Let me see if I've got this right . . .' Once you have grasped the patient's problem, summarise it back. This checks your own understanding, and reassures the patient that they've been understood.

The past medical history

• The past medical history is essential background to the presenting problem. The GP may not need to explore it in a familiar patient, or if the records are to hand.
• *'Have you had any serious illnesses?'* *'Have you seen a specialist or been in hospital?'* Don't list random diseases, ask general questions about the past, and . . .
• Ask specific questions relevant to the presenting complaint. Ask *'Ever had migraine?'* to the patient with headaches.

The treatment history

• *'Can you bring all your medicines to the surgery with you?'* Drug side effects and interactions cause huge amounts of iatrogenic illness and many hospital admissions. A secure drug history will allow you to spot current problems and prevent your own prescribing causing future ones.
• The drug history is a back door route to past medical history. You may only discover that your patient is hypertensive from the drug history.
• Ask about over-the-counter drugs and recreational drugs. Remember, the most important of these are alcohol and tobacco.

Family history

Enquire about illness in relatives rather than a list of conditions. Ask for anything that has come up as a possibility in the patient's history – like diabetes in the family of a patient presenting with thirst and weight loss.

Where next?

From the history you should now have a good idea of what's going on. If you haven't, sit back and think what else you need to fill out the picture. Use the history to make sure you find out all you need to help you make a diagnosis and plan management. If that takes time, it's time well spent. Remember 80% of diagnoses are made on the history and in many conditions (e.g. epilepsy, migraine) a secure diagnosis can only be made from the history, so use it well.

The 10-minute consultation: managing your patient

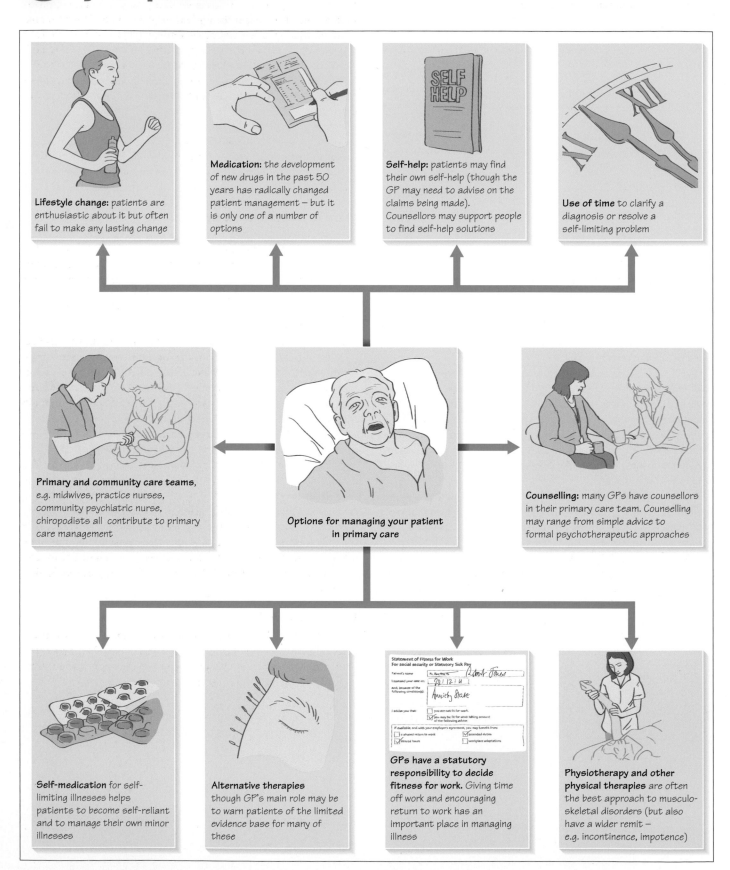

Lifestyle change: patients are enthusiastic about it but often fail to make any lasting change

Medication: the development of new drugs in the past 50 years has radically changed patient management – but it is only one of a number of options

Self-help: patients may find their own self-help (though the GP may need to advise on the claims being made). Counsellors may support people to find self-help solutions

Use of time to clarify a diagnosis or resolve a self-limiting problem

Primary and community care teams, e.g. midwives, practice nurses, community psychiatric nurse, chiropodists all contribute to primary care management

Options for managing your patient in primary care

Counselling: many GPs have counsellors in their primary care team. Counselling may range from simple advice to formal psychotherapeutic approaches

Self-medication for self-limiting illnesses helps patients to become self-reliant and to manage their own minor illnesses

Alternative therapies though GP's main role may be to warn patients of the limited evidence base for many of these

GPs have a statutory responsibility to decide fitness for work. Giving time off work and encouraging return to work has an important place in managing illness

Physiotherapy and other physical therapies are often the best approach to musculo-skeletal disorders (but also have a wider remit – e.g. incontinence, impotence)

General Practice at a Glance, First Edition. Paul Booton, Carol Cooper, Graham Easton, and Margaret Harper.
© 2013 Paul Booton, Carol Cooper, Graham Easton, and Margaret Harper. Published 2013 by Blackwell Publishing Ltd.

The previous chapter went into some detail about effective history-taking. This chapter shows how to use the information you gained to plan the management of your patient.

What's next?

Having taken a careful history, you may have all the information you need, but more likely you may find yourself in a situation where you have some ideas about what's going on but not all you need to know. The big question now is not 'what's the diagnosis?' but 'what's next?' What do you need to do to take management to the next stage?

Examining your patient

Most clinical skills guides think of the history and examination as one item, but it's worth thinking of the examination as part of your investigations and plan it on the basis of what you've discovered in the history.

• As with the history, the **focused examination** explores areas chosen because they are likely to be important based on what you have found in the history.

• It's more revealing to do a thorough examination of the system where you believe the problem lies than a 'fishing trip' which skims over everything.

• Always do the examination that the clinical situation demands. Patients who need a rectal exam in surgical outpatients need it just as much in general practice.

Investigations

Investigations are of two main sorts – for diagnosis and for management. For instance, a random blood sugar test is very useful to confirm the diagnosis of diabetes, but of little use in diabetes management while glycosylated haemoglobin is the opposite. Choose investigations on the basis of how they will help you in each of these two areas. Why not a long list of investigations like on *ER*? Because every investigation you do has false positive potential. If you test for something that is clinically unlikely the risk of a false positive may be higher than the likelihood of a true positive.

Managing your patient

If you've taken a careful history and chosen your examination and investigations well you will have a good idea of what's going on with your patient. That is not necessarily the same as having a formal diagnosis. In general practice you often don't have a complete diagnosis but manage uncertainty through reducing risk by 'safety netting'. For instance, in a patient who presents with mild flu symptoms, it's not particularly helpful to patient or doctor to confirm the diagnosis of flu through virological testing, so the patient is advised on the basis of diagnostic probability of suitable management. Acknowledging that they might (rarely) develop a life-threatening viraemia or (more commonly) a bacterial pneumonia, one also advises the patient of what to do if they become more ill, what specific warning symptoms to look out for and what to do if these arise. (There may be other reasons for being sure about a diagnosis: in 2009 when the H1N1 flu epidemic appeared in the UK with real concerns about its virulence, exact diagnosis became extremely important and extensive virological testing was carried out.)

Tools for management

Ordering pathology tests is not the only way forward. Reviewing a non-critical problem after a week or so may give time for the clinical picture to evolve or the patient to find better ways of explaining the symptoms. This is particularly useful in primary care where patients tend to present early, before the clinical picture has recognisably evolved. 'Come back in a week' must be for a reason and not just prevarication! A second opinion from another GP colleague or other member of the primary care team often helps: the practice nurse or community midwife may be the best person to help you plan care.

Treatment

Writing a prescription at the end of each consultation suggests bad practice. Often explaining to your patient the nature of their symptoms and how to live with them, giving health advice on exercise, diet or smoking offers your patient a better chance to manage their own health. Figure 2 shows some of the different options available to you and your patient.

Negotiation

We've moved a long way from the doctor giving orders to the patient to follow. Patients who haven't understood or engaged with the importance of the treatment, or who don't trust the doctor or believe in his or her diagnosis are unlikely to comply with it. Careful explanation of your plan and taking on board the patient's ideas and expectations (yes, ideas, concerns and expectations once again!) is crucial to acheiving **concordance**, a negotiated plan that both you and the patient believe is the best way ahead in this particular situation.

Documentation

Once you've finished your consultation you should carefully document what you've discovered, planned and agreed. Your patient's future management and safety and your own medico-legal survival depends on the quality of these notes.

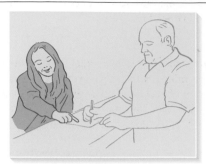

Receptionist, secretaries and admin staff: The receptionists have a challenging task which requires excellent interpersonal skills; they are in the front-line, dealing with appointments, prescriptions and test results, either face to face or on the phone, with people who may be anxious or unwell. Secretaries and clerks also look after paperwork and medical records

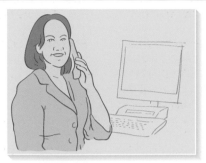

Practice manager: Most practices employ a practice manager to oversee the practice administration including the management of staff, practice systems, finance and pay, premises, and complaints. Some are practice partners

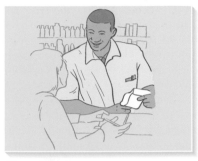

Pharmacist: The community pharmacist who runs the local dispensing chemist provides primary care advice and over-the-counter (OTC) medication as well dispensing the medications prescribed by doctors. They will fill dosette boxes for patients to assist with compliance, especially helpful for elderly patients. Some pharmacists perform medication reviews with patients

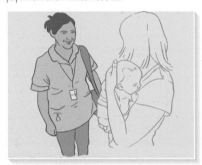

Community midwife: Midwives are usually General Nurses with at least one year's special training. They are involved in ante-natal and post-natal care in patients' homes, community based clinics or the GP surgery. They have a statutory responsibility to attend all home births (around 1% of all births) and monitor all mothers and babies until ten days post-partum whether at home or in hospital

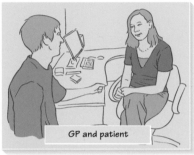

GP and patient

Other members of the primary healthcare team:

Community Psychiatric Nurse (CPN): Registered Mental Health Nurses who visit, support and supervise the care of people with mental health problems in the community. **Physiotherapist, dietitian, specialist nurses:** e.g. diabetic, respiratory, **Macmillan nurses** (palliative care), **Admiral nurses** (dementia care) and **Chiropodists**, who are available to patients in the Community Clinics, the GP surgery or in patient's own home. **Social Workers:** Can provide advice, support and counselling for vulnerable people such as the disabled, those with mental health problems and their carers. **Home Carers:** Take on domestic responsibilities such as personal care, washing and dressing when, for example, an elderly person becomes housebound. **Meals-on-wheels and laundry services:** Are amongst the other support services available to the very needy

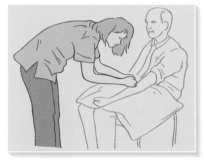

Healthcare assistant: Many surgeries employ healthcare assistants (HCAs). They are not trained nurses, but have received some formal training and perform tasks such as venepuncture, dressings, and blood pressure checks, measurement of height & weight and urine testing

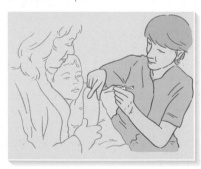

Practice nurse: Practice nurses are usually Registered General Nurses who work in the practice. In larger practices, there may be several sharing duties. The work of the practice nurse includes: new patient health checks, blood and urine tests, injections, immunisations, dressings, monitoring blood pressure, assisting with minor surgery, syringing ears and sterilising all practice equipment. Increasingly practice nurses are taking on special clinics managing cervical screening and family planning or chronic diseases such as diabetes or asthma. An increasing number of practices are employing **nurse practitioners** with extra training to undertake a broader range of clinical duties which may include diagnosis and management of minor illness

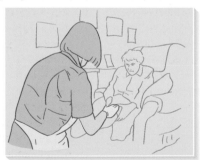

District nurse: District nurses are Registered General Nurses with an additional one year's training. They work predominantly in patients' homes where their tasks include dressing operation sites and ulcers, giving injections and eye drops to the housebound, looking after catheters, incontinence, pressure sores and syringe drivers etc. Some nurses are now able to prescribe a small range of medicines from the nurses' formulary

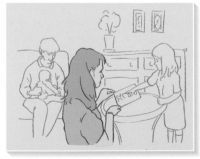

Health visitor: Health Visitors are Registered General Nurses with a one-year specialist training in health education and child development. They visit new babies soon after birth, and are responsible for ensuring that s/he receives regular health supervision and full immunisation as well as undertaking developmental screening. They also offer health education for parents. They see children at home, in the GP surgery or in a Community Child Health Clinic. The health visitor continues to have responsibility for the well being of children until the age of five especially those children considered to be 'at risk'

General Practice at a Glance, First Edition. Paul Booton, Carol Cooper, Graham Easton, and Margaret Harper.

16 © 2013 Paul Booton, Carol Cooper, Graham Easton, and Margaret Harper. Published 2013 by Blackwell Publishing Ltd.

Continuity of care

A major benefit of our primary care system is to be able to provide care continuously over a number of years, building a history of the health of the patient and developing a trusting relationship. In urban practices it is common to have a population of about 30% lifelong patients, 30% staying only a year and the rest staying somewhere in between.

Patients register with a practice, ideally as a family. The records of the patient and the rest of the family are available to all the professionals in the practice. This knowledge of the family can add unique value to the doctor–patient relationship and quality of care. For example, the GP will be attuned to any significant genetic predispositions or be aware of the stresses that may be occurring in family life.

In some practices patients can see the same doctor at each visit, but increasingly there will be several doctors working on a shift system so this may not be possible. Patients are encouraged to see the same doctor for a particular illness or condition, and communication between doctors becomes central to maintaining continuity of care.

Primary care team

Primary care doctors work in teams which vary from practice to practice (see Figure 3): nurses, dietitians, counsellors, physiotherapists, phlebotomists and others. They will be supported by a practice manager, receptionists and secretaries. Completing the team are externally employed primary care professionals such as district nurses, including specialist nurses for mental health, palliative care and a range of other specialist services. Effective care depends on good communication through meetings, notes and discussion. In most practices the doctor is the pivotal member of the team. This requires recognition of the skills of all the other members as they all play a vital part in the successful provision of patient care.

Appointments

Most patients are seen by appointment at the practice. Patients will be seen on the same day if their medical condition requires it. The initial appointment may be with a nurse or a doctor. Increasingly, patients are choosing to see a nurse where the request is for a procedure (e.g. a dressing or an injection). Nurses have demonstrated their particular training in developing and adhering to protocols of care. Some nurses have academic qualifications or special training and are recognised as nurse practitioners. They are able to demonstrate a high degree of knowledge and skill, especially in some well-defined areas such as managing minor illness including prescribing certain medications and increasingly in managing chronic illness such as hypertension.

Use of time

The supreme advantage of primary care is the ability to see a patient as often as necessary. The diagnosis may be unclear at the initial appointment but the patient may be seen again later. It is now easy to organise investigations at the hospital with the results sent back to the practice as rapidly as if requested by a hospital doctor. It has been shown that providing these facilities to primary care is economical.

Preventive medicine

Primary care is in a prime position to promote the prevention of disease and ill health. This may be by the administration of vaccination programmes or the recognition of early factors leading to chronic ill health such as the management of obesity, smoking or high blood pressure (see Chapter 5).

Special interests

Some GPs develop an interest and extra training in a particular area of medicine, such as minor surgery, gynaecology, management of drug addiction or diabetic care and accept referrals from other practices or from GPs within their own practice. Most GPs with a special interest (GPSIs) see this as only part of their work.

Chronic diseases

Chronic conditions are well managed from primary care. Most patients with diabetes or hypertension need not be referred to a hospital clinic. It is in this area the practice team comes into its own (see case study).

Case study: diabetes and the primary care team

A 52-year-old woman presents with increasing fatigue and thirst. The doctor or nurse confirms a diagnosis of diabetes using the facilities of the local laboratory. The doctor carries out a full examination and starts treatment for diabetes, including lifestyle advice and medication. Arrangements are made to see the patient in the practice at regular intervals when their health is monitored by the practice team. The practice dietitian gives advice and support and the practice phlebotomist takes the necessary blood samples. Over time the patient may become housebound and her medication changed to insulin which can be administered by the district nurse. The community podiatrist may be required to give foot care.

Home visits

Home visits are increasingly rare in modern urban primary care because of increased mobility of patients, easier access to appointments and the awareness that three or four patients can be seen at the medical centre in the time it takes to carry out a single visit. However, they do occur when patients are genuinely unable to attend the clinic. This may be for an acute condition but more commonly for disabling chronic conditions – or in rural practices where distance and transport make it difficult for patients. Occasionally a visit is necessary because a mentally ill patient needs to be examined with a view to organising a 'section' prior to compulsory admission to hospital. On such occasions a joint visit may be carried out by the GP, a psychiatrist and an Approved Mental Health Professional (AMHP).

Other visits will be to elderly patients, patients in need of palliative care and occasionally when the doctor feels that knowledge of the patient's living conditions would be helpful. Visits to the elderly will often be in support of the district nurse, and palliative care visits may be in conjunction with a specialist (e.g. Macmillan) nurse who is trained to give support to the patient and advice to the GP and the district nurse.

Why do patients consult?

(a) **The Symptom Iceberg** *(data from 'BTS recommendations for the management of cough in adults.' Thorax 2006:61 (suppl) i1-i24)*

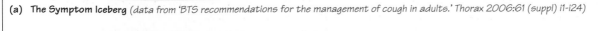

Hospitalisation	?
GP consultation	12
Self-medication	24 million
Acute cough	48 million
URTI	120 million

(b) Biopsychosocial model of health

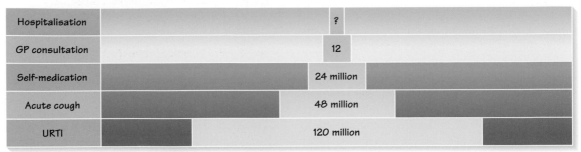

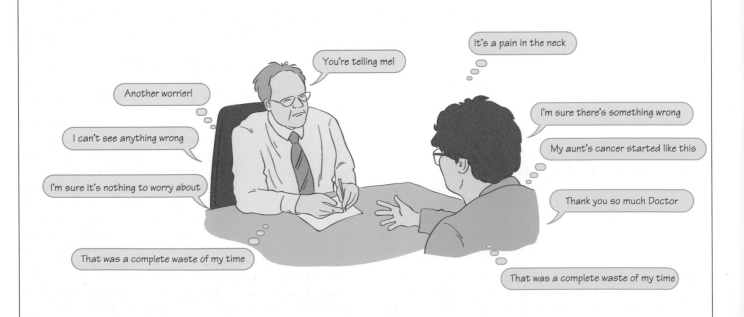

General Practice at a Glance, First Edition. Paul Booton, Carol Cooper, Graham Easton, and Margaret Harper.

18 © 2013 Paul Booton, Carol Cooper, Graham Easton, and Margaret Harper. Published 2013 by Blackwell Publishing Ltd.

As a GP this is a fascinating question. Some patients seem to come in with trivia while others sit at home with chest pain determined not to worry the doctor. An understanding of medical sociology helps explain why this might be happening. What is seen in the consulting room really is the 'tip of the iceberg'. This phenomenon was described by Hannay in 1979 and illustrates the fact that most people self-treat at home.

Figure 4a from the British Thoracic Society illustrates the symptom iceberg well, taking the example of cough. Of an estimated 120 million episodes of upper respiratory tract infection (URTI) in the UK each year, about one-third have a cough, of those half choose to self-medicate and one-quarter see their GP. So, overall, only 1 in 10 patients with a URTI actually makes an appointment with their GP.

Lay referral system

So what makes some people attend and others not? Sociologists have developed many different models.

Friedson described the *lay referral system* in 1970. He said 'the whole process of seeking help involves a network of potential "consultants" from family members through successively more select, and authorative laymen until the "professional" is reached.'

How many lay contacts the patient makes before they reach us has been found to depend on the degree of congruence between the subculture of the potential patient and that of the doctor. That is higher socio-economic backgrounds require less 'permission' from others to attend.

Zola's triggers

In 1972, Zola noted that symptoms alone were often not a sufficent reason to decide to see the doctor: something else had to happen. He identified five types of trigger:

1 The occurrence of an interpersonal crisis (e.g. a death in the family)
2 Interference with social or personal relations ('I can't look after the children')
3 Sanctioning – pressure or advice from others to consult ('The wife told me to go')
4 Interference with vocational or physical activity ('I can't go to work')
5 Temporalising – the setting of a deadline ('If I am no better in one week I will make an appointment')

This is something frequently observed in our patients' lives. Good examples are the mother who struggles on with symptoms of post-natal depression attending only when she is unable to look after her baby or the student with disfiguring acne, back from university, who finally attends after pressure from his mother.

Ideas, concerns and expectations

Looking into why people attend helps us tailor treatment to their particular need. Pendleton argues that patients bring their 'ideas, concerns and expectations' to each consultation. Patients come with their own ideas as to what is wrong with them, concerns about what this might mean for them and their expectations of the GP as to what the GP will do (which may be positive or negative). For example, a man who attends with headaches may think it is caused by stress but be concerned about an underlying brain tumour and need his doctor to reassure him about this. If his doctor identifies and addresses this issue he will:

• Be more likely to go away satisfied
• Be more likely to be compliant with his newly prescribed anti-hypertensive medication, and
• Leave with a healthy ongoing doctor–patient relationship.
    If not he may leave with a correct diagnosis but with:
• His fears not addressed
• He will remain worried and unsatisfied, and
• Probably not take medication that he doesn't believe in.

Biopsychosocial model of health

Health cannot be seen purely in terms of absence of pathology. The World Health Organization (WHO) describes health as 'a state of complete physical, mental and social wellbeing and not merely the absence of disease'.

Obviously we cannot guarantee mental well-being for all our patients but we do well to take into account the effect of psycho-social factors on our patients' health and the interplay between all these factors.

In 1977, American psychiatrist George Engel introduced the concept of the biopsychosocial model of health (see Figure 4b). The model proposes that biological, psychological and sociological factors form interconnected spectrums, each like a system of the body. Engel's work accompanied a shift in focus from disease to health, recognising that psychosocial factors (e.g. beliefs, relationships, stress) greatly impact not just how we cope with disease, but the disease process itself.

Doctors in general and GPs in particular need to view patients holistically and treat all aspects of their health.

Diversity and language difficulties

With increasing diversity in Britain we also see many different cultural beliefs about health which can be very different from our own and not always easy to identify. A study by Trisha Greenhalgh found that British Bangladeshis with diabetes had a variety of folk health beliefs. Some felt that lack of sweating in the British cold weather was bad for the metabolic system and that if they could only return to warmer climates they would be cured.

Other countries organise healthcare very differently: primary care does not exist in many countries and we can find ourselves spending time educating our patients about the role of the British GP. On the one hand they may be surprised that they do not need to pay directly for a consultation, on the other that they do not need to see a gynaecologist for a smear test or a paediatrician for childhood immunisations.

In inner city multi-ethnic communities language is an important issue. Consultations can be in pigeon English with a lot of pointing to 'problem' areas. Refugee patients may have special health needs relating to backgrounds which can be hard for 'sheltered western-ers' to understand. Parents often use their child to interpret. This can be an ethical minefield especially when sensitive issues of con-traception or mental health are discussed. Local arrangements to provide translators via telephone or in person and allowing extra time for the consultation is a solution of sorts, but many of the subtleties of communication are lost and at significant expense and time. Overcoming these difficulties allows the GP an opportunity to improve the medical and psychological wellbeing of some of the most needy people in our society, and for the GP gives fascinating insights into other lives and cultures.

Health promotion activity	Rationale	Intervention

Physical activity	• Prevents obesity
	• Lowers risk of coronary heart disease
	• Lowers blood pressure
	• Improves insulin sensitivity
	• Maintains function in musculo-skeletal problems
	• Reduces risk of hip fracture in elderly
	• Improves mental health
		• **Opportunistic advice**
		  – counselling patients to undertake 30 minutes of moderate-intensity physical activity on 5 or more days a week. Patient information leaflets, posters or useful websites:
		    – Change4Life, Let's Get Moving, Keep Fit Association, Walking the Way to Health
		• **'Exercise on prescription'**
		  – referring patients with at least one cardiovascular risk factor to a local leisure centre or gym for supervised physical activity

Smoking cessation	• Smoking cessation:
	  – halves the risk of cardio-and cerebrovascular disease
	  – is the most effective management for COPD
	  – reduces risk of smoking related cancers
	• Smoking is the main cause of preventable disease and premature death in the UK
		• **Opportunistic advice**
		  – counselling all smokers to quit, especially if presenting with a smoking-related illness. Information leaflets and posters around the GP surgery
		• **Pharmacotherapy**
		  – nicotine replacement therapy – gum, patches, inhalators
		  – varenicline (Champix)
		  – bupropion (Zyban)
		• **Behavioural support**
		  – self-help material and referral for intensive support such as the NHS Stop Smoking Services

Dietary advice and tackling obesity	• Obesity is associated with:
	  – insulin resistance
	  – hypertension and stroke
	  – hyperlipidaemia
	  – some cancers e.g. liver
	
	Eating at least 5 pieces of fresh fruit a day can:
	• Lower the chance of developing cardio-and cerebrovascular disease
	• Reduces risk of bowel and lung cancer
	• Prevents constipation
		• **Opportunistic Advice**
		  – counselling patients about healthy eating. Providing self-help information, websites
		  – encouraging young mothers regarding the health benefits of breast-feeding for first 6 months of life for mother and baby
		• **Referral** to NHS dietitian for patients who are obese or at risk of developing diabetes
		• **Bariatric surgery**
		  – available for adults over 18 with BMI >35 and co-morbidities that would improve with weight loss, or BMI>40
		  – thorough psychological assessment to assess readiness for change
		  – examples include jaw wiring, gastro-jejunal by-pass or vertical banded gastroplasty
		• **Pharmacotherapy**
		  – considered for patients who have not reached target weight loss with dietary and lifestyle changes
		  – orlistat (Xenical). Available for adults with BMI >28 and risk factors, or BMI >30. NICE guidelines advise to continue only if after 3 months there has been >5% weight loss

Accident and injury prevention	• For children and young people, accidents are the greatest threat to life	• **Opportunistic advice**
		  – counselling parents about hazards at home and steps that can be taken to prevent accidents e.g. stair gates, keeping chemicals out of reach, bicycle helmets etc.
		  – counselling on fitness to drive and consider reporting to DVLA patients who fail to comply if deemed a serious risk to the public
		  – identify, treat and monitor conditions that are associated with increased risk of accident or injury for example obstructive sleep apnoea, diabetes, epilepsy, alcohol dependence

NHS Screening programmes Visit: http://cpd.screening.nhs.uk/timeline

Antenatal and newborn screening

There are 6 antenatal and newborn screening programmes and these screening tests need to be carried out at set times. Please see the antenatal and newborn timeline for full details of the optimum times for testing. Visit: http://cpd.screening.nhs.uk/timeline

• Linked antenatal and newborn Sickle cell and thalassaemia
• Infectious diseases in pregnancy
• Down's syndrome and fetal anomaly ultrasound screening
• Newborn hearing
• Newborn and infant physical examination
• Newborn blood spot

Other screening

Abdominal aortic aneurysm (AAA) screening	Offered to all men in their 65th year. Men over this age are able to self-refer
Bowel cancer screening	Offered to men and women aged 60–69 every 2 years. Those aged 70+ can request screening by ringing 0800 707 6060
Breast screening	Offered to women aged 50–70 every 3 years. Women aged 70 or over can self-refer
Cervical screening	Offered to women aged 25–49 every 3 years and to women aged 50–64 every 5 years
Diabetic retinopathy	Screening offered annually to people with diabetes from the age of 12

General Practice at a Glance, First Edition. Paul Booton, Carol Cooper, Graham Easton, and Margaret Harper.
20 © 2013 Paul Booton, Carol Cooper, Graham Easton, and Margaret Harper. Published 2013 by Blackwell Publishing Ltd.

Preventive medicine in general practice

Preventive medicine focuses on the prevention of illness, promotion of health and prolongation of life. GPs have a crucial role in all three processes and, because half the mortality from the 10 leading causes of death in the UK can be traced to lifestyle and behaviour, preventive medicine is of utmost importance.

Many GP consultations are for relatively minor ailments which create opportunities to discuss healthy living and the early detection of illness. Also, the trust that builds within the doctor–patient relationship over time allows GPs to motivate their patients to change their behaviour in order to maintain good health. GPs do not work alone here – the entire primary care team, including practice nurses, midwives and health visitors, is geared to promoting health in their patients and local community. In addition, GPs work alongside public health specialists to prevent illness at a **community** level, which requires a broad knowledge of the socio-economic characteristics and disease epidemiology of their local practice population.

Primary prevention

This is the prevention of the **onset** of disease and can also be termed health promotion – defined by the WHO as 'the process of enabling people to increase control over their health and its determinants, and thereby improve their health'.

GPs have an active role in promoting health in their day-to-day practice, and some examples of health promotion are summarised in Figure 5. Cardiovascular disease accounts for a huge proportion of primary care morbidity and mortality and GPs have a key role in preventing (or delaying) its development. Population strategies include anti-smoking campaigns, promotion of physical activity and dietary advice to reduce obesity and individual strategies are summarised in Figure 5 (see also Chapter 37).

Secondary prevention

This is the detection and management of disease in its earliest stages or the detection of asymptomatic disease – which is also known as screening. In general practice, screening takes place on two levels.

Opportunistic screening

Individual asymptomatic patients are screened on an informal or ad hoc basis in clinic. Examples include:
• Registration 'health checks' of new patients which measure body mass index (BMI), blood pressure, urinalysis, smoking status and alcohol consumption.
• Annual review of patients on chronic disease registers such as diabetes or ischaemic heart disease, which involves screening for disease complications and depression.

NHS population screening programmes

Screening involves targeting apparently healthy people and offering them information to make informed choices about undergoing tests for specific diseases, while causing the least harm (see Figure 5 for NHS screening programmes).

Before embarking on a screening programme, there are a number of criteria to be met – these are known as **Wilson's screening criteria:**

• The condition should be an important health problem
• The epidemiology and natural history of the condition should be well understood
• There should be a detectable risk factor, disease marker or early asymptomatic stage
• There should be a simple, acceptable, safe, precise and validated screening test
• There should be an accepted treatment for the disease and this should be more effective if started early
• The risks of the screening programme, both physical and psychological, should be less than the benefits
• Diagnosis and treatment should be cost-effective
• Case-finding should be a continuous process and intervals for repeating the test should be agreed.

Even if these are met, screening still has its limitations. No screening tool is perfect – there will always be false positives and negatives, which means that while the screened population as a whole benefits, a few patients with the disease will slip through the 'screening net' (**false negative**) and some healthy patients will be wrongly suspected of having the condition (**false positive**). GPs need to be familiar with these concepts and make sure patients have realistic expectations of what the screening programme can deliver.

Tertiary prevention

This is the halting of the progression of already established disease. In conjunction with their secondary care colleagues, GPs have a prominent role in tertiary prevention of disease. This involves 'optimising' risk factors in patients with pre-existing disease – for example, ensuring that all patients with ischaemic heart disease are taking aspirin and encouraging them to stop smoking.

Quality and Outcomes Framework

The government has introduced measures to incentivise GPs to participate in prevention programmes. In England, this was formalised by the introduction of the Quality and Outcomes Framework (QOF) in 2004, in which GPs are paid for meeting a range of performance targets.

QOF aims to promote evidence-based medicine, standardise the delivery of primary care and reduce health inequalities. It accounts for about 25% of general practice income. It is divided into a number of indicators, against which practices score points according to their level of performance and disease prevalence. The higher the score, the larger the financial reward for the practice.

QOF has four main components:
1 **Clinical standards:** chronic disease management
2 **Organisational standards:** primary care records, patient information, staff training and medicines management
3 **Patients' experience**
4 **Additional services,** whereby practices can opt to provide more advanced patient services (e.g. family planning).

Although there is evidence that QOF has improved and standardised many aspects of primary care in England, the quality of care across the country is still variable. The benefits for the individual patient to be derived from QOF are still to be determined – and some evidence suggests that while financial rewards improve the quality of documentation, the effect on standards of care is more limited.

6 Significant event analysis, audit and research

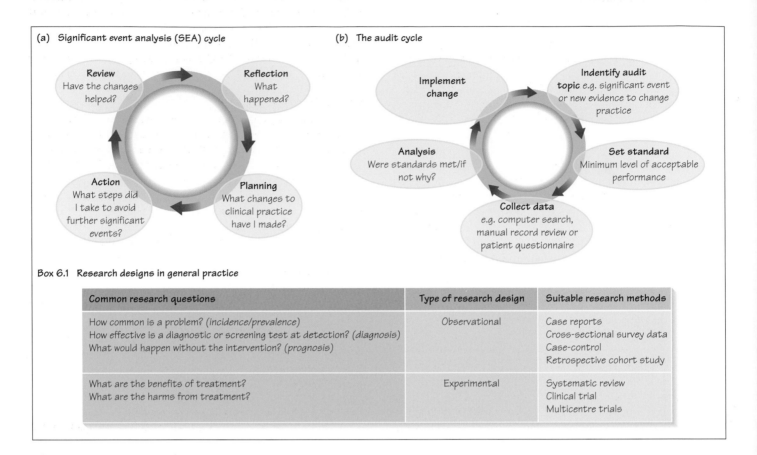

(a) Significant event analysis (SEA) cycle

Review Have the changes helped?

Reflection What happened?

Action What steps did I take to avoid further significant events?

Planning What changes to clinical practice have I made?

(b) The audit cycle

Implement change

Indentify audit topic e.g. significant event or new evidence to change practice

Analysis Were standards met/if not why?

Set standard Minimum level of acceptable performance

Collect data e.g. computer search, manual record review or patient questionnaire

Box 6.1 Research designs in general practice

Common research questions	Type of research design	Suitable research methods
How common is a problem? (incidence/prevalence) How effective is a diagnostic or screening test at detection? (diagnosis) What would happen without the intervention? (prognosis)	Observational	Case reports Cross-sectional survey data Case-control Retrospective cohort study
What are the benefits of treatment? What are the harms from treatment?	Experimental	Systematic review Clinical trial Multicentre trials

These three related activities have the common goal of improving practice for the benefit of patients. Significant event analysis (SEA) gives you a structure to ask questions about and learn from a single event. Audit is research that lets you ask questions of your own practice, comparing it with best practice to make beneficial changes. Research asks questions and chooses tools to answer it in ways that are generalisable to wider situations.

What is significant event analysis?

Case review is one of the oldest principles in medicine; by looking at cases where things have gone wrong you try to learn for the future. This has been formalised in official inquiries like the Bristol children's heart surgery inquiry, and is based on the principles of case review.

GPs (and other specialties) use this to review their practice when something significant happens (not necessarily involving an undesirable outcome for the patient). SEA is now a requirement of the Clinical Governance provisions of the GP's contract. It is part of the training of GP registrars and required for the Appraisal and Revalidation of qualified GPs.

Example of an SEA

You see a 4-year-old child with a headache and fever and reassure them they have flu and will get better but then subsequently that patient becomes seriously unwell and is admitted to hospital with meningitis.

Analysing a case like this should start the process of reflection (see Figure 6a), changing practice, for example reviewing guidelines for feverish illness in children and reviewing the case with colleagues and 'safety netting' to improve the outcome next time. Documentation is important, otherwise all the lessons learnt are lost, and there should be an action plan of recommended changes to practice and procedures. The final step is to set a deadline for reviewing whether the changes have been implemented and if this has averted similar events.

As a student you may be asked to identify a significant event as part of your practice attachment. This may be anything that raised questions in your head or perhaps made you feel uncomfortable. For example, a patient suddenly storms out of a consultation or you feel uneasy about the way the doctor has responded to an abortion request. Reflecting on the issues raised in a structured way may help to change your own thinking, or allow you to make suggestions to change the way the practice approaches the issue.

What is audit?

Audit is a systematic way of reviewing how you practise (process audit) or what happens as a result of your practice (outcome audit)

and comparing this with how others practise using professionally recognised standards. There are several key steps that make up the 'audit cycle' (see Figure 6b).

Example of an audit

The National Institute for Clinical Excellence (NICE) publishes a new guideline stating that there is now good evidence that all patients who have had a confirmed thrombo-embolic stroke should be receiving aspirin and dipyridamole or clopidogrel to prevent further cardiovascular events. Your GP tutor suggests that as part of your attachment you conduct an audit of this for the practice.

Stage 1: identifying the question

A good audit question evolves from problems noticed in the practice, often coming from ideas from patients or the practice staff. It requires a good evidence base: you can't see if best practice is being followed if it is not clear what best practice is. There should be a clear potential for improving service delivery. In the example, because the guideline is new, it is likely that not all patients will be on the correct treatment.

Stage 2: defining criteria and standards

You should write an evidence-based statement that will form the audit criteria; for example 'Patients who have had a stroke should be on antithrombotic therapy for secondary prevention.' 'Standards' define the threshold of compliance for each criterion you are measuring. These should be explicit and measurable. In the example this could be 'Ninety-eight per cent of all patients who have had a thrombo-embolic stroke should be taking aspirin–dipyridamole combination or clopidogrel if eligible within the past year.' **Not** 'Are patients who have had a stroke on antithrombotics?'

Stage 3: data collection

GPs have electronic databases that can be used to search for patients with coded diagnoses and prescribed medications. Often the notes will need to be examined manually to verify reasons why some clinical decisions were made. For example, some patients may be taking warfarin for a coexisting condition and therefore giving them clopidogrel would not be appropriate. Because audit involves direct contact with patient records, it must be conducted ethically and respect patient confidentiality.

Stage 4: compare performance with criteria and standards

How well were the standards met in your audit? Is this acceptable? If not, how could this be improved? This should be discussed with the practice team to produce an action plan.

Stage 5: implementing change

Recommendations should be written as clear action points and a named person who has responsibility for making it all happen with a timescale for review. Often audits will change practice for a short while then everyone goes back to doing what they were before the audit happened. Re-auditing the same topic or 'completing the audit cycle' can sustain the changes, although ideally you refine your criteria with new emerging evidence or lessons learned.

What is research?

Most clinical research aims to improve scientific knowledge which can be directly fed back to improve heath or to change existing practice. It is less concerned with generating (or disproving) scientific theories in the way that basic science research does (Box 6.1). Like SEAs and audit it usually begins with defining a problem, examines the current evidence and then, rather than applying this (like audit), identifies gaps where new knowledge or theory is needed (exploratory) or tests the hypotheses that the gaps in current understanding expose (empirical or experimental research).

The research process

Most research follows a series of steps:

1 Observation and identification of a problem needing an answer
2 Generating a hypothesis
3 Defining an answerable research question
4 Predicting findings
5 Collecting data
6 Analysing data
7 Interpreting results
8 Repeating the test (often by other researchers).

The most suitable research method depends on the question but includes the following:

• Qualitative research methods (for understanding human behaviour)
• Quantitative research methods (for quantifying differences in systematic empirical study; Box 6.1).

It's good to be involved in research as a student, but easy to do bad research. Getting involved with your academic department of primary care will help you plan good research: design, statistics, ethical approval, etc. With the limited time available to you as a student you may be better joining in with an existing project rather than trying to manage a whole project yourself. Involvement in research will help you gain experience of academic writing and publication, and can be useful for your future career.

HEALING HEALTH CENTRE 14 Caring Street, Healing, UR GR8 Tel 020 11119999, Fax 020 11118888

Dr Feelgood
Elderly Care Consultant
St Elsewhere Hospital
Healing
_____

ROUTINE NHS REFERRAL

- **This guidance on referral letters is based on:**
  Scottish Intercollegiate Guidelines Network (SIGN) report on a recommended referral document. 1998 (SIGN publication no. 31) Available from url – http://www.sign.ac.uk/guidelines/fulltext/31/index.html
- The recommendation is divided into two sections, **patient** information and then **clinical** information

19.6.2010
NHS number: 0101
RE: Mr Mickey Mouse
     DOB: 14.8.1930
     18 Disney Street
     London MM1
     Tel 00000 00000

Patient information should include at least the patient's full name, date of birth, address, telephone number, details of the referrer, registered general practice, urgency of the referral and special requirements (transport requirements, interpreter)

Reason for referral: Assessment of recurrent falls

Problems:

1. Ataxia and falls
2. Transient hypoglycaemia
3. Mild cognitive impairment – MSE 23/30
4. Intermittent bradycardia – pacemaker

Clinical information history, investigations, reason for referral, past medical history, medication including allergies, social history and clinical warnings (e.g. blood borne viruses, history of violence to staff)

Additional relevant information should be attached to the referral to provide the recipient with a global assessment of the patient's health

Dear Dr Feelgood,

I would be very grateful for your expert assessment of Mr Mouse, an 81-year-old former accountant with a 6-year history of intermittent presyncope, ataxia and occasional falls. He has no symptoms of vertigo, and no episodes of loss of consciousness, weakness, paraesthesia, visual loss or headaches. He has been investigated by cardiology with a 7-day event recorder which revealed only minor runs of bradycardia for which he had a pacemaker fitted. He has also been diagnosed with transient hypoglycaemia by endocrinology, which he manages with frequent small meals. He has been seen by the neurologists and a CT brain revealed only minor age-related changes.

Examination:
key positive and negative findings

On examination he has a broad-based gait and is mobile independently at home but uses a stick when walking outside. He has an otherwise normal neurological examination, normal heart sounds, no bruits and no postural hypotension.

Investigations: relevant positive and negative results

All relevant blood tests are normal including FBC, ESR, iron studies, U+E, LFT, TFT, random glucose, syphilis screen, B12 and folate (attached).

Social history: relevant information that builds a useful picture of the patient's life and how any health problems affect him

He takes aspirin and occasional paracetamol, has no allergies, has never smoked and does not drink alcohol.

Medication: including over-the-counter remedies, and any allergies

He lives alone in a warden controlled flat. He has two sons, the elder is an eminent diplomat in the West Indies. His youngest son lives in Spain and he has little contact with him. He is fearful that his sons will force him into a nursing home to sell his flat. He has twice daily carers for bathing, washing and cleaning and has had frequent falls assessments by OT and physiotherapy who confirm his property is as safe as possible for him. Despite his daily fear of falling he still manages to visit White Hart Lane to see his beloved Tottenham Hotspur and visits an old friend weekly in Islington.

Reason for referral outlining your specific hopes/ expectations for what the specialist team will be able to help with

We have been unable to find a cause or reduce the frequency of his episodes of presyncope, ataxia and falls and wondered whether a fresh perspective might reveal an alternative diagnosis or facilitate an additional intervention.

Kind regards,
Dr P Centred

By far the most important information is the reason for the referral
- If there is diagnostic doubt then suggest a differential to help the recipient understand your thinking
- If you would like the recipient to perform a specific task then make it clear
- If you do not expect to find pathology but wish for 'specialist assessment' to reassure your patient then make that obvious in the letter

General Practice at a Glance, First Edition. Paul Booton, Carol Cooper, Graham Easton, and Margaret Harper.

24 © 2013 Paul Booton, Carol Cooper, Graham Easton, and Margaret Harper. Published 2013 by Blackwell Publishing Ltd.

Why communication matters

Despite efforts to make their journey smooth and seamless, patients often end up navigating their way across a dangerous chasm between primary and secondary care. Without clear communication between professionals and patients, it is very easy for them to fall through the gap. So whether you are working in general practice or hospital, communicating with your colleagues elsewhere in the health system is essential to good patient care. It will also make your professional life run more smoothly.

Key features of effective communication

• **Be clear about what you want.** If you are asking for professional advice or support, be clear about how you are hoping your colleagues might help. For example: 'Could you help with establishing the diagnosis?', 'Please could you advise on the next steps in management?' or 'Please could you consider taking over this patient's care?'

• **Communicate with the right person or team.** Referrals made to the wrong specialty or member of the team can get lost and result in mistakes or poor patient care. For example, an ENT registrar accepts an outpatient referral by telephone from the accident and emergency department (A&E) but the team in A&E are not aware of the correct pathway for referral. They fax it to the wrong department as a result. No appointment is made and the patient is lost to follow-up.

• **Give clear and relevant information.** Poorly presented, illegible or irrelevant information can often cause confusion and lead to unnecessary or ineffective treatment. Writing everything you know about the patient is not usually helpful: too much irrelevant information can mean your main message gets lost.

• **Ensure two-way communication.** Make sure you leave clear contact details and make yourself available for discussions. Your opinion or knowledge of the patient may well be required at a later date.

Referral letters

Document concisely the history of the relevant illness, any investigations and interventions (including what has worked and what has not), and outline any plans for future management. Be clear about what you are asking of your hospital colleagues (see Figure 7). Include relevant past history and medication details. Unfortunately, referrals can easily get lost, so advise patients to contact the practice if they do not hear from the hospital about an appointment within a reasonable time frame.

Discharge summaries

Discharge summaries (sent from hospital to general practice when the patient is discharged) are often the only reliable information a GP will have about a patient's hospital stay and any plans for future management. So, although it may seem like a time-consuming chore for a busy junior doctor, the discharge summary is central to good patient care. Evidence suggests GPs appreciate discharge summaries written in a clearly structured format. As a minimum they should contain details about:
• Reason for admission and/or diagnosis
• Date and details of discharge

• Investigations and treatments
• Complications
• Changes to medication
• Follow-up arrangements (e.g. when stitches should come out or referrals that need to be made)
• Community services involved in ongoing care (e.g. Social Services or occupational therapy)
• Further action required by the patient's GP (e.g. any checks that need doing after starting new treatment)
• Prognosis
• Functional ability
• Contact details of the admitting team.

Ideally, email or fax an immediate discharge summary to the surgery, and give the patient a copy to keep with them or to drop into the surgery as soon as they can. A more detailed letter can be sent later (see link to SIGN guidelines on immediate discharge document in further reading).

Phoning hospital colleagues

• Follow the key features of effective communication above.
• Introduce yourself first. Give your full name, location and job title.
• Ensure you are speaking to the correct person ('Hi, is this the neurology registrar on call?') and that you record their full name in the records.
• Ensure you have given them your direct contact details; this makes any further communication easier.
• Be clear about your reason for calling early in the conversation.
• Begin with the most effective discriminators first. These are usually age, sex, employment, ethnicity, followed by key symptoms, acute/chronic, mild/severe, risk factors and relevant negatives.

For example: 'This is a 35-year-old male Somali refugee presenting with a 3-month history of cough, weight loss, night sweats and haemoptysis. He has never smoked' suggests TB as a likely diagnosis. But if the history had been: 'This is a 65-year-old male heavy smoker with a 3-month history of cough, haemoptysis, weight loss and night sweats' the most likely diagnosis is bronchial carcinoma. In the second case the smoking history is more important and is therefore mentioned earlier. Smoking and age are the discriminators that help the listener formulate a diagnosis.

Getting patients seen or admitted

Patients are usually referred for assessment or admission because they need rapid secondary care intervention (e.g. an angiogram), or they have severe symptoms, worsening symptoms with no clear diagnosis or they cannot be cared for at home (although hospital at home teams are reducing this burden on secondary care). When you want your patient to be seen that day, decide how urgently the patient should be transferred to hospital (e.g. a well patient with suspected early appendicitis may go by taxi but a patient with acute cerebrovascular accident [CVA] should go by 999 ambulance). For 999 emergencies, call the ambulance and stabilise the patient first, then inform the admitting team only when the patient is en route to hospital.

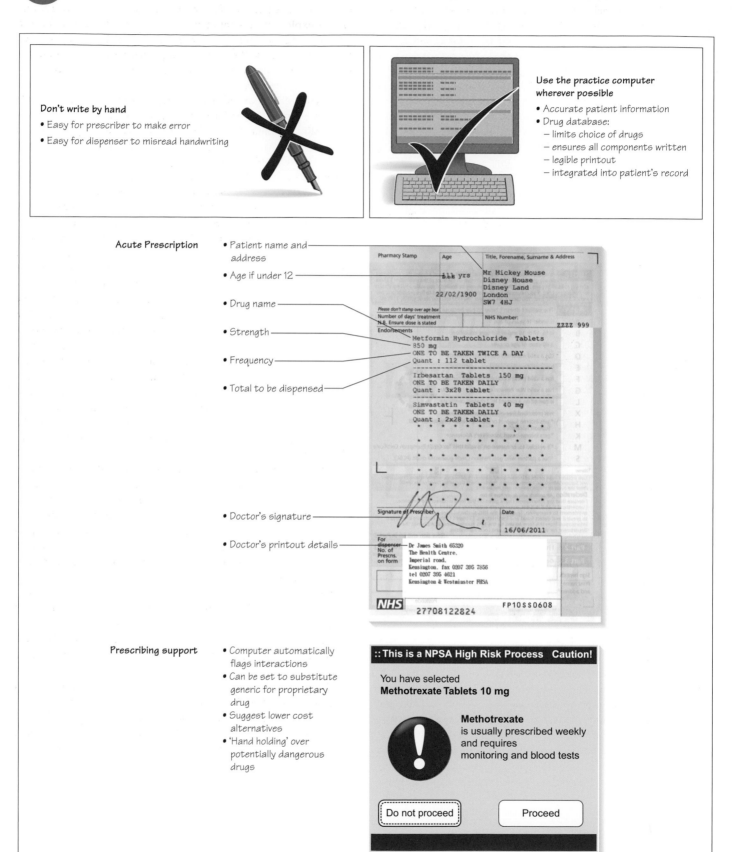

Don't write by hand
- Easy for prescriber to make error
- Easy for dispenser to misread handwriting

Use the practice computer wherever possible
- Accurate patient information
- Drug database:
  - limits choice of drugs
  - ensures all components written
  - legible printout
  - integrated into patient's record

Acute Prescription
- Patient name and address
- Age if under 12
- Drug name
- Strength
- Frequency
- Total to be dispensed
- Doctor's signature
- Doctor's printout details

Pharmacy Stamp | Age | Title, Forename, Surname & Address

111 yrs

22/02/1900

Mr Mickey Mouse
Disney House
Disney Land
London
SW7 4HJ

Please don't stamp over age box

Number of days' treatment
N.B. Ensure dose is stated

NHS Number:

ZZZZ 999

Endorsements

Metformin Hydrochloride Tablets
850 mg
ONE TO BE TAKEN TWICE A DAY
Quant : 112 tablet

Irbesartan Tablets 150 mg
ONE TO BE TAKEN DAILY
Quant : 3x28 tablet

Simvastatin Tablets 40 mg
ONE TO BE TAKEN DAILY
Quant : 2x28 tablet

Signature of Prescriber | Date

16/06/2011

For dispenser
No. of Prescns. on form

Dr James Smith 65320
The Health Centre,
Imperial road,
Kensington. fax 0207 305 7856
tel 0207 305 4621
Kensington & Westminster PHSA

NHS

27708122824

FP10SS0608

Prescribing support
- Computer automatically flags interactions
- Can be set to substitute generic for proprietary drug
- Suggest lower cost alternatives
- 'Hand holding' over potentially dangerous drugs

:: This is a NPSA High Risk Process   Caution!

You have selected
Methotrexate Tablets 10 mg

!

Methotrexate
is usually prescribed weekly and requires monitoring and blood tests

| Do not proceed | | Proceed |

General Practice at a Glance, First Edition. Paul Booton, Carol Cooper, Graham Easton, and Margaret Harper.
26   © 2013 Paul Booton, Carol Cooper, Graham Easton, and Margaret Harper. Published 2013 by Blackwell Publishing Ltd.

As a GP, a solid understanding of the principles and practice of drug use is essential. At the same time, you must also be aware that often drugs are neither the only nor the best solution to many of your patients' problems. You need to have a good working knowledge of the range of drugs used to treat the common and important conditions for which GPs take primary responsibility and which are discussed in the chapters of this book. But you also need to be aware of the much broader range of drugs that your patients will be on following various secondary care interventions. As the doctor responsible for coordinating the patient's overall care, you need to be aware of the potential for interaction between drugs prescribed by different specialties perhaps working in ignorance of each other. Nowhere is this more common than in prescribing for the elderly, where multiple pathologies often require multiple therapeutic interventions and an enhanced risk of problems.

Before you reach for your prescription pad, consider the following seven questions.

1 Is a drug necessary? The 'pill for every ill' culture has caused more problems than solutions. Treating social problems with diazepam (popular in the 1960s) produced addiction without resolving the underlying problems. Be clear about the nature of the problem you are treating and the potential for a drug to solve it. Medication may be used to cure an underlying problem (e.g. antibiotics), control a chronic problem (e.g. antihypertensives) or manage symptoms (e.g. opiates in end stage breathlessness). Non-drug approaches involve **physical therapy** (e.g. physiotherapy for musculoskeletal problems, exercise for mild depression), **psychological therapies** (of which brief intervention by the GP is one example), **self-help** through support groups or individual exertion (often helped by books or other written information – pretentiously labelled 'bibliotherapy') often with the aim of **lifestyle change**.

2 Is the drug effective? The rise of evidence-based medicine has made a large body of evidence available to GPs on the effectiveness of therapy. Persuading patients of the ineffectiveness of favoured remedies (which may have been promoted by other doctors) is a challenge (e.g. the lack of benefit of antibiotics in minor infections such as otitis media). At the same time, applying evidence to individual patients who may not conform to the exclusions and inclusions of the original trials requires clinical judgement, which may sometimes be little more than an educated guess.

3 Is the drug safe? All medications carry a risk of adverse reactions, or interactions with other drugs. All the more reason to be sure the drug is really required. Reactions may be **predictable** (diarrhoea from antibiotics, which on occasion can be life-threatening), **idiosyncratic** (thrombocytopenia from quinine – commonly given for leg cramps in the elderly), **end of use** from drug withdrawl (e.g. discontinuation of steroids producing Addisonian symptoms – remember, the patient who has apparently successfully been weaned off steroids, but an acute infection produces an Addisonian crisis as the recovering adrenals fail to respond adequately to the need for increased steroids). Beware of **wrongly identified side effects:** when a patient tells you they are allergic to a medication, always explore fully what they mean and whether this is likely to be a true allergy – this may prevent a potentially life-saving drug being withheld in the future. **Drug interactions** are common, important and frequent cause of hospital admission, especially in the elderly – see Chapter 9.

4 Is therapy economical? Drug companies are keen to persuade GPs to prescribe their latest expensive patented product, often with little therapeutic justification (beware of industry-sponsored drug trials and selective reporting in glossy brochures). Generic prescribing of well-established drugs is not only economical, but the safety profile is better known.

5 Have you agreed on the plan? Studies show only one-third of patients comply with prescribed treatments, perhaps because they are unconvinced of the need (e.g. antihypertensives), afraid of side effects (e.g. MMR) or cannot afford them (several drugs each with a prescription charge of around £8 can be a real issue for some patients). Negotiating and agreeing the management plan and the drugs to be taken is a critical part of patient management. Assess the **patient's expectations** – did they expect to get a drug? Are they confident it will work? Do they expect a course will cure them? Are they afraid of side effects? Explain **your expectations** to the patient (e.g. it won't work straight away, may give these side effects). This 'concordance' approach has replaced doctor-centred 'compliance' and offers better outcomes. Think about how you would negotiate a new prescription of antihypertensives with a patient: they need to be taken for life, they may have side effects, the patient will need regular check ups but will not feel any direct benefit from the medication. Ensuring patient and doctor agree the plan is crucial to its success.

6 Does your patient know how to take the medication? Studies show patients do not recall much of what has happened in the consulting room. Ensure your patient understands what they are meant to do (writing it down helps), keep the number of drugs to a minimum and keep the regime simple (as few times a day as possible, preferably all tablets taken together). 'Polypills' containing common drug combinations help compliance and have demonstrably improved outcomes.

7 What's next? Never prescribe without having a follow-up plan. This may be quite simple ('If it's not better in a week, come back') or more complex, but in all situations you need to:

- Agree a plan with the patient, 'Once you've done the urine sample, take 2 pills the first day then one a day for the rest of the week.'
- Include success or failure criteria, 'You should start to feel better after 3 or 4 days, if not ring me.'
- Plan any follow-up arrangements, 'Let's meet in 10 days to look at the tests and decide whether it's an enlarged prostate gland leading to these infections.'

(a) Use a dosette box

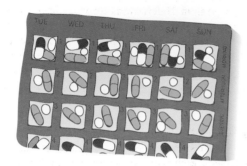

(b) Brown bag review

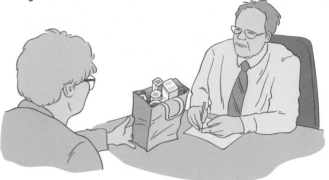

- Chemist makes up box
- Easier to understand
- Easier for carer or clinician to monitor if tablets are taken

- Ask patient to bring all tablets and medicines to surgery (whether prescribed or OTC)
- Look at each medication with patient:

  What symptoms does patient have? Could these be attributable to medication (e.g. cough: ACE inhibitors; falls: antihypertensives; dizziness: psychotropics

  – is it correct dose/frequency/in date?

  – does the patient understand how to take it/what it is for?

  – is there a sensible quantity? (too many – ?compliance; too few – adjust prescription)

  – is it their own medication? (patients often take their partner's accidentally or intentionally)
- What interactions could these cause (e.g. think about OTCs)?

  – can some of them be dropped? (not needed, not taken, potential adverse effects outweigh benefits)

  – plan next review

(c) Calculating children's drug doses

Rough and ready:
Calculate from child's age but does not allow for bigger/smaller child than average

Better:
Calculate from weight but may overdose an obese child

The above methods are adequate for 'ordinary' doses of 'safe' drugs with 'normal' children

Best:
Base calculation on surface area from normogram of height vs weight: not normally necessary in GP situation

General Practice at a Glance, First Edition. Paul Booton, Carol Cooper, Graham Easton, and Margaret Harper.

28 © 2013 Paul Booton, Carol Cooper, Graham Easton, and Margaret Harper. Published 2013 by Blackwell Publishing Ltd.

Prescribing for special groups

Children and elderly patients comprise a large proportion of the GP's workload and have very particular prescribing requirements. Fifteen per cent of the population is over 65 years but consume around 45% of all prescriptions. Elderly people with several co-morbidities often require multiple medications but cope less well with them. Calculating dosage in children can be problematic and the effect of drugs idiosyncratic. Most medication information relates to people between these age groups but the bulk of your work will be at these two extremes where particular care is needed in prescribing. As in Chapter 8, we consider necessity, effectiveness, safety and concordance for each group.

Prescribing for children

Children are not small adults; they respond differently. Attention deficit hyperactivity disorder (ADHD) is treated with amphetamine in children where it functions as a sedative – in adults it is a stimulant.

• **Necessity.** Most children seen in general practice have minor self-limiting illness. Parents are understandably concerned and may exert considerable pressure on the doctor to prescribe antibiotics. These will rarely be appropriate. You need to understand the patient's concerns (the child and the parent) and deal with them. You need to develop a safe management plan with the parents so they feel reassured and know what to look for and what to do if things take a turn for the worse (safety netting). Patients requesting antibiotics may do so because 'that's want the last doctor did' or because of particular concerns like high fever (and the dangers they worry it poses). Remember: good communication prevents unnecessary medication.

• **Effectiveness.** While antibiotics have no place in viral illness, there are common bacterial illnesses where one might imagine antibiotics to be useful. This is often not the case in minor infections. Otitis media is painful, acute and bacterial but antibiotics do not affect its natural history. Around 40% of pharyngitis is bacterial, but antibiotics have a very minor effect on its symptoms (in one study decreasing duration of symptoms by just 8 hours). Moreover, available evidence does not suggest that giving antibiotics prevents progression to a more serious disease (e.g. otitis media to mastoiditis or pharyngitis to quinsy).

• **Safety** is a major concern in children. Children are not adults and their relative proportions of body fat give different volumes of distribution to adults (see Figure 9c for dose calculations in children). Giving drugs of questionable necessity is particularly risky as the chance of benefit from the drug is low (e.g. antibiotics for otitis media) but the risk of side effects remains the same. While many side effects are minor, some are serious and even fatal. Another aspect of safety is that it may be difficult to differentiate side effects of the drug from effects of the infection. So a child who develops a skin rash a few days after starting antibiotics probably has a viral rash, but possibly has a drug allergy. Precautionary labelling of a child as drug allergic may limit drug choice for the rest of their life.

• **Concordance.** Negotiating the treatment plan with the parents (and child if they are old enough) is crucial. While some parents push for medications (e.g. antibiotics), others are reluctant to use them – fears over immunisation is a case in point. Understanding concerns and anxieties and spending time addressing these can have lifelong implications (e.g. the young man who does not get polio during his gap year in Nigeria because you alleviated his mother's immunisation fears when he was a few weeks old). Practical considerations, such as offering children a choice of formulation (e.g. tablets, liquid, dispersible) or giving the parents a syringe to use rather than the traditional teaspoon will help parents medicate a reluctant child (pharmacists supply these anyway for certain medications).

Prescribing for the elderly

Elderly patients may have several co-morbidities (and several specialists attending to each), each requiring a variety of medications. Patients may be mentally less able to cope with understanding and taking prescribed medication. Patients have physically different metabolisms with slower absorption or metabolism of drugs and slower excretion.

• **Necessity.** Drugs are often necessary in the elderly to manage chronic disease, but elderly people often have many symptoms and you should take care not to chase minor symptoms with powerful medications (e.g. NSAIDs for aches and pains followed by proton pump inhibitors [PPIs] for indigestion), elderly people often sleep poorly; hypnotics have equivocal benefits and contribute to falls and confusion.

• **Effectiveness.** Be clear about what you are trying to achieve in treatment and realistic about whether drugs can achieve this. Try to ensure there is a good evidence base for your interventions (although beware trial data that exclude the elderly population most likely to benefit).

• **Safety.** There is a relation between polypharmacy (defined as taking four medications or more) and under-utilisation of medication (although confusion can equally cause overuse). Simple drug regimens (e.g. all tablets once a day), minimising drugs or combining them as 'polypills' all contribute towards correct use. Regular 'brown bag review' is helpful. Drugs are often more potent in the elderly. It is a good rule of thumb to start with half the adult dose and titrate as necessary.

• **Concordance.** Good communication with patients is vital. Perhaps 50% of elderly people do not take drugs as the doctor intended. Clear dosage labelling on the packet (avoid 'as directed'), consistent quantities (3 months' supply of everything) and written instructions (which carers not present at the consultation may also find helpful) all help. Make use of carers (both professional and family and neighbours) and the community pharmacist to help you achieve your aims. Pill devices, such as the 'dosette' box, can help both patients and carers cope with a tricky drug regimen.

Good communication between primary and secondary care is equally important: a 50% error rate has been observed in transferring medication information both from primary to secondary and from secondary to primary care (see Chapter 7).

10 Law and ethics

(a) Consent – the three 'pillars'

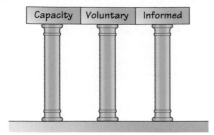

Capacity | Voluntary | Informed

(b) Elements of capacity

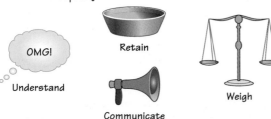

OMG!

Understand

Retain

Communicate

Weigh

Box 10.1 Principles of the Mental Capacity Act 2007

The law **presumes that a person has capacity** unless there is evidence otherwise (so just because a person has Down's Syndrome it does not automatically mean they lack capacity)

There are two steps in demonstrating **lack of capacity**
- There is a disturbance of the brain or mind
- The abnormality must be sufficient to impair capacity

Both of these steps must be demonstrated and supported by evidence

NB: An **unwise decision** is not evidence of lack of capacity

If the patient lacks capacity:
- Any decision made on behalf of a person who lacks capacity must be made in their **best interests**
- If there are more than one option then the one that is **least restrictive** to the person's freedom must be chosen

Capacity relates to **each individual decision** to be made (you may be able to consent to having your blood pressure taken but not to starting renal dialysis)

People need to be supported in making decisions (e.g. using appropriate tools such as pictures if necessary)

Table 10.1 The 'Four Quadrants' approach to ethical problems

Medical indications
The principles of Beneficence and Non-maleficence

1. What is the patient's medical problem? Is the problem acute? Chronic? Critical? Reversible? Emergent? Terminal?
2. What are the goals of treatment?
3. In what circumstances are medical treatments not indicated?
4. What are the probabilities of success of various treatment options?
5. In sum, how can this patient be benefited by medical and nursing care and how can harm be avoided?

Patient preferences
The principle of Respect for Autonomy

1. Has the patient been informed of benefits and risks, understood this information and given consent?
2. Is the patient mentally capable and legally competent and is there evidence of incapacity?
3. If mentally capable, what preferences about treatment is the patient stating?
4. If incapacitated, has the patient expressed prior preferences?
5. Who is the appropriate surrogate to make decisions for the incapacitated patient?
6. Is the patient unwilling or unable to cooperate with medical treatment? If so why?

Quality of life
The principles of Beneficence and Non-maleficence and Respect for Autonomy

1. What are the prospects with or without treatment for a return to a normal life and what physical, mental and social deficits might the patient experience even if treatment succeeds?
2. On what grounds can any one judge that some quality of life would be undesirable for a patient who cannot make or express such a judgement?
3. Are there biases that might prejudice the provider's evaluation of the patient's quality of life?
4. What ethical issues arise concerning improving or enhancing a patient's quality of life?
5. Do quality-of-life assessments raise any questions regarding changes in treatment plans, such as forgoing life sustaining treatment?
6. What are the plans and rationale to forgo life sustaining treatment?
7. What is the legal and ethical status of suicide?

Contextual factors
The principles of Justice and Fairness

1. Are there professional, interprofessional or business interests that might create conflict of interest in the clinical treatment of patients?
2. Are there any parties other than clinicians and patients, such as family members, who have an interest in clinical decisions?
3. What are the limits imposed on patient confidentiality by the legitimate interests of third parties?
4. Are there any financial factors that create conflicts of interest in clinical decisions?
5. Are there problems of allocation of scarce health resources that might affect clinical decisions?
6. Are there religious issues that might influence clinical decisions?
7. What are the legal issues that might affect clinical decisions?
8. Are there considerations of clinical research and education that might affect clinical decisions?
9. Are there issues of public health and safety that might affect clinical decisions?
10. Are there conflicts of interests within institutions and organisations (e.g. hospitals) that might affect clinical decisions and patient welfare?

(Jonsen AR, Siegler M and Winslade WJ; Clinical Ethics: A Practical Approach to Ethical Decisions in Clinical Medicine, 7th edition, McGraw-Hill 2010)

General Practice at a Glance, First Edition. Paul Booton, Carol Cooper, Graham Easton, and Margaret Harper.

30 © 2013 Paul Booton, Carol Cooper, Graham Easton, and Margaret Harper. Published 2013 by Blackwell Publishing Ltd.

What should a GP do when he or she believes that a patient with dementia is no longer safe to drive, or is faced with a mother asking what took place in a recent consultation with her 15-year-old daughter who came in requesting a termination of pregnancy?

These are the sorts of dilemmas that a typical GP can expect to encounter regularly. To be able to practise effectively, safely and on the right side of the law requires a good understanding of the basic principles of ethics and of the law relating to medicine.

Consent to treatment

Before performing any procedure involving a patient, even a simple blood test, the GP must ensure that an adult patient has the **mental capacity** to give consent (see Figure 10a), that their decision is free from coercion and that they have been given sufficient information to make the decision. Without proper consent such procedures could result in a charge of battery.

Of these, assessing mental capacity can be the least straightforward. Since the Mental Capacity Act (MCA) came into force in 2007, doctors have a clear framework to work with. The Act covers adult patients in England and Wales.

To assess capacity the patient must be able to:
• Understand the information being given
• Retain the information in their mind
• Use or weigh the information in considering the decision
• Communicate the decision using any means (see Figure 10b).

The Act also covers the legal basis for decisions made for patients who lack capacity. These are summarised in Box 10.1.

Children under 16 years

Although most consultations with children under 16 years will be with an adult, there are situations where the GP will be faced with a child requesting treatment in the absence of a parent or adult. This may be because the child does not wish his or her parents to be present, for example, a request for contraception.

Treatment relating to children is covered by the **Children Act 1989**. This defines those with 'parental responsibility' who may make decisions on behalf of a child patient. If, say, the child minder brings a child to surgery they would not be able to give consent for the child unless the parent has given their explicit permission. This means it is normally necessary to contact the parent before proceeding. In an emergency, if it is not possible to get hold of a parent, a child can be treated under the Act if it is 'reasonable' to do so.

In certain circumstances children can give consent without the need of a parent or adult. There is no age limit that determines this, instead it is determined by the child's ability to demonstrate 'sufficient understanding and intelligence to enable him or her to understand fully what is proposed' (also known as 'Gillick' or 'Fraser' competence). Where the GP relies on the child's consent in the case of contraception, the GP must also ensure that:
• He or she has sought to persuade the child to involve her parents
• That the child is likely to engage in sexual activity, and
• That the treatment is in her best interests.

Finally, although children with sufficient maturity may consent to treatment, even a competent child may have a refusal of treatment overturned by his or her parents or the courts in the case of life-saving treatment.

Confidentiality

Keeping information gained from patients secret has been a fundamental part of medical ethics as far back as Hippocrates. Doing so serves to protect patient autonomy and trust in the doctor–patient relationship.

In certain circumstances a GP may be permitted or even have a duty to breach patient confidentiality, if:
• It is required by law (e.g. notification of certain infectious diseases; Public Health Act 1984).
• It is justified in the public interest where others may be at risk of serious harm. For instance, a patient with epilepsy who insists on driving.
• The patient consents. Express consent is necessary if identifiable information is to be disclosed. Consent may be implied when sharing information within the healthcare team.

Data protection

GP records hold large amounts of sensitive personal information and are regulated under the Data Protection Act 1998. GPs are responsible for ensuring that data are accurate, secure and accessible to patients.

Confidentiality and the student

As a medical student you also carry confidential information from clerking and examining patients and from seeing the patient's records. You should always take care to protect your patient's confidentiality. Do not talk with colleagues about your patient in a public place (e.g. the hospital lifts). Do not write identifiable details in your patient clerkings (they might get left on the bus). Equally, beware of what you put on Facebook or other social networking sites.

Ethics

The ability to recognise, analyse and resolve ethical dilemmas in clinical practice is a crucial skill for any doctor. There are many tools or frameworks that can be used to help in this process. None are perfect but with a thorough understanding of the clinical issues, the non-medical factors and context of a case, these frameworks help resolve the ethical issues involved.

The **Four Principles** approach is widely used in medical ethics. Although it looks easy to apply, problems can occur when any of the principles conflict, which is all too common in practice. As the approach does not tell us how to resolve such conflicts one is still left with difficult decisions to make.

1 Autonomy. Ensure the principle of self-determination is given due weight, and that patients who have capacity are enabled to make informed choices.

2 Beneficience. Treatment decisions should be aimed at maximising patient welfare. This involves balancing the risks and burdens of treatment.

3 Non-maleficence. Most medical treatment have risks, but any such harm should be minimised and not disproportionate to the benefits of treatment.

4 Justice. The fair distribution of benefits, risks and costs of treatment. Treating patients in a similar position equally.

The **Four Quadrants** approach (Table 10.1), specifies some of the practical questions you should ask in considering the above principles. It is a practical approach which is a useful framework in considering issues in general practice.

11 # Child abuse, domestic violence and elder abuse

(a) Child abuse

What to look for on your physical examination:	• Undress the child and do a full examination. If you don't you will miss important signs • Ask consent • The pattern of bruises relate to the developmental stage	• Remember the only sign of abuse in a baby/toddler may be a crying unhappy baby – difficult to settle • If you suspect abuse and the patient or carers do not speak English always use an independent interpreter

Physical examination
• Bruises – note pattern and compatibility with child's age
• Eyes – bruising/eye injuries
• Ears – look behind the ears
• Mouth – frenulum, dental injuries
• Neck
• Trunk and limbs
• Signs of intracranial injury
 – look for intracranial signs
 – remember the shaken baby syndrome
• Slap marks
• Scalds
• Bite marks
• Cigarette burns
• Bilateral scalds
 – immersion?
• Fractures
• Abdominal injuries
 – spleen/small bowel

Sexual abuse
• Bruising inner thighs
• Genital injury
• Abnormal vaginal discharge/bleeding/genital warts/STI
• Anal injury
• Pregnancy in a child
• Often no physical signs

Neglect
• Poor general appearance
• Poor hygiene/dirty inappropriate clothing
• Failure to thrive
• Poor parental management of chronic conditions e.g. neglected eczema
• Failure to attend or engage with child health promotion
 – immunisations, checks etc.
• Failure to keep hospital appointments

Emotional abuse
• Withdrawn/watchful/passive/over affectionate
• Evidence of self-harm
• Low growth for age

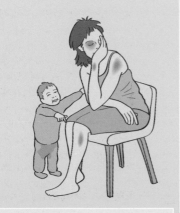 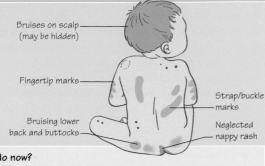

Bruises on scalp (may be hidden) — Fingertip marks — Bruising lower back and buttocks — Strap/buckle marks — Neglected nappy rash

What to do now?
Consult local guidelines and discuss with a senior colleague
– Record in the notes
Serious injury – at immediate risk
• If medical:
 – refer hospital paediatrician. Phone first.
 – discuss who will inform Children's Social Care (that day)
 – check child has arrived at hospital
• If non-medical:
 – inform Children's Social Care that day or if indicated police
Suspected abuse
• Discuss with senior colleague/named doctor/nurse in child protection
• If indicated refer to Children's Social Care
• Remember the siblings. Check parental history
• Inform HV (under fives)

(b) Domestic violence

Common: ¼ of all violent crimes
• Accounts for ⅓ of all female homicides
• 30% start in pregnancy
• Occurs across the social spectrum
• Men can be victims

Symptoms and signs may be:
• Injuries at different times
• History of injury not consistent with story and examination
• Self neglect and low self-esteem
• Reluctant to talk in front of a partner
• Depression and anxiety
• History of self-harm

Children at risk
• 60% witness abuse
• Have an increased risk of physical abuse
• Psychological and emotional damage
 – can occur into adulthood
• Behaviour problems
• Self-harm
• Risk of harm to the unborn child

Action to take
• Focus on her and the children's safety
• Refer to Children's Social Care (Social Services) if indicated
• Give information
• Advice helplines
• Refuges offer places of safety and support
• Police domestic violence units
• Domestic violence Freephone helplines
• Liaise with other health colleagues

(c) Elder abuse

What to look for:
May occur in their own home, care home, hospital or day centre.
Be alert to:
• *Physical abuse*
 – unexplained or frequent injuries, misuse of medication, restraint or inappropriate sanctions
• *Psychological abuse*
 – emotional abuse, verbal abuse, threats of harassment, isolation
• *Financial abuse*
• *Neglect*
 – failure to provide adequate care, withdrawal of care and acts of omission

Action to take
– must be with the patient's consent (if patient is capable to give it – see Chapter 10)
• Make the care home aware of what is happening
• Contact Social Services Care of the Elderly. Explain to the carers they are there to help
• Put the patient in touch with advice and care lines
• Arrange support for the carers
• If a criminal offence has been committed inform the police

Child abuse, domestic violence and elder abuse are all under-recognised. There are about 46,705 children subject to a child protection plan or on a child protection register (NSPCC 2011). Many vulnerable children are unreported. Older children aged 15–18 years are also vulnerable. Be prepared to **think the unthinkable**.

Abuse can happen in any family, across the social spectrum. This means GPs need to think in a different way to the usual approach to patients and have a high index of suspicion, appreciating that abuse can happen in families that they may know well and like. Objectivity is essential. The carer or parent is often able to deceive the GP as to how injuries occurred. Child abuse most commonly occurs in babies under 1 year or in toddlers who are unable to tell what has happened. In the older child they may be too afraid to give the real account of how they came by their injuries, especially if the perpetrator is sitting by them, is someone they know or another member of the family. This applies equally to domestic violence and elder abuse, both of which are under-diagnosed, with the victims unable, afraid or ashamed to report the abuse. It is essential to:
► **Recognise abuse**
► **Know what to do – be familiar with local guidelines**
► **Act on it.**

Child abuse

The welfare of the child is paramount. The usual concept of confidentially may have to be breached. Communication with other agencies is vital in establishing that abuse has taken place. You may only see part of the jigsaw which, put together with pieces from other agencies, adds up to a clear picture of abuse. One of the advantages of being a GP is easy access to the child's medical records and probably those of the siblings and carers.

You may suspect abuse from your examination of the child, information from an outside agency or relative, or from the child.

Risk factors

Child: Under 1 year and pre-term babies.
Adult:
• Domestic violence
• History of drugs and/or alcohol
• Learning disability or mental health problem
• Registered child sex offender or serious violent offender
• Single parent or teenage mother who is isolated

Types of abuse (often overlap)

• **Physical.** This may be bruising, biting, burning, scalds, fractures, head injury, suffocating or other physical harm.
• **Sexual.** Forcing or persuading a child to take part in sexual activity ranging from watching pornography to full penetrative sex.
• **Emotional.** Persistent emotional ill treatment making the child feel worthless and unloved, unrealistic expectations leading to low self-esteem. This includes domestic violence.
• **Neglect.** Persistent failure to fulfil the child's basic needs (e.g. inadequate feeding, clothing, supervision), leading to health-, developmental, emotional and educational problems.

History

If a child comes to the surgery and you suspect abuse has taken place:
• Take a detailed account of the incident.
• Identify who has brought the child. Who is the main carer? Who lives at home?

► Was there any delay in reporting the incident or inconsistency in the history?
• Is the injury compatible with the child's age and development?
► If there are bruises or injuries do they fit in with the story? Be particularly alert if the injury is in an unusual place.
► Any other injury?
• Full past medical history, social and developmental history especially checking for previous injury. Check notes for any A&E visits.
• Check your records to see if the child or the siblings are known to Social Services.
• Check parents and siblings notes for any risk factors.
• Talk to the health visitor and/or school nurse.
• Do they attend nursery or school? If so where?
• If the child is older try and talk to them alone. Remember you cannot offer them full confidentiality.
• **Document** fully and carefully the history and your findings – they may be produced in court. Take any allegation as seriously as with medical problems.
• Consult the local guidelines. Discuss with a senior colleague.

What to tell the parents and child

Explain what you are going to do, for example contacting Children's Social Care (Social Services) or referring to hospital, that they are there to help and give support. The exception to informing the carer or parent is if this puts the child at increased risk of current sexual abuse or forced marriage.
► **Remember the welfare of the child overrides anything else.**

Domestic violence

► **The GP may be the first and only contact by the victim.** About 89% of victims of domestic abuse are women. The attacks are usually part of a repeated pattern. Abuse may be physical, sexual (rape can occur within marriage) or emotional. Victims are often ashamed about what has happened, may think it their fault and be frightened to report it for fear of repercussions.

History

Always see the patient alone. Give her the opportunity to talk. Note non-verbal cues and hidden agendas. Does she seem to have low self-esteem or self-neglect? Ask open then closed questions. If necessary you may have to say 'Did someone do this to you?'
Explain the limits of confidentiality.
Ask about self-harm, depression, anxiety, drug or alcohol abuse, all often related to domestic violence.
► **Ask about the children.** They may be at risk.

Elder abuse and vulnerable adults

This is under-diagnosed. 'Vulnerable is defined as any adult needing community services because of mental or other disability, age or illness' (Select Committee on Health). The GP may be the only person who is aware that abuse is happening. It is estimated there may be 500,000 incidents of elder abuse a year which may be physical, emotional, sexual or financial. It is important to recognise and take action, which may be difficult as the victim is often dependent on the abuser and afraid or unable to complain. Take a careful history; do not be afraid to ask direct questions. The GP's role is often that of an advocate.

The abusers may be family, carers or staff in the care home.

- If the child is a toddler examine on the parent's lap. Examine babies on the couch
- Take your time do not rush the child; use the parents to help you
- Use toys to distract the child. Be systematic and note any red flags in the table below
- Ask yourself – 'does this child look ill?'

Causes of childhood fever includes

- URTI-sore throat, otitis media, croup (mainly viral)
- Viral illnesses e.g. chickenpox, measles, influenza, infectious mononucleosis
- Chest infections
- Urinary tract infections
- Meningitis, encephalitis
- Septic arthritis, osteomyelitis
- Septicaemia
- Kawasaki disease
- Tropical diseases
- Rarely non-infectious causes – malignancy, autoimmune disorders

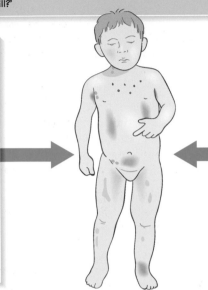

Assessment of a child with a fever can be difficult. The table below is based on the NICE Guidelines and is for guidance only. Finally your clinical judgement should determine your course of action. If in any doubt about underlying serious pathology refer

Look for:

- **Signs of URTI** – common
- **Rashes** – blanching, non-blanching
- **Hydration** – see table
- **Signs of sepsis** – lethargy, tachycardia, cold peripheries/poor capillary return
- **Lymphadenopathy** – localised, general
- **Eyes** – jaundice, conjunctivitis, peri-orbital cellulitis
- **ENT** – best left until last. Throat, mouth, tympanic membranes. Any stridor? – croup, signs of epiglottitis
- **Chest** – tachypnoea, rib recession, tracheal tug Listen to the chest – any abnormal breath sounds, signs of consolidation. (Infants may have a chest infection and no abnormal chest sounds)
- **CVS** – pulse rate – listen to the heart
- **Abdomen** – any pain – site, radiation, guarding; any masses, supra-pubic tenderness Diarrhoea – any blood e.g. shigella
- **Joints** – tender, swollen – septic arthritis, osteomyelitis
- **CNS** – alert, playing, normal movements
- **Signs of meningitis:** (maybe non-specific signs in infants) drowsy, floppy, irritable, bulging fontanelle, neck stiffness, positive Kernig's sign, purpuric rash, any fits
- **Check the urine-dipstick**
- **Take the temperature**

Assessment of the febrile child

	Green (low risk)	Amber (intermediate risk)	Red (high risk)
Colour	• Normal colour of skin, lips and tongue	• Pallor reported by parent or carer	• Pale/mottled/ashen/blue
Activity	• Responds normally to social cues • Content – smiles • Stays awake or wakes quickly • Strong normal cry	• Not responding to normal social cues • Wakes with prolonged stimulation • Decreased activity • No smile	• No response to social cues • Appears ill to a healthcare professional • Unable to rouse, or if roused does not stay awake • Weak high-pitched or continuous cry
Respirations	• Normal	• Nasal flaring • Tachypnoea • RR >50 breaths/minute 6–12 mths • RR >40 breaths/min >12 mths • Oxygen saturation <95% in air • Crackles	• Grunting • Tachypnoea • RR >60/minute • Chest indrawing
Hydration	• Normal skin and eyes • Moist mucous membranes	• Dry mucous membranes • Poor feeding in infants, • CRT >3 seconds (capillary refill time) • Reduced urinary output (ask about wet nappies)	• Reduced skin turgor
Other	• None of the amber or red symptoms or signs	• Fever for longer than 5 days • Swelling of limbs or joints, not weight bearing, or not using an extremity • A new lump >2 cm	• Fever aged 0–3 mths >38 • Status epilepticus • aged 3–6 mths >39 • Focal neurological signs • Non blanching rash • Focal seizures • Bulging fontanelle • Bile stained vomiting • Neck stiffness

(Source: Feverish Illness in Children. (2007) RCOG Press, London. © Royal College of Obstetricians and Gynaecologists; reproduced with permission)

General Practice at a Glance, First Edition. Paul Booton, Carol Cooper, Graham Easton, and Margaret Harper.

Children often have fevers. Most have a self-limiting illness needing only advice and do *not* need a course of antibiotics. However, in some the diagnosis is serious, with potentially catastrophic outcomes if missed. An added challenge for GPs is that children with a serious illness may present in the early stages when there are few symptoms or signs. In babies and infants, features of life-threatening illnesses are frequently non-specific (e.g. irritability or lethargy).

Assessment of the child with a fever

History
Listen to the parents; take their concerns seriously. If the child can answer don't forget to ask the child about the symptoms.
- Ask about the symptoms and duration of the illness.
- Are there any signs of a URTI (e.g. coryza, cough)?
- Ask about diarrhoea or vomiting, rashes or symptoms suggesting a urinary tract infection (UTI) or meningitis.
- What treatment or management including medication have they tried? Has it helped?
- Have they taken the temperature or subjectively assessed the fever?
- Is the child deteriorating?
- Ask about foreign travel and contact with infection.
- Check their immunisation history.
- Take a past medical history, social and developmental history including risk factors such as poor immunity, sickle cell disease.
- Has there been a fit (seizure)? Febrile fits are associated with fever in children aged 6 months to 5 years. While often caused by a URTI you must exclude the possibility of a serious illness.

Management and advice for non-serious fever
- Keep the child or baby cool – do not wrap up or sponge down.
- Give fluids. Continue breast-feeding.
- Use paracetamol or ibuprofen. Both are effective; either can be used. If one is not effective then try the alternative. A fever is a normal physiological response and the well child may not need medication. Ask about allergies, any contraindication (e.g. asthma with NSAIDs) (see BNF for Children).
- Keep the child away from nursery.
- Give the parents clear advice about what to look for if there is deterioration and what to do if the child does not improve.

Indications for referral
- Any baby under 3 months who has a temperature of >38°. They have a poor immune system, and may rapidly deteriorate.
- Any infant over 3 months who has a persistent fever >39.9° or any red flag signs.

Meningococcal disease
▶ Infants may present with non-specific signs such as drowsiness, lethargy or poor feeding.

Children over 2 years can present early before the signs evolve.

Fifty per cent of children are not diagnosed on the first consultation. **Always think of meningococcal disease in an ill child. Remember children can deteriorate rapidly over a few hours.**

Important early signs: cold hands and feet, skin changes, leg pains.

Look for:
▶ A purpuric rash, neck stiffness, lethargy, positive Kernig's sign. Ask about vomiting, headache, photophobia, altered consciousness.

Tell the parents what to look for.

▶ If you suspect meningococcal disease do not wait. Refer urgently. Give antibiotics in the surgery (see BNF) and call 999.

Urinary tract infection
Most UTIs occur in the first year of life; 4% of girls and 1% of boys will have a UTI before they are 11 years.

UTIs often present with non-specific symptoms, especially in infants. **Always suspect a UTI in a child with an unexplained fever, recurrent fevers or symptoms and signs of a viral or minor infection that does not respond to treatment.**

▶ Over 30% of children, particularly infants presenting with a UTI, have an underlying renal abnormality such as vesicoureteric reflux (VUR), posterior urethral valve or other congenital renal abnormalities. Missing these can lead to serious renal damage.

Other risk factors for UTI include a family history of congenital renal problems, spinal lesions, constipation and poor hygiene.

Differential diagnosis
- In girl vulval irritation, in boys balanitis.
- Threadworms.
▶ Remember the rare possibility of sexual abuse.

History
- Symptoms may be non-specific in infants. **Ask about: irritability, lethargy, poor feeding, vomiting and even jaundice.** Parents may have noticed offensive urine.
- Those over 6 months may present with a febrile fit.
- Older children may have fever, frequency, dysuria, haematuria, abdominal pain, diarrhoea, vomiting, secondary enuresis or noticed offensive urine.
- Take a past medical history (PMH) and ask about any risk factors.

Examination
- Exclude other causes of fever.
- Feel the abdomen for tenderness, renal mass or large bladder.
- Inspect the external genitalia if indicated for evidence of a congenital abnormality, vulvitis or balanitis.

Investigations
Take a urine sample (if possible clean catch) before treating, and send the sample for culture to confirm the diagnosis. Explain to the parents the importance of a sterile sample. Whether you treat based on the dipstick or wait for the results of a mid stream urine (MSU) depends on the child's age and the clinical picture.

Management
Refer urgently: if the child is less than 3 months and you suspect a UTI or is ill with any of the red flag symptoms.

Otherwise treat with antibiotics (usually trimethoprim).

In view of the incidence of underlying renal abnormalities there is a case for referring all children for renal ultrasound after their first UTI. NICE guidelines suggest referral based on the child's age, the severity of the infection and risk of renal damage.

Advice to parent
- Give fluids and treat fever and pain
- Stress the importance of completing the course of antibiotics
- Avoid constipation
- Return if the symptoms don't resolve or if the child has any recurrent episode of unexplained fever
- Encourage complete voiding
- Give advice on hygiene, wiping front to back for a girl.

13 Cough and wheeze

Cough and wheeze

Most coughs in children are caused by URTI and are self-limiting, but cough and/or wheeze can herald serious illness. Causes may overlap but in your differential diagnosis consider those in Table 13.1.

Table 13.1 Causes of cough, stridor and wheeze.

Cough	Stridor	Wheeze
Acute	**Acute**	Respiratory tract
URTI	Croup, 6 months to	infection
Croup	6 years	Bronchiolitis, 1–9
Pneumonia	Epiglottitis, 1–6	months
Pertussis	years	Atopic asthma
	Bacterial tracheitis	Asthma – non-atopic
Chronic	FB, toddler	Transient wheezing in
Post-bronchiolitis or	Acute allergic	infancy – usually
pertussis	reaction	resolves by 5 years
Aspiration of feed		Croup
Gastro-oesophageal	**Chronic**	Gastro-oesophageal
reflux	Usually congenital	reflux
	causes (e.g.	Inhaled foreign body,
Recurrent	laryngomalacia)	typically toddler
Asthma		Heart failure
Cystic fibrosis		
Bronchiectasis		

History

Find out if symptoms are **acute or chronic**. Consider the child's age.
- If there is a wheeze, clarify what the parents mean by this.
- Ask about duration of symptoms.
- What is the timing? Asthma and croup are worse at night.
- Are symptoms recurrent? Think cystic fibrosis, bronchiectasis and asthma.
- What is the type of cough?
- If there is fever, infection is likely, either viral or bacterial. Remember specific infections (e.g. pneumonia, TB).
- Are there any feeding difficulties? Or any weight loss?
- Was there choking? Think of a foreign body (FB).
- Take a PMH and a family history (e.g. cystic fibrosis, asthma).
- Ask about smoking in the household, family or other carers.
- Check the growth and immunisation record.

Examination

Ask yourself: is this an ill child? Look for:
► Respiratory distress, cyanosis, intercostal recession, tracheal tug, tachypnoea, lethargy, low oxygen saturation, dehydration.
- Take the temperature, pulse and respiration rate.
- Listen to the cough. Is it barking or spasmodic? Is there stridor?
- Assess severity of stridor (at rest or only when the child is active?).
- Distinguish between croup and epiglottitis (see below).
► If you suspect epiglottitis or an inhaled foreign body do not examine the throat or you may precipitate complete obstruction.
- Listen to the chest for wheezes, other sounds or evidence of consolidation. Unilateral wheeze suggests a FB.
- If you suspect asthma, perform a peak flow test if possible.

Croup and epiglottitis

Stridor is a noise that occurs on inspiration because of partial upper airways obstruction; it can be acute or chronic. Croup is a common cause and often seen in general practice.

Croup is a laryngo-tracheal infection usually caused by para-influenza virus. It is more common in winter and starts with URTI. The typical barking cough and stridor develop later. Most episodes can be managed at home. Refer to hospital if:
► Ill child with cyanotic spells
► Respiratory distress, feeding difficulties or dehydration
► Parents not confident in managing at home
► Poor access to hospital
► If you suspect epiglottitis or an FB dial 999.

If you decide to manage at home, explain to the parents this is a self-limiting illness. Give them clear advice:
- Keep calm and reassure the child who may be frightened.
- Sit the child upright to help breathing.
- Treat fever and give plenty of drinks to maintain fluid intake.
- Inhaling steam has **not** been shown to be of any benefit.
- Dexamethasone and nebulised steroids can reduce severity.
- Do not give cough mixtures as they may cause drowsiness.
- If breathing worsens or child deteriorates get urgent medical help. Make sure the parents know what to look for.

Epiglottitis is now rare since *Haemophilus influenzae* type B (HiB) immunisation. **It is a medical emergency.** Unlike croup the onset is rapid over a few hours. The child is ill with a soft stridor and may lean forwards, drooling because of extreme difficulty in swallowing.

Bronchiolitis

Bronchiolitis is mostly caused by respiratory syncytial virus (RSV) and occurs mainly in winter in babies under 12 months. Many infections are mild, but it can be a life-threatening illness.

Initially there is a cough and URTI. Later respiratory symptoms develop and there may be difficulty in breathing, feeding or dehydration and apnoeic attacks.

Examination

Look for dehydration and respiratory distress. The chest may be hyper-inflated with widespread wheeze and fine crackles. The differential diagnosis includes heart failure and pneumonia. The management is mainly supportive. Admit to hospital if:
► Baby under 3 months
► High risk (e.g. prematurity or any co-morbidity)
► Dehydration, poor feeding, lethargy or cyanosis
► Respiratory rate >70 or severe recession
► Parental difficulty in coping or accessing medical help.

Many babies can be managed at home with careful follow-up. Give advice on hydration, fever management, what to look for if the baby deteriorates and how to get help urgently.

Pertussis

Immunisation gives 95% protection. The cough is paroxysmal, followed by prolonged inspiration when a whoop may be heard. Vomiting can then occur. The cough can last months. Refer if the child is under 6 months, dehydrated or has apnoeic attacks.

14 Asthma

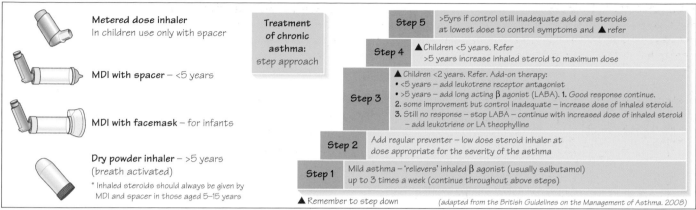

Treatment of chronic asthma: step approach

Step 5 >5yrs if control still inadequate add oral steroids at lowest dose to control symptoms and ▲ refer

Step 4 ▲ Children <5 years. Refer
>5 years increase inhaled steroid to maximum dose

Step 3 ▲ Children <2 years. Refer. Add-on therapy:
• <5 years – add leukotrene receptor antagonist
• >5 years – add long acting β agonist (LABA). 1. Good response continue.
2. some improvement but control inadequate – increase dose of inhaled steroid.
3. Still no response – stop LABA – continue with increased dose of inhaled steroid – add leukotriene or LA theophylline

Step 2 Add regular preventer – low dose steroid inhaler at dose appropriate for the severity of the asthma

Step 1 Mild asthma – 'relievers' inhaled β agonist (usually salbutamol) up to 3 times a week (continue throughout above steps)

Metered dose inhaler
In children use only with spacer

MDI with spacer – <5 years

MDI with facemask – for infants

Dry powder inhaler – >5 years
(breath activated)
* Inhaled steroids should always be given by MDI and spacer in those aged 5–15 years

▲ Remember to step down   (adapted from the British Guidelines on the Management of Asthma. 2008)

Asthma is an inflammatory disease of the airways with reversible outflow obstruction, associated with bronchial hyper-responsiveness. About 15% of children have asthma. Many have symptoms that affect their education and quality of life, and each year about 40 die. Persistent symptoms and poor control are linked with lack of information, poor compliance or poor inhaler technique.

Chronic asthma is managed almost entirely in primary care. Management is a team approach aimed to keep the child symptom-free with normal quality of life.

The diagnosis of asthma is clinical, resting on history and signs.

History
Remember not all wheezes and chronic coughs are due to asthma.
The key features for the diagnosis of asthma are:
• **Recurrent wheeze** – expiratory and high pitched, often worse at night or early morning.
• **Tightness of the chest and breathlessness.**
• **Recurrent cough** – dry, non-paroxysmal, often worse at night.
• **Trigger factors** (e.g. URTI, pets, dust, cold, exercise, smoke).
• **Family history of atopy.**
• **Other atopic symptoms** (e.g. eczema, hay fever).
• When taking the history, establish what is meant by a wheeze.
• Ask about frequency of episodes. When was the last? What happened? Have there been hospital visits?
• Ask about time off school, effect on sport, walking or running.
• If taking bronchodilators – how often? Response to therapy.
• Ask about smoking – older child or passive smoking at home.

Examination
• There may be no signs.
• Note any chronic features: poor growth, Harrison's sulci (a depression at the base of the thorax), a hyper-inflated chest.
• Plot the growth.
• Check for other signs of atopy (e.g. eczema).
• Look for finger clubbing to exclude other chronic conditions.
• Note the respiratory rate, pulse rate.
• Listen to the chest. Is there any wheeze?
• If the child is >5 years perform spirometry or peak flow (PF).
• Note any improvement after bronchodilator therapy.
• Plot the growth.

Acute asthma
Acute asthma can be life-threatening. Clinical signs are poor indicators and the severity of the attack may not be recognised. The following is adapted from the British Thoracic Society (BTS) and SIGN guidelines. It refers to children over 2 years. Under 2 years diagnosis is difficult – assess and refer urgently.

Acute severe asthma
► Unable to complete sentences or feed, agitation, altered consciousness, use of accessory muscles of respiration
• Pulse rate >120 if over 5 years, >140 if aged 2–5 years
• Respiratory rate >30 if over 5 years, >40 if 2–5 years old
• SpO2 <92%
• Peak flow in older children <33–50% of best or predicted PEFR
► Give beta-agonists as first line treatment up to 10 puffs, if no improvement refer urgently to hospital. Give beta-agonist while waiting for the ambulance.

Life-threatening asthma
► Hypotension, exhaustion, confusion, poor respiratory effort or 'silent chest'. Pulse rate, respiration rate, SpO2 as for acute severe asthma PF <33%. Refer urgently to hospital giving beta-agonist and oxygen via a face mask while waiting for the ambulance.

If it is not asthma, what is it?
Consider any of the causes of a wheeze in Table 13.1 including cystic fibrosis and rarer causes, e.g. bronchopulmonary dysplasia, bronchiectasis or a developmental abnormality.

Management of chronic asthma
Routine follow-up is usually carried out by the practice nurse:
• Monitor growth.
• Peak flow and/or symptom diary, ensuring the child knows how to use it.
• **Check inhaler technique on each visit** and check compliance.
• Ask about breakthrough attacks, use of short-acting beta-agonists, and any exercise-induced asthma.
• Ask about sleep disturbance and time away from school.
• Choose an inhaler that is suitable for the child's age and is acceptable to the child and the family (Figure 14).
• Consider allergen avoidance.
• Advise about active/passive smoking and flu vaccination.
• **Written management plan acceptable to the child and parents.**

General Practice at a Glance, First Edition. Paul Booton, Carol Cooper, Graham Easton, and Margaret Harper.
© 2013 Paul Booton, Carol Cooper, Graham Easton, and Margaret Harper. Published 2013 by Blackwell Publishing Ltd.

Causes of acute abdominal pain

- **Surgical**
  - appendicitis
  - Meckel's
  - intestinal obstruction e.g. malrotation (consider if bile stained vomiting)
  - Intussusception (2 months – 2 years) (screaming episodes, redcurrant jelly stools)
  - strangulated hernias
- **Medical**
  - gastroenteritis
  - UTI/pyelonephritis
  - tonsilitis
  - mesenteric adenitis
  - Henoch–Schönlein (HSP) purpura
  - diabetic ketoacidosis, sickle cell crisis, inflammatory bowel diseases
- **Extra-abdominal**
  - torsion of the testis, lower lobe pneumonia, referred pain from the hip or spine
  - in girls – ovarian cyst, pelvic inflammatory disease, ectopic pregnancy
- **Causes of recurrent abdominal pain**
  (occurs in 10% all school children)
  - functional – in 90% of the above no organic cause found
  - abdominal migraine
  - irritable bowel syndrome
  - non-ulcer dyspepsia
  - inflammatory bowel disease
  - coeliac disease
  - mesenteric adenitis
  - giardia
- **Extra-abdominal**
  - gynaecological (e.g. dysmenorrhoea, ovarian cyst, pelvic inflammatory disease)
  - psychosocial
  - referred pain from hip or spine
  - urinary tract infections
  - sickle cell disease

Examination of abdominal pain

- Take the pulse rate and temperature
- Note rashes – systemic illness, HSP
  - purpuric rash on extensor buttocks and legs
- Any scars?
- Feel for lymphadenopathy – ? mesenteric adenitis
- Mouth – any foetor
- Look for jaundice
- Listen to the chest – ? lower lobe pneumonia

Causes of acute diarrhoea

- Infective gastroenteritis
- Food poisoning
- Diarrhoea associated with a febrile illness (e.g. URTI, UTI, chest infection)

Causes of vomiting in infants

- Overfeeding, posseting
- Gastro-oesophageal reflux
- Gastroenteritis
- Surgical causes – pyloric stenosis (1–4 mths), malrotation
- Intussusception
- Extra-abdominal causes of infection

Causes of chronic diarrhoea

- Toddler diarrhoea
- Post-infective gastroenteritis, parasites (e.g. giardia)
- Over-flow from constipation
- Malabsorption – ulcerative colitis or Crohn's, cystic fibrosis

Causes of vomiting in older children

- Gastroenteritis
- Viral illness
- Systemic infection (e.g. UTI, meningitis)
- Migraine
- Bulimia
- Raised intracranial pressure
- Pregnancy, drugs

Examining the child with diarrhoea and/or vomiting

Does the child look ill?
- Any lethargy?
- Take the temperature, pulse rate, capillary refill time
- Weigh
- Assess hydration
- Look for signs of meningitis – bulging fontanelle, rash
- Exclude raised intracranial pressure – fundi
- Look for other systemic disease

With chronic diarrhoea plot height and weight
Look for finger clubbing. Test the urine

Assessment of hydration
- Note any lethargy
- Sunken fontanelle
- Dry mucous membranes and sunken eyes
- Reduced skin turgor
- Increased capillary refill time
- Tachycardia/tachypnoea
- Ask about urine output

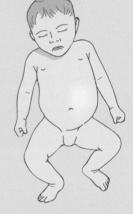

Abdomen
- Any distension – ? intestinal obstruction
- Feel for masses (e.g. pyloric stenosis)

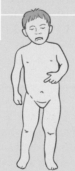

Abdomen (warm hands, look at the child's face for pain)
Look for:
- Any scars, abdominal distension
- Ask where pain is
- Note any radiation, guarding or rebound, pain on coughing
- Feel for masses, an enlarged liver or spleen – (may be significant in recurrent abdominal pain), remember faecal masses and constipation
- Listen to the bowel sounds
- Feel the testes
- Examine hernial orifices
- If appropriate measure height and weight
- Test the urine to exclude infection or diabetes

There is a wide range of gastrointestinal illnesses in children. Many are rare but these too often first present to the GP so you must be able to recognise them. Do not forget gynaecological pain in girls, testicular pain in boys and child abuse.

Consider the child's age: many conditions are age related. Check the growth and look at the growth chart. Poor growth is always significant.

Abdominal pain
History

- Establish if this is the first episode of pain or if there have been recurrent attacks, if so, over what period of time?
- Ask about the site of the pain, its frequency, quality and timing (e.g. SOCRATES). How does pain affect the child? Are they reluctant to move? **Do they appear ill?**

General Practice at a Glance, First Edition. Paul Booton, Carol Cooper, Graham Easton, and Margaret Harper.

- Is there vomiting? **Bilious vomiting with abdominal pain is always abnormal and should be considered a malrotation until proved otherwise.**
- Ask about constipation or diarrhoea. Ask parents to describe the stools. Blood may indicate Henoch–Schönlein purpura, intussusception (associated with bouts of severe pain, drawing up of the legs and pallor), inflammatory bowel disease or gastroenteritis.
- Is there fever? This may be present with appendicitis or indicate non-gastrointestinal cause of the pain. Ask about urinary symptoms and other signs of systemic infection.
- Is there weight loss? If the pain is recurrent ask about interference with activities or school or psychological factors.
- Explore the past medical history, including any previous surgery.
- Take a family and social history.

Management of acute abdominal pain

This depends on the cause. All should have a urinary dipstick. The majority will have self-limiting abdominal pain with no abnormal finding. If there is doubt or signs of a serious cause admit.
► Children with an acute abdomen can deteriorate rapidly. If you suspect an organic cause for the pain refer urgently.

Management of recurrent abdominal pain

Causes such as constipation and irritable bowel syndrome (IBS) can be treated in primary care but others such as malabsorption and inflammatory bowel disease need referral. The most common cause of recurrent abdominal pain is functional. Parents want the reassurance of a definitive diagnosis. Be sympathetic, explaining to child and parents that although no specific cause has been found the pain is real and not 'all in the head'. Try to identify trigger factors and together form a management plan that aims to minimise any disruption to the child's activities.

Diarrhoea and vomiting

Diarrhoea and vomiting are usually caused by viral gastroenteritis which is mostly self-limiting.

History
Vomiting
In infants, vomiting is common and you must distinguish between true vomiting and that caused by overfeeding or posseting. These babies usually regurgitate small amounts, are well and gaining weight. Ask about:
- The size of the vomit, frequency and relation to meals (gastro-oesophageal reflux [GOR] occurs after meals and when lying flat).
- Take a detailed feeding history to exclude overfeeding in babies. Ask about **fluid intake and signs of dehydration.**
- Is the vomit projectile as in pyloric stenosis or bile stained suggesting obstruction?
- Is there fever? Vomiting or diarrhoea can occur with non-gastrointestinal infections like otitis media, UTIs or meningitis.
- Ask about signs of raised intracranial pressure – lethargy and raised fontanelle in the baby, headache in the older child who may also have papilloedema.
- In older children consider migraine, infection and bulimia.

Diarrhoea (frequently coexists with vomiting)
- Ask how the stools have changed, and their frequency. Distinguish between acute and chronic symptoms.

- Is there any blood in the stool? Are symptoms associated with weaning (?coeliac). Undigested food in the stool in a well child suggests toddler diarrhoea.
- Is there vomiting, weight loss or abdominal pain? ► **Weight loss is always significant.**
- In acute diarrhoea ask about fluid intake.
- Are there any symptoms suggesting a systemic cause?
- Enquire about foreign travel or contact with anyone with diarrhoea.
- Exclude constipation with overflow.

Management
Management depends on the cause. Treat mild dehydration at home with glucose electrolyte mixture. Continue breast-feeding.

Acute gastroenteritis does not usually need investigation but send a stool sample if you suspect a bacterial cause or to exclude parasites. Admit a child if unwell or dehydrated, or you suspect an acute surgical cause or an underlying medical cause.
► Chronic symptoms usually need referral for diagnosis.

Constipation

Constipation usually presents with large hard stools (<3 stools per week), 'rabbit droppings' or constipation with overflow but there is enormous variation. Breast-fed babies may pass infrequent stools.

Constipation is stressful for child and family. The child is reluctant to pass painful stools and withholding leads to further constipation with overflow or megacolon.

History
Establish if the cause is organic (uncommon) or idiopathic. Ask about the type of stool, frequency, any pain (?anal fissure), soiling, straining or bleeding. Ask about abdominal pain, toilet training and diet. Have there been any precipitating factors such as a febrile illness or hot weather leading to fluid depletion? What about stress or emotional problems? When did it start?

Examination
- Exclude underlying medical conditions (e.g. hypothyroidism)
- Feel the abdomen for any faecal or other masses
- Examine the spine and legs for any neurological causes
- Examine the anus gently looking for fissures
- Access faecal impaction (overflow soiling, palpable mass)
- Measure growth.

Management of idiopathic constipation
The aim is to restore normal bowel functioning.
- Explain it may take months to resolve. The first step is to clear the bowel. Treat with an osmotic laxative (e.g. lactulose) and/or a bowel stimulant (e.g. Senokot®). Continue treatment several weeks after resolution and reduce gradually.
- Identify triggers (e.g. the toilet at school, pressure at home).
- Give lifestyle advice – exercise, fluids and diet. Give encouragement and support.
- Liaise if appropriate with the school nurse or health visitor.
- Refer if treatment is unsuccessful or if there are any red flags:
► Constipation from birth or the first few weeks of life
► Ribbon stools in babies <1 year (?Hirschsprung's disease)
► Delay in passing meconium
► Distended abdomen and/or vomiting
► Poor growth? Hypothyroid or coeliac
► Neurological symptoms.

Below are some common behaviour problems. The list is not complete. Be aware of depression in children

Eating problems in younger children

– mealtimes often a nightmare with refusal to eat/faddy eating/throwing food on floor

• **Causes** – parenting, snacks, temperament

• **Management** – be supportive
– discuss trigger factors and dietary history
– measure height and weight, examine to exclude an organic cause
– refer to health visitor or dietitian if indicated
– parental advice
– no force feeding or focusing on the child during meals
– no alternative
– ignore food refusal
– no snacks
– try and eat together

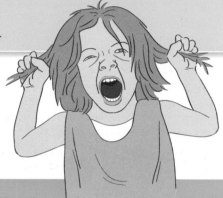

Bedwetting

– 1 in 5 children wet the bed at 5 years. Male>females
– *primary enuresis* – delay in normal sphincter control
– *secondary enuresis* – child previously dry – often psychological

• **Causes**
– usually no organic cause
– strong family history
– organic causes e.g. diabetes or renal disease, constipation
– consider stress factors – family/child e.g. new school, bullying
– sexual abuse

• **Examination**
– test the urine (glucose, protein, infection), check height and weight, feel for faecal masses and exclude neurological or congenital abnormality

• **Management**
Explain
– common, usually no underlying cause, not the child's fault. There is a high rate of spontaneous resolution
– <7 years reassure unless an organic cause is suspected
– discuss bladder maturation
– involve the child in management
– refer to enuresis clinic if treatment fails. Eneursis alarm has been shown to be the most effective treatment
– medication – desmopressin for short term (see Children's BNF)
Parental advice
– keep calm, no punishments
– allow drinks – avoid fizzy or caffeinated drinks
– environmental changes (e.g. accessibility of the toilet, fear of the dark)
– practical measures (e.g. waterproof cover on bed)
– rewards for dry nights – star charts, stickers

Crying baby

– mostly part of a normal spectrum
– stressful for the family ▶ and can lead to risk of abuse

• **Causes** – hunger, wet or dirty nappy, hot or cold, noise, illness e.g. URTI, UTI, any pain – reflux oesophagitis, infantile colic, intussusception

• **Management**
Exclude an organic cause
– ask about change in the nature of the cry, poor feeding, weight loss, signs of infection, pain
– plot the weight and assess development
– examine to exclude underlying illness. Refer to secondary care if indicated
If non-organic
– explain normal crying and sleep patterns (crying usually worse at 6 weeks resolving by 3 months)
Parental advice
– discuss changes in routine like walks, playing with the baby, feeding, sleep routine
– consult health visitor, support groups

Temper tantrums (2–3 years)

• *Normal* – frustrated child trying to control his environment, may be associated with head banging, breath-holding

• **Causes** – hunger, tiredness, frustration, temperament

• **Management**
Parental advice
– keep calm – try not to get cross
– consistent approach
– prevention – avoid triggers, distract, offer restricted choices
– ignore bad behaviour, reward good
– time out – remove from the situation and audience
– comfort and reassure

Sleep problems

– 40% children have sleep problems – maybe settling, waking, nightmares, night terrors
– ▶ Impacts on the parents who often become tired and stressed

• **Causes** – poor night time routine, daytime activities, noisy environment, fear or anxiety, school or family problems, physical illness e.g. asthma

• **Management:**
– get parental agreement on the management plan
Parental advice
– consistent bedtime routine – quiet play, bath, story
– address any anxieties or fears
– sleep diary for 1 week
– modified extinction – leave for agreed time – check – do not pick up or feed
– medication – not recommended (maybe helpful with children with special problem e.g. cerebral palsy, learning/behaviour difficulties)
– refer for management – consider referral to sleep clinic

• **Night terrors** – common in toddlers, differ from nightmares as child semi wake screaming, disorientated, unable to remember the dream and taking time to recover. Usually resolve spontaneously. Reassure parents

General Practice at a Glance, First Edition. Paul Booton, Carol Cooper, Graham Easton, and Margaret Harper.

40 © 2013 Paul Booton, Carol Cooper, Graham Easton, and Margaret Harper. Published 2013 by Blackwell Publishing Ltd.

Most behaviour problems in general practice are common, self-limiting and part of a spectrum of normal behaviour which can be managed in primary care. It is important to recognise more serious problems and take the right action. While secondary care leads the treatment of complex disorders like autism and attention deficit hyperactivity disorder (ADHD), the GP has a significant role in **early recognition**, supporting a family under pressure, and guiding them through the system.

Whatever the problem, **early intervention** is important. By the time the parents attend they may be stressed and exhausted, arguing about managing the child plus dealing with the impact on siblings.

History

• Your history needs to be tailored to each patient but always ask what exactly happens and how long the problem has existed.
• Take a past medical and developmental history to exclude any possible causes.
• The parents' own experience of being parented is important in developing their own skills.
• Have there been any precipitating factors such as illness in the child or family, a new house/school, family crisis or depression in the parents?
• Are there triggers at the time (e.g. tiredness or hunger)?
• Does the behaviour only happen at home?
• How do the parents or carers manage the problem? What have they tried? Be specific (e.g. do they get angry, give in or offer bribes?)
• Do the parents **agree** on their management and are they consistent?
• Evaluate how much disruption is being caused to the family.
➤ Explore any underlying fears or worries the child may have.
➤ Are there any parental problems, e.g. alcohol or drug misuse?
• Do the parents have support?
• If the parents come alone ask them to return with the child.
Ask yourself:
➤ Is the behaviour age appropriate for the child? For example, temper tantrums are common in a 2-year-old but abnormal in a 10-year-old.
Remember the possibility of child abuse or neglect.
➤ Remember depression can occur in children.

Range of problems

Common problems in under-5-year-olds include **crying, feeding, sleep problems, temper tantrums, aggressive behaviour and bed-wetting**. Health visitors are experienced in helping parents handle this age group but you must be familiar with how to manage common behaviour problems and work with the health visitor.

Behaviour problems in the older child include **bed-wetting, school refusal, bullying, hyperactivity and anxiety, depression, self-harm, eating disorders and aggression.**

School refusal

This often presents when the child is stressed, typically on starting school, or transfer to secondary school. Take a detailed history including a past medical history. Ask about possible precipitating factors such as bullying, new teacher, change of class, school journey or friendship problems. The child may avoid school by complaining of illness. If indicated perform a physical examination to exclude this and to reassure the parents.

Liaise with the teacher or nurse and encourage the child to return to school either gradually or immediately. The longer the absence the harder it is for them to return. If this is not effective, refer to the Child and Adolescent Mental Health Service.

The hyperactive child and attention deficit hyperactivity disorder

Parents may be concerned their child is hyperactive. Establish what they mean. This may depend on their perception of how a child should behave. Many children are excitable, overactive and rowdy at times and the behaviour may be normal for their age and stage of development. The parents may simply need advice on how to manage.

ADHD is thought to be a combination of genetic and environmental factors. There are three key factors for diagnosis: **1. impulsivity, 2. hyperactivity, 3. inattention.**

These must be persistent (not episodic), occur in different situations and lead to social and educational impairment. Typically, the child is difficult to control in the classroom, unable to sit still, has poor concentration and impulsive inappropriate behaviour. Other features are sleep disturbance, aggression, temper tantrums, mood swings and low self-esteem. Friendships are often difficult. ADHD continues into adult life but with changes and can coexist with other conditions (e.g. learning disability).

Take a full past medical history, social and developmental history to exclude any other cause for the behaviour.

Assess the impact on the child and family.

Management

NICE guidelines recommend that GPs make the initial assessment but **the diagnosis should only be made by a specialist in secondary care**. They recommend that GPs identify possible ADHD. If symptoms are severe, refer to secondary care. If moderate, 10 weeks of watchful waiting, offering an education–support programme before formal diagnosis. If the behaviour persists, refer. Led by secondary care, management includes:
• Specific advice to parents and school about behaviour modification, encouraging the child and establishing clear boundaries with a consistent management plan.
• Ongoing support and information about self-help groups.
• Structured routine.
• Drug treatment prescribed by secondary care.

Autistic spectrum disorder

Parents often notice early that something is wrong. The disorder has a wide spectrum of symptoms, disability and severity:
• Major impairment in verbal and non-verbal communication
• Poor social interaction, lack of empathy, eye contact, no interest in other people
• Repetitive ritualistic behaviour with impairment of imagination and imaginative play.

Autism can be associated with developmental delay and learning disability. In classic autism there is regression from 18 months and severe learning disability. Exclude other causes of learning disability, deafness or language disorders. Refer to secondary care for diagnosis. Interdisciplinary cooperation helps ensure the parents, siblings and child get maximum support and guidance. Put in touch with self-help groups (e.g. National Autistic Society).

Asperger's falls at the other end of the spectrum and often presents later. The IQ is usually normal but there is impaired social interaction with obsessive behaviour and poor imagination. A diagnosis enables the patient to take advantage of therapy and gives an explanation for their difficulties.

17 Childhood rashes

When a child presents with a rash a careful history helps to establish the cause. Ask if the rash is acute or recurrent, if there is any fever preceding the rash as in the viral exanthems. Are there any other systemic symptoms? **Is the child ill?** In an ill child with a rash consider serious illness such as meningococcal meningitis. Is the rash itchy? Enquire about any impact on the child's quality of life. Eczema can cause intense itching, disrupting sleep and affecting daytime activities. Ask what treatments have already been tried. This is particularly important in chronic conditions like eczema or psoriasis when parents may seek alternative therapies. Ask about immunisations.

Examination

Note the distribution of the rash and the characteristics of the lesions – the size, shape and type. Whether it is papular, macular, maculo-papular, vesicular or purpuric, does it blanch on pressure? Look at the mucosal surfaces. Note any crusting, excoriation or lichenification. Do a general physical examination.

Rashes and spots in babies

Rashes and spots in babies are common, particularly in the newborn infant. Erythema toxicum and milia each occur in 50% of babies. You must be aware of benign self-limiting rashes and give the parents appropriate reassurance. Common rashes include the following:

Erythema toxicum. A benign rash with unknown aetiology, presenting in the first 48 hours in a **well** infant. There are erythematous patches with yellow papules often covering the whole body. If the infant is ill consider the possibility of herpes which is a life-threatening illness.

Nappy rashes. See Figures 17a–c.

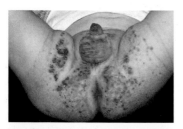

a. Ammoniacal dermatitis. Erythematous papular/vesicular lesions. Contact with irritants, usually dirty nappies. Sparing of the skin folds. Look for secondary infection (bacterial or Candida). Treatment: frequent nappy changes, protective creams. Treat infection.

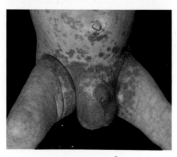

b. Candida nappy rash. Bright red, well-demarcated rash. The rash occurs in skin folds and there may be satellite lesions. Look for oral thrush. Treatment: topical antifungal creams.

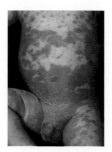

c. Seborrhoeic nappy rash. Yellow, scaly, greasy lesions. May also have cradle cap. Treatment: mild topical steroids or combined steroid antifungal/antibacterial cream if secondary infection suspected. (Treat cradle cap with olive oil/combing or antiseborrhoeic shampoo.)

Common birthmarks These include Mongolian blue spots (benign; more common in black children; occur in the sacral area; resolve spontaneously; do not confuse with bruises), haemangiomas and port-wine stains (Figures 17d,e).

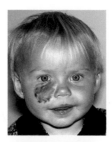

d. Strawberry naevus (haemangioma) appears at 1–3 months increasing in size. 70% resolve by 7 years. Consider referral if the lesion is near the eyes, resulting in obstructed vision, which can lead to amblyopia. If the lesion is situated near other orifices (e.g. anus or lips) it may lead to problems.

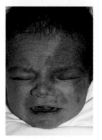

e. Port-wine stain. Present from birth (due to dilated dermal capillaries). Be alert to the association with **Sturge–Weber syndrome** if the lesion is in the distribution of the ophthalmic division of the trigeminal nerve with an underlying meningeal haemangioma and possible subsequent CNS problems like epilepsy/learning difficulties. All should be referred for laser treatment and to exclude underlying abnormalities.

Exanthems

Exanthems are mostly caused by a viral infection (occasionally by drugs or toxins). With immunisations the incidence has markedly decreased. The rashes are typically macular or maculo-papular, associated with a prodromal phase and fever.

Roseola infantum. Sixth disease (herpes virus 6). Incubation 5–15 days. Occurs in children <2 years old. High fever in well child. Macular rash over the trunk. Associated rhinitis, fever and malaise.

Kawasaki disease. From 6 months to 5 years. It is a systemic vasculitis. Fever > than 5 days. Clinical signs: bilateral conjunctivitis, strawberry tongue, morbilliform rash, dry and fissured lips, red hands and feet becoming swollen followed by desquamation. The disease carries significant morbidity with complications of coronary artery aneurysms.

General Practice at a Glance, First Edition. Paul Booton, Carol Cooper, Graham Easton, and Margaret Harper.

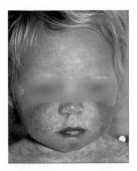

f. Measles. Incubation period 10–14 days (paramyxovirus). Rash begins behind the ears spreading down the trunk. Discrete papulomacular rash becoming blotchy. Followed by desquamation. Koplick spots on the buccal mucosa. Associated symptoms: fever, cough, coryza and conjunctivitis. Rare serious complications include chest infection, encephalitis.

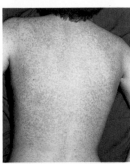

g. Rubella. Mild illness. Incubation 14–21 days. Fine macular rash on the face spreading down the body. Occipital and post-auricular nodes. Associated with serious congenital abnormalities in the first trimester of pregnancy.

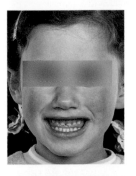

h. Fifth disease. Parvovirus B19. Incubation 13–21 days. Mild illness. Well-defined red rash on cheeks – 'slapped cheek' – later a fine lacy rash on the arms and legs. Beware of complications of aplastic anaemia in children with sickle cell or thalassaemia If contracted in first trimester of pregnancy – fetal hydrops.

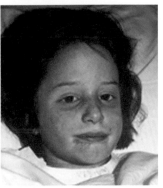

i. Scarlet fever. Group A B haemolytic Streptococcus toxin. Incubation 2–4 days. Punctate red rash starting in the neck. Strawberry tongue. Circumoral pallor. High fever, sore throat, abdominal pain.

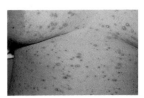

j. Chickenpox. A herpes virus. Incubation 10–14 days. Prodromal phase. Rash progresses from papules to vesicles, pustules and crust. Look for ulcers in the mouth and vulva. Rash very itchy with cropping. Complications include secondary infection, scarring, chest infection, encephalitis. Management: supportive, management of itching and fever.

Purpuric rashes

Purpuric rashes cause anxiety both to the parents and doctor because of fear of meningococcal disease. In your diagnosis consider the following:

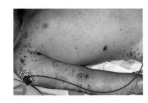

k. Meningococcal septicaemia. Petechial or morbilliform rash later typical purpuric rash. No blanching on pressure. Ill child. It is a medical emergency requiring immediate action. (See Chapter 12.)

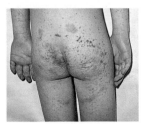

l. Henoch–Schönlein purpura. Auto-immune vasculitis. Children 3–10 years. Purpuric rash over extensor surfaces of buttocks, thighs and legs. Associated features include abdominal pain, painful swollen joints, haematuria. Look out for renal complications.

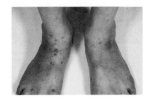

m. Idiopathic thrombocytopenic purpura (immune thrombocytopenia). Often follows viral infection. Petechiae, bruising, purpura. Low platelet count. Note mucosal bleeding. Look for hepatosplenomegaly to exclude other causes.

Other common rashes

Other common rashes seen in children by the GP include herpes simplex infection, which is often asymptomatic. The primary clinical presentation is usually gingivostomatitis (usually 10 months–3 years). There are painful lesions on the lips, tongue and hard palate making eating and drinking difficult. Management is symptomatic with aciclovir in severe cases. Remember more serious presentations like eczema herpeticum, eye involvement or CNS infection. Molluscum contagiosum, impetigo, warts and scabies are also common and are described in Chapter 56.

Atopic dermatitis is a common and important condition seen in general practice and affects 15–20% of school children, often first presenting under 2 years. There is usually a family history of atopy. Diagnosis is made on the history and typical distribution of the rash. In infants the rash usually affects the face and scalp, sometimes the trunk. Later the rash occurs in the skin flexures and in areas of friction. While up to 50% will develop hay fever or asthma, in most children the eczema will resolve by their mid-teens. In some children the eczema can be severe. A crucial part of the management is to give the child and family support, information and encouragement. (See Chapter 55 for further details.)

You should know the basic developmental stages, when they occur and when to refer. In your routine consultation with children be aware of any developmental problems. Always take parental concern seriously. In assessing a child's development you should look at four areas:

Gross motor,   Vision and fine motor,   Hearing and language,   Behaviour, emotional and social development

Remember to:
1. Adjust for prematurity until 2 years of age
2. Allow for normal variation in development
3. Always ask yourself if the child has any impairment in vision or hearing
4. Delay in one area may not be significant but delay in several areas is
5. Notice how the child interacts with his parents and other people
6. Environmental factors, lack of stimulation and physical illness can cause developmental delay as can child abuse
7. Ask to see the red book.
8. Measure the growth and plot it. Check the height and weight.
9. Examine the four areas systematically. Avoid any distractions. The most useful equipment is bricks and crayons

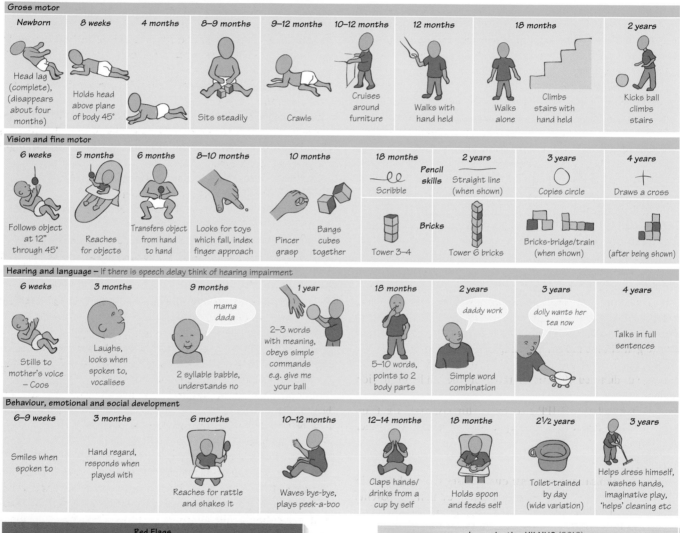

Gross motor

Newborn	8 weeks	4 months	8–9 months	9–12 months	10–12 months	12 months	18 months	2 years
Head lag (complete), (disappears about four months)	Holds head above plane of body 45°		Sits steadily	Crawls	Cruises around furniture	Walks with hand held	Walks alone / Climbs stairs with hand held	Kicks ball climbs stairs

Vision and fine motor

6 weeks	5 months	6 months	8–10 months	10 months	18 months	2 years	3 years	4 years
Follows object at 12" through 45°	Reaches for objects	Transfers object from hand to hand	Looks for toys which fall, index finger approach	Pincer grasp / Bangs cubes together	Pencil skills – Scribble / Bricks – Tower 3–4	Straight line (when shown) / Tower 6 bricks	Copies circle / Bricks-bridge/train (when shown)	Draws a cross / (after being shown)

Hearing and language – If there is speech delay think of hearing impairment

6 weeks	3 months	9 months	1 year	18 months	2 years	3 years	4 years
Stills to mother's voice – Coos	Laughs, looks when spoken to, vocalises	mama dada / 2 syllable babble, understands no	2–3 words with meaning, obeys simple commands e.g. give me your ball	5–10 words, points to 2 body parts	daddy work / Simple word combination	dolly wants her tea now	Talks in full sentences

Behaviour, emotional and social development

6–9 weeks	3 months	6 months	10–12 months	12–14 months	18 months	2½ years	3 years
Smiles when spoken to	Hand regard, responds when played with	Reaches for rattle and shakes it	Waves bye-bye, plays peek-a-boo	Claps hands/ drinks from a cup by self	Holds spoon and feeds self	Toilet-trained by day (wide variation)	Helps dress himself, washes hands, imaginative play, 'helps' cleaning etc

Red Flags

6 weeks	– persistent squint
10 weeks	– not smiling
3 months	– no eye contact
6 months	– persistent primitive reflexes
	– not reaching for objects
10 months	– not sitting unsupported
	– no double syllable babble
12 months	– no pincer grasp
18 months	– not walking
	– does not have 6–8 words with meaning
2½ years	– no 2–3 word sentences
Any regression of skills acquired	
Parental concern	

Immunisation UK NHS (2010)

Birth	– BCG in selected infants
	– Hep B if indicated
2 months	– diphtheria, tetanus, polio, Haemophilus influenzae type B (DTaP/IPV/Hib+Pneumococcal (PCV))
3 months	– DTaP/IPV/Hib+meningitis C (MenC)
4 months	– DTaP/IPV/Hib+MenC+PCV
12–13 months	– Measles, Mumps, Rubella (MMR), Hib+MenC+PCV
3–5 years	– DTaP/IPV+MMR
12–13 years	– Human Papilloma Virus (HPV) 3 injections over 8 months
13–18 years	– Td/IPV (tetanus/low dose diphtheria/polio)

General Practice at a Glance, First Edition. Paul Booton, Carol Cooper, Graham Easton, and Margaret Harper.

44   © 2013 Paul Booton, Carol Cooper, Graham Easton, and Margaret Harper. Published 2013 by Blackwell Publishing Ltd.

The primary health team is ideally placed for its major role in the Child Health Promotion Programme (CHPP). In the first year of life a baby will be seen on average nine times, the GP is likely to have looked after the mother during her antenatal care and known her before she became pregnant. There are opportunities to foster child health promotion during antenatal checks, paediatric surveillance and immunisations but opportunistic health promotion is just as important. **When a child attends surgery for a minor illness always ask yourself if this child is developing normally, had their immunisations and if there are any areas of concern.**

The aim of the CHPP is that all children reach their maximum physical, mental and emotional potential. Prevention and early identification of potential problems, with effective intervention, underpins the programme. There is a strong connection between disadvantage and a poor outcome for children. It is therefore important to identify and focus on vulnerable families (e.g. those with low income, unemployment, poor housing, single parents, physical or mental illness, drug or alcohol misuse, domestic violence and safeguarding issues). These aims are delivered by:

• **Antenatal care.** This provides an opportunity to explore the individual needs of the parents, give them support and spot any problems or risk factors early. It is a time when parents are receptive to education and parenting programmes.
• **Prevention of illness** (e.g. immunisations).
• **Education** e.g. accident prevention (the most common cause of death in children aged 1–14 years), obesity, behavioural management and dental health.
• **Early detection** of disability and illness in screening programmes and paediatric surveillance.

To achieve these goals the CHPP offers a universal core programme. This includes core screening, the surveillance programme, immunisation and advice. After the initial assessment there are:
1 Those who do not need additional input unless they make contact
2 Those who need additional structured help from the health visitor (e.g. first time mothers, feeding or mental health problems)
3 Those needing intensive input with structured inter-agency support (e.g. disabled children or those on the Child Protection Register).

The delivery of the CHPP (led by health visitors) is a team approach which includes a wide spectrum of health and other professionals and organisations.

Immunisations

Thanks to immunisations many serious diseases are rarely seen in the UK. This can breed an air of complacency making parents vulnerable to the media promoting the latest immunisation scare. It is important that GPs are familiar with these diseases and their potential to cause serious illness and death. We know from past experience that when immunisation rates fall the diseases return.

Child surveillance programme

Most of this is carried out by the GP and health visitor. The parents' viewpoint about their child's progress is important in detecting abnormality. They are often the first to notice if something is wrong. Listen to what they have to say – they are usually right. Their opinion on hearing, language and vision is an essential part of the assessment.

Examination of the newborn infant

A midwife and doctor carry out a complete physical examination to identify any congenital or physical abnormality. Weight and head circumference are plotted. The baby is screened for vision (red reflex), and the cardiovascular system, hips (for developmental dysplasia of the hip [DDH]), spine, genitalia and CNS examined. Breast-feeding is encouraged. Advice is given on immunisations, home safety and preventing sudden infant death syndrome (SIDS). Any relevant family history or risk factors are identified. The personal child health record is given (Red Book).

First 5 weeks

• The Newborn Hearing Screening Programme.
• 4–7 days. Biochemical screening (heel prick).
• Midwife visits: check the health of the mother and baby, and identify new problems. It is an opportunity to give health promotion, feeding advice and encourage breast-feeding.
• New baby review by 2 weeks: health visitor identifies new problems including any mental health problems in the mother, giving advice on feeding and home safety and encouraging parent–baby interaction.

8-week check by the GP and health visitor (includes the first immunisation)

This aims to assess how the first 8 weeks have gone, identifies any concerns including the mother's health, any postnatal depression (Edinburgh questionnaire) and to ensure the baby is healthy and progressing developmentally.

Perform a full physical examination. This includes:
• Plotting the weight and head circumference.
• Checking the fontanelle and sutures, tone and head control.
• Look for jaundice and any dysmorphic features.
• Vision. Is the baby is fixing, following and smiling?
► Look for the red reflex to exclude any opacities such as cataracts or retinoblastoma (ophthalmoscope at approximately 30 cm from the infant's eyes).
• Examine the heart, femoral pulses, hips, spine and palate. Check the genitalia and feel for hernias.
• Ask about hearing and if the baby is vocalising.

Use the checks as an opportunity for health promotion including immunisations, breast-feeding, nutrition, obesity, accident prevention and safety in the home.

A new mother often feels isolated so ask about her support. The health visitor will be able to put her in touch with local groups (e.g. National Childbirth Trust or Sure Start).

8–9 months to school age

Health visitor clinics (usually at the GP surgery): when the child comes for immunisations their progress and development are reviewed at the same time. It is an opportunity to discuss diet, obesity, dental problems, common behaviour problems and accident prevention at the appropriate stages. Encourage parents to come to the clinic if worried about any part of their child's health, development or behaviour. Vision should be checked by the orthoptist by the time the child is 5 years old.

Primary and secondary schools

Sweep test for hearing on school entry plus identification of any children who have fallen through the net. Formal reviews are not carried out but health promotion remains important covering sexual health, smoking, drug and alcohol misuse, exercise and diet. The school nurse is available for advice. Children with disability often remain in mainstream school and their care coordinated by the specialist team.

Assessing musculo-skeletal symptoms in children is simple with pGALS (paediatric Gait, Arms, Legs, Spine) and quick, taking no more than 2 minutes. Originally developed for school-age children, it can also be used for pre-school children, but not babies and toddlers

Figure	Screening manoeuvres (note the manoeuvres in bold are additional to those in adult GALS)	What is being assessed?
	Observe the child standing (from front, back and sides)	• Posture and habitus • Skin rashes (e.g. psoriasis) • Deformity (e.g. flat feet)
	Observe the child walking and 'walk on your heels' and 'walk on your tiptoes'	• Ankles, subtalar, midtarsal and small joints of feet and toes
	'Hold your hands out straight in front of you'	• Elbow extension • Wrist extension • Extension of fingers
	'Turn your hands over and make a fist'	• Wrist supination • Elbow supination • Flexion of fingers
	'Pinch your index finger and thumb together'	• Manual dexterity • Coordination
	'Touch the tips of your fingers'	• Manual dexterity • Coordination of fingers and thumbs
	Squeeze the metacarpophalangeal joints for tenderness	• Metacarpophalangeal joints
	'Put your hands together palm to palm' and 'put your hands together back to back'	• Extension of small joints of fingers • Wrist extension • Elbow flexion
	'Reach up, "touch the sky"' and 'look at the ceiling'	• Elbow extension • Wrist extension • Shoulder abduction • Neck extension
	'Put your hands behind your neck'	• Shoulder and elbow function
	'Try and touch your shoulder with your ear'	• Cervical spine lateral flexion
	'Open wide and put three (child's own) fingers in your mouth'	• Temporomandibular joints (and check for deviation of jaw movement)
	Feel for effusion at the knee (patella tap, or cross-fluctuation)	• Knee effusion
	Active movement of knees (flexion and extension) and feel for crepitus	• Knees
	Passive movement of hip (knee flexed to 90°, and internal rotation of hip)	• Hip flexion and internal rotation
	'Bend forwards and touch your toes'	• Forward flexion of thoracolumbar spine (and check for scoliosis)

(reproduced by kind permission of Arthritis Research UK [www.arthritisresearchuk.org])

General Practice at a Glance, First Edition. Paul Booton, Carol Cooper, Graham Easton, and Margaret Harper.

Children often have musculoskeletal symptoms. Most are benign and many occur after trauma. The GP's duty is to distinguish these from more serious conditions.

Here are just some conditions that affect children. They are included because they are common, or because primary care has a pivotal role in prevention and/or management.
- Children may deny pain, or claim to have pain when they don't.
- Observe the child's relationship with the parent. Benign pains are more common if the child gains attention from them.
- Your careful history and examination must take into account the child's developmental progress for his or her age.
- A child's job is to play.
▶ The child who does not play is ill until proven otherwise.

Developmental dysplasia of the hip
Formerly known as congenital dislocation of the hip, this affects around 1% of infants. In developmental dysplasia of the hip (DDH), the acetabulum is too shallow for the femoral head, which can sublux or dislocate. The aim is to diagnose it as early as possible.

DDH is more common in:
- Girls
- Breech deliveries
▶ Spina bifida
▶ Families with a history of DDH (ask about hip problems).
 Look for:
▶ Asymmetric skin creases in the thigh
▶ Any leg length discrepancy.

Tests for DDH can be performed from birth. In both tests, flex the knees:
- Barlow's test – feel for a clunk as you abduct the hip and push it backwards.
- Ortolani's test (rarely positive) – feel for a clunk as the abducted and dislocated hip slips back into place when you push the femur forwards.

Refer promptly for assessment if you suspect DDH as splinting (or occasionally surgery) can be curative. Uncorrected DDH rarely delays walking, but it can cause a limp and lifelong problems.

Limping
▶ A limp is always significant. Causes include:
- Transient synovitis of the hip (common and benign)
- Septic arthritis or osteomyelitis (rare but serious)
- Perthes' disease
- Slipped upper femoral epiphysis
- Rickets
- Acute lymphoblastic leukaemia
- Trauma, including non-accidental injury (see Chapter 11).
 Always assess the whole child, and remember that hip pain can be referred to the knee (and vice versa).
▶ Look for sepsis.
▶ Check for signs of injury, especially injuries of varying ages.

Consider full blood count (FBC), erythrocyte sedimentation rate (ESR), C-reactive protein (CRP) and X-rays. Refer if there are red flags or the limp persists.

Growing pains
While a convenient shorthand term for benign limb pain in childhood, 'growing pains' may not be caused by growth.

History
- The child is usually aged 3–12 years, and may be athletic.
- Pain is usually symmetrical, in the lower limbs below the knees.
- It often occurs at night, especially after an active day, but never in the morning.
- Ask about limping. Growing pains do not cause a limp.
- Ask about limitation of activities.
▶ Persistent night pain or asymmetrical pain can be caused by osteosarcoma.

Examination
Assess the child carefully, including general health and developmental milestones.
▶ Can you see a limp?
▶ Is there any joint abnormality (see Figure 19)?
▶ Are there signs of injury? Always think of non-accidental injury.
- Is the child very hypermobile? While not a red flag, this suggests an orthosis may help.
- Is the child well? Refer if there are any red flags, including the following:
▶ Fever
▶ Fatigue
▶ Weight loss
▶ Loss of appetite
▶ Limitation of activities.
 Consider FBC, ESR, CRP, thyroid function tests, muscle enzyme tests and X-rays.

Management
Reassure parents and child that pains fluctuate but settle eventually. Tell the parents not to fret unless the child appears ill or limps.
- Advise comfortable sensible shoes (e.g. trainers).
- Massaging or rubbing the leg may relieve night pain.
- Occasional bedtime analgesic is useful after very active days.
- Follow-up can reassure both you and the family.

Flat feet, bow-legs and knock-knees
Flat feet can be normal up to age 6, but usually disappear when walking on tip-toe. Flat feet may persist in hypermobile children.

Bow-legs are normal from birth to age 18 months.

Knock-knees are common between 3 and 6 years. The feet may point inwards too (intoeing gait).
▶ Refer if signs occur outside these age limits, or there are other signs or symptoms.

Rickets
The childhood equivalent of **osteomalacia**, rickets results from severe vitamin D deficiency, usually brought about by poor intake either from lack of sunlight, poor diet, or both. Rickets itself is uncommon, but some 50% of children are deficient in vitamin D.
- Few children have vitamin D supplements even though the Department of Health recommends them for all under-5-year-olds.
- Pregnant women who lack vitamin D are most likely to have infants also deficient in the vitamin.
- As with adults, pigmented skin needs more sunlight to synthesise vitamin D.

There are also long-term conditions linked with low vitamin D levels, including cancer, multiple sclerosis and metabolic syndrome.

Suspect rickets if a baby under 6 months old has:
► Convulsions
► Tetany or impaired growth.

Suspect rickets if a child over 6 months has bony abnormalities, typically:
► Bow-legs or knock-knees
► Chest deformities ('rickety rosary')
• Delayed dentition
► Poor growth
► Fractures or bone pain.

Investigations
Low serum calcium and phosphate together with a raised alkaline phosphatase. X-rays may show typical changes, but the diagnostic test is a low serum vitamin D level (25-OH D below 25 nmol/L or 10 µg/L).

Management
Refer to a paediatrician for treatment (usually vitamin D supplementation, and calcium in the first weeks of treatment).

Check siblings and the mother as they are likely to lack vitamin D too.

Juvenile idiopathic arthritis
Juvenile idiopathic arthritis (JIA) is any chronic arthritis in under-16-year-olds. It is rare, but vital to recognise in the one child in 1000 who has it. There are three main patterns:

1 Mono-articular or oligo-articular – one or a few joints are affected
2 Poly-articular – many joints are affected
3 Systemic – with features such as fever, rash, enlarged lymph nodes and hepatomegaly.

Suspect JIA and refer promptly if a child has:
► Synovitis, or is
► Unwell with musculoskeletal symptoms.

Consider FBC, ESR, CRP and rheumatoid factor tests before referring.

(a) Vacuum device or pump

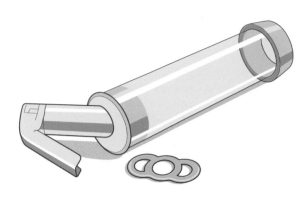

(b) Penile implants

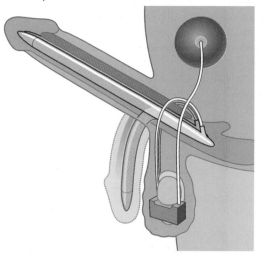

Vacuum devices or pumps offer an alternative to medication for erectile dysfunction. With the penis placed inside the cyclinder, a pump creates a partial vacuum around the penis. This causes it to fill with blood, leading to an erection. An elastic band is then placed around the base of the penis to maintain an erection

In men with persistent ED, a penile implant can restore sexual function. The inflatable implant consists of two cylinders that are surgically inserted inside the shaft of the penis. When the man wants an erection he uses a pump (in the scrotum) to fill the cylinders (in the penis) with pressurised fluid from a reservoir (in the abdominal wall). An alternative method is a malleable implant, which bolsters erections with surgically implanted rods

Possible causes of dyspareunia

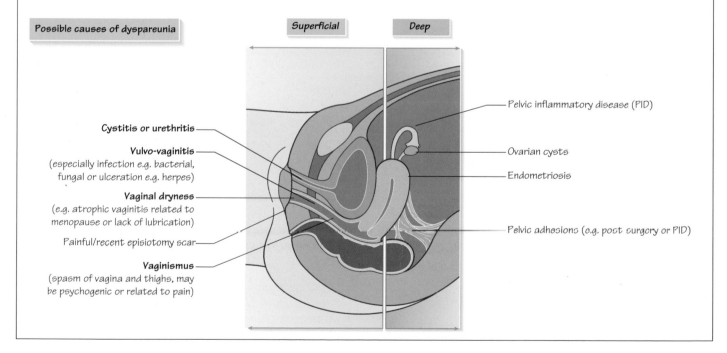

Superficial   Deep

Cystitis or urethritis

Vulvo-vaginitis
(especially infection e.g. bacterial, fungal or ulceration e.g. herpes)

Vaginal dryness
(e.g. atrophic vaginitis related to menopause or lack of lubrication)

Painful/recent episiotomy scar

Vaginismus
(spasm of vagina and thighs, may be psychogenic or related to pain)

Pelvic inflammatory disease (PID)

Ovarian cysts

Endometriosis

Pelvic adhesions (e.g. post surgery or PID)

Around 10% of men and up to 50% of women experience sexual difficulties at some point, and although some will need specialist advice, the GP should be able to help with most problems. When dealing with any sexual problem, bear in mind the following:
• Some sexual problems have a physical origin and some a psychological origin, but many are a mix of both.
• Sex is usually a two-way activity; consider the couple (and don't make assumptions about sexuality).
• Don't forget that sexual problems can be a sign of serious organic disease.
• Explore the patient's **ideas** (e.g. what the patient thinks the problem is, and what they think is 'normal'), **concerns** (e.g. something seriously wrong, effects on relationship) and **expectations** (e.g. likely outcome or treatments).
• GPs can make a big difference to patients using quite basic techniques – for example, providing information, reassurance or the chance to talk to someone with non-directive counselling skills.

Erectile dysfunction (impotence)

Erectile dysfunction (ED) is the inability to get or maintain an erection that is sufficient for satisfactory sexual intercourse. Sustained ED affects about 8% of 20- to 40-year-olds and half of men over 70. Causes include **organic** (e.g. atherosclerosis, neurological disease, diabetes, hypertension, medications) and **psychological** (e.g. depression or anxiety, or relationship problems). ED is mostly psychological in nature in one-third of patients, mostly physical in one-third and a mix of both in the remaining third.

History

Take a full history, especially:
• Medications (e.g. antihypertensives such as beta-blockers, antidepressants, anticonvulsants)
• Alcohol and smoking
• Sudden onset, morning erections maintained and reduced sex drive suggest psychological causes
• Gradual onset, absence of morning erections and normal sex drive suggest physical cause.

Examination

Examination should include: full cardiovascular examination including BP, peripheral pulses (ED shares many risk factors with cardiovascular disease [CVD]), genital exam for hypogonadism or anatomical problems, neurological exam (e.g. for spinal cord lesions or peripheral neuropathy).

Investigations

Consider: urine dipstick, fasting lipids and blood glucose, U&E, LFT, endocrine (if reduced sex drive or secondary sex characteristics (e.g. testosterone, prolactin, FSH/LH), prostate specific antigen (PSA). Doppler flow studies probably in secondary care.

Management

Management will depend on the likely cause.
• Modify any obvious lifestyle causes, address medication issues and tackle any CVD risk factors.
• Psychogenic ED can respond well to psychosexual therapy.
• First line drug treatment is phosphodiesterase inhibitors (e.g. sildenafil or Viagra®) which relax smooth muscle but are contrain-dicated in patients taking nitrates or in whom vasodilatation or sexual activity is inadvisable (e.g. recent stroke or MI).
• Other approaches include prostaglandins either inserted into the urethra or injected into the corpora cavernosa; vacuum devices (see Figure 20a); or penile prostheses (see Figure 20b).

Premature ejaculation

Descriptions of 'premature' vary from 30 seconds to 4 minutes – so a useful definition is 'inability to control ejaculation enough to allow both partners to enjoy sexual intercourse'. It can cause significant upset in relationships and can dent self-confidence in men. It is often anxiety-related and is common in young men or early on in a new relationship, when the problem usually settles down with time. Drugs such as amphetamine and cocaine can cause premature ejaculation, as can neurological causes such as multiple sclerosis or peripheral neuropathy, and urological problems including prostatitis.

Management

Management in general practice includes advice to increase frequency of sex, use condoms or anaesthetic gels to reduce sensation, or to use the 'squeeze' technique which involves squeezing below the tip of the penis when climax is imminent for 10–20 seconds (this can delay ejaculation). Other approaches include medications such as selective serotonin reuptake inhibitors (SSRIs), antidepressants or sildenafil, and psychosexual therapy.

Loss of libido

This is loss of sexual desire or drive. There are many possible causes: depression, overwork, excess alcohol, tiredness, relationship difficulties, ill health, hormonal (e.g. climacteric in women or prostate cancer treatment in men), pregnancy, postpartum and breast-feeding, medications (especially antihypertensives) and other sexual problems such as dyspareunia.

History

The history is very important.
• What does the patient mean by loss of sex drive? What is normal for them?
• What do they think is the cause (men often think it's a hormone problem – it rarely is)?
• Do they feel depressed or stressed at work or at home?
• Are there any other sexual problems?
• How is their relationship and whose idea was it to come to the doctor?
• What medications is the patient taking?
• Are there any major health problems?
• For women (if appropriate), are they still having regular periods, are they using contraception?

Examination

Examination isn't usually very fruitful but may help to reassure the patient that there is no physical abnormality and that you are taking the problem seriously.

Investigations

Investigations include blood tests: FBC (raised mean cell volume [MCV] in alcoholism), U&E (renal and/or adrenal disease), LFT (alcohol), thyroid function test (TFT) (hypothyroidism), FSH, LH, prolactin, oestradiol (to detect hormone deficiencies).

Management

Counselling for relationship difficulties or alcohol problems, and treatment for depression. Treat physical problems such as hypothyroidism or sexual problems and review medication if relevant. HRT may be appropriate to boost libido in women where low sex hormone levels are implicated, but always balance benefits and risks. Testosterone patches are controversial in men and even more so in women.

Dyspareunia

Dyspareunia is pain during or after sexual intercourse and usually applies to women (see Figure 20). It affects about 20% of women at some point in their lives. Many women find it difficult to talk about, so may mention a vague 'soreness down below' or present with a different problem such as stress or infertility.

History

Ask whether the pain is deep or superficial, and when it started. Ask about urinary symptoms or any signs of sexually transmitted diseases. Enquire about the relationship and keep in mind trauma or abuse.

Examination

Examination should include abdominal exam followed by gentle vulval and vaginal examination, checking for skin changes, lubrication, vaginismus or cervical excitation (may accompany pelvic inflammatory disease [PID]).

Investigations

These include high vaginal swab (HVS) and endocervical swabs, urinalysis, MSU, pelvic ultrasound or laparoscopy (in secondary care).

Management

Depends on findings and is tailored to the couple. For example, treat infections (often best assessed at a genito-urinary medicine [GUM] clinic); psychological problems may respond to psychosexual counselling; HRT and lubricants can help with menopausal vaginal dryness; vaginismus responds to a combination of behaviour modification, counselling and vaginal dilatation techniques.

▶ Be familiar with the local guidelines. Offer high risk patients screening. Explain the benefits of screening, reassuring them about confidentiality. If the tests are positive have clear plan with the patient about informing them of the results and make sure you know how to contact them

High risk patients

- Young age group
- Unsafe sex
- Frequent sexual relationships
- Early sexual activity
- Previous STI or attendance at GUM
- Men who have sex with men
- Social deprivation and poor access to health promotion
- Alcohol or drug misuse
- Learning disability /mental ill health
- Sex workers
- Those visiting countries with a high incidence HIV and STIs

Tests

Tests vary locally; check what your local microbiology lab offers, their policy on taking the test, transport of the specimen and time for the results

- **Nucleic acid amplification tests** – (NAAT) for chlamydia and gonococcus (GC)
  – in some labs herpes simplex virus (HSV). NAAT advantage is:
  Not invasive
    – can be self-taken from first catch urine (FCU) men or vagina for women
    – is stable at room temperature **but** does not give culture and sensitivities
    – does not test for TV (Trichomonas)
- **If GC is suspected** – refer for microscopy for immediate diagnosis and C and S to identify resistant strains
- **Other Swabs** – e.g TV and HSV contact local lab for their policy BASHH recommend confirmation and typing for HSV in newly diagnosed patient for diagnosis and prognosis

Also offer blood tests for HIV, and hepatitis B, if the patient is at high risk for syphilis, and if indicated hepatitis C (explain the importance and benefit to the patient of the tests)

Physical examination for symptomatic STIs (make the patient comfortable and explain what you are going to do)

Symptomatic female

- General examination look for – rashes, lymphadenopathy. Look in the mouth for ulcers or lesions
- Examine the external genitalia for:
  – trauma
  – rashes
  – ulcers, warts
- Speculum examination – note discharge – is it offensive or frothy (TV) – is it blood stained?
- Look for warts and ulcers. Look at the cervix – is it inflamed?
- Take swabs for chlamydia and GC (NAAT)
- If discharge take swabs for candida TV and bacterial vaginosis
- Do a bimanual for tenderness/masses. Don't forget pregnancy
- Blood test as above

Symptomatic male

- Examine standing or lying
- General examination as for female
- Feel scrotum/penis – look for sores or rashes – note any discharge. If discharge present +/– dysuria think of chlamydia, gonorrhoea, NSU
- Ask the patient to pull back his foreskin
- Examine the anus
- Take FCU for chlamydia or GC (NAAT)
- If indicated dipstick to exclude UTI
- If suspect GC refer for urgent microscopy
- Blood tests as above

Management: your options are:

- Treat in the surgery if applicable
- Refer to GUM
- Make an immediate referral for HIV, syphilis or hepatitis (▶rectal infection of GC, chlamydia or syphilis carry a high risk for HIV)
- Take swabs and refer to GUM for further sexual screening management, and contact tracing
- Have details of communication of the results

If the swabs are positive and you decide to treat (e.g. chlamydia) first consult the local guidelines

- Explain management plan to the patient and give written information.
- Refrain from sex including oral sex until both partners are treated. If the sexual contact was within the last 2 weeks retest in 2 weeks
- Contacts – with contact- tracing patients may do this themselves or prefer someone else, which is usually the GUM clinic. Advise all contacts of chlamydia or TV to have treatment OR to abstain from sex until their results are known, and to have screening for STIs
- Give information on safer sex including oral and anal sex and reinfection. Offer support and follow-up

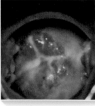

(a) Mucopurulent cervical discharge with cervicitis

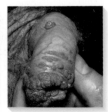

(b) Penile warts

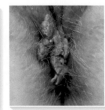

(c) First episode of genital herpes

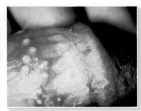

(d) Vulval warts

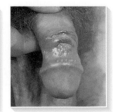

(e) Primary syphilis

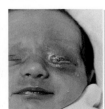

(f) Ophthalmia neonatorum
Develops within 21 days of birth. Likely to be chlamydia or gonococcal

General Practice at a Glance, First Edition. Paul Booton, Carol Cooper, Graham Easton, and Margaret Harper.
52 © 2013 Paul Booton, Carol Cooper, Graham Easton, and Margaret Harper. Published 2013 by Blackwell Publishing Ltd.

Sexually transmitted infections (STIs) are common. Young people account for nearly half of all infections. Many are asymptomatic and unreported, so the real incidence is much higher, increasing the spread of disease. Patients attend either general practice or go direct to GUM clinics. General practice should:

- Raise awareness of and give information about STIs.
- Provide early diagnosis and treatment to decrease transmission and the risk of complications.
- Screen high risk asymptomatic patients.
- Look for other sexually transmitted diseases. **A patient with one STI often has others.**
- Provide a clear management plan.
- Provide adequate follow up and advise about contact tracing.

Much depends on the facilities the practice offers and on patient preference. Many prefer the anonymity of the GUM clinic, the free prescriptions provided and the fact that the consultation will not be recorded in the GP notes. However, many practices can confidently treat common STIs within local guidelines and the surgery is a familiar place where patients may feel more comfortable.

Sexual history

This can be challenging. It is awkward asking intimate sexual questions particularly of someone already known well. The patient may be embarrassed so it is important to take the history in a non-judgemental way, putting the patient at ease and reassuring them that the consultation is confidential (where appropriate).

Listen to what the patient has to say, noting non-verbal clues and hidden agendas. The presenting complaint may be a trivial illness if the patient finds it hard to say what the real problem is. Be aware of and sympathetic to cultural differences. **Above all, don't make assumptions about type of sex, sexual orientation or age.**
- Start with the least uncomfortable questions rather than immediately asking detailed questions about sex. Explain that the more intrusive questions are **routine questions** to assess their risk and plan appropriate investigations and treatment.
- Review general health and past sexual health particularly any past history of STIs.
- Ask about the last sexual encounter. What type of sex was it – vaginal, anal or oral? Does their partner have any symptoms?
- Was it a same-sex encounter?
- Were condoms used?
- Ask about the partner's history and past partners.
- Be aware of the possibility of child abuse and rape.

Chlamydia

Chlamydia trachomatis is the most common STI. Some 5–10% of females under the age of 24 years may be infected, many asymptomatically. If untreated, there is a 20–40% incidence of PID and subsequent fertility problems. Other complications include Reiter's syndrome, epididymo-orchitis and ectopic pregnancy. Transmission to the newborn baby can cause conjunctivitis and pneumonia.

If there is a history of persistent inflammatory or inadequate smears this may be due to chlamydia.

Gonococcus

Gonococcus (GC) has declined in the West but is still the second most common bacterial STI in the UK, remaining high in Africa and Asia. It occurs most frequently in the age group 15–29 years, and in men who have sex with men where one-third have coexisting HIV. Mother-to-child transmission can cause neonatal conjuncti-vitis. Primary sites of infection are the urethra, endocervix, rectum, pharynx and conjunctiva. Patients may present with urethral or vaginal discharge. Follow local protocols for investigation and management.

Trichomonas vaginalis

This usually presents with an offensive frothy discharge or non-specific urethritis (NSU). Up to 50% may be asymptomatic. Complications include PID and epididymo-orchitis.

Herpes virus (type 1 or 2)

Transmission is by close contact and is usually sexually acquired. Primary infection can be asymptomatic or present with painful ulcers. After the primary infection, the virus is latent in the sensory ganglion leading to recurrent infections.

Diagnosis is mainly clinical (see Figure 21 for swabs for first infection). Management aims to relieve symptoms, and antiviral drugs may not be needed. Counselling is important, advising about the natural history, reducing the risk of transmission during recurrences, asymptomatic shedding, safe sex and awareness of potential problems in pregnancy.

Genital warts: human papilloma virus

Human papilloma virus (HPV) is transmitted by direct sexual contact. There are over 100 strains. Ninety per cent of genital warts are due to types 6 and 11 which are not associated with neoplastic change. Types 16 and 18 have a high risk of neoplastic change in the cervix, vulva, vagina and penis. Incubation period is 2 weeks to 8 months. HPV can be passed on to the neonate.

Diagnosis is clinical. If there is any doubt about the diagnosis, especially any concerns about possible malignancy, refer for confirmation. Otherwise treatment is topical or ablative. If topical, the patient can be shown how to self-administer at home.

Syphilis

Syphilis is a spirochete which is spread by close physical contact. It enters through breaches in the epithelium. It is uncommon in primary care but you must be aware of the possibility. The disease is known as the 'great mimicker' because of its many presentations. It causes significant morbidity. Co-infection with HIV is common. Congenital syphilis remains important worldwide (see British Association for Sexual Health and HIV [BASHH]).

HIV

Anti-retroviral therapy has transformed the outcome and quality of life for patients. Testing should be treated as any other test. The UK National Guidelines for HIV advise that those at risk should be encouraged to have HIV testing because:
- Early diagnosis increases life expectancy and quality of life
- 24% of all deaths with HIV are due to late diagnosis
- Undiagnosed patients are a risk to themselves and others.

Explain the benefits of testing, that the test is voluntary and confidential, how the results will be given and the management if the test proves positive.

HIV testing is recommended:
- As part of a routine sexual health screen to patients attending antenatal clinics, GUM and drug dependency clinics and for termination of pregnancy
- All patients with STIs
- All men who have sex with men and their female contacts
- High risk or clinical indication (e.g. hepatitis B).

Type of contraception	What it looks like	When to start	Contraindications	Potential problems	Failure rate (% unintended pregnancy within 1st year)
Combined Oral Contraceptive Pill (COCP), patch or vaginal ring		• Start at onset of menstrual period • Can be started at any time in cycle if no risk of pregnancy but must wait 7 days for efficacy	Relative C/I • Age above 35 • Smoker • BMI >35 • BP >140/90 Absolute C/I • Previous DVT • Thrombogenic mutation • Migraine with aura	• Breast tenderness • Mood changes • Breakthrough bleeding • Strongly user dependent	0.3% Efficacy reduced when taking broad spectrum antibiotics, enzyme inducing drugs, St John's Wort
Progestogen only pill (POP)		Start at onset of menstrual period up to and including day 5	• Breast cancer • Liver problems • Use of liver enzyme inducing medication	• Hormonal side effects e.g. skin changes, breast tenderness, mood changes • Irregular bleeding	0.3%
Contraceptive Injection im		First 5 days of menstruation	• Breast cancer • Liver problems	• Acne, breast tenderness, mood changes • Amenorrhoea • Irregular bleeding	0.3%
Intrauterine system (IUS)		• Any time in the menstrual cycle if certain woman is not pregnant • Licensed for 5 years	• Ovarian cancer • <4 weeks postpartum • Unexplained vaginal bleeding • Distortion of pelvic cavity	• Irregular bleeding • Amenorrhoea • Risk of PID and perforation	0.1%
Copper IUD		• Any time in the menstrual cycle if certain woman is not pregnant • Licensed for 5 years	• Ovarian cancer • <4 weeks postpartum • Unexplained vaginal bleeding • Distortion of pelvic cavity Caution: risk factors for CVD/VTE, breast masses, migraine	• Irregular bleeding • Heavier/more painful periods • Risk of PID and perforation	0.6%
Implant		• Ideally days 1–5 of cycle but can be inserted any time if certain that woman not pregnant • Licensed for 3 years	• Previous VTE • Arterial disease • Migraine with aura • Unexplained vaginal bleeding • Breast disease • Liver disease • Enzyme inducing drugs	• 20% of users will have no bleeding, while almost 50% will have infrequent, or irregular bleeding • Insertion may cause bleeding/infection	<0.1% over 3 years
Barrier methods – condoms		• Cap should stay in place for 6 hours afterwards • Condoms easy to obtain • Offer protection against STIs		• Personal preference • Most contain latex and are unsuitable for latex-allergy sufferers	• Male condom 2%, • Female condom 5%, • Diaphragm/cap with spermicide 4–8%
Levonorgestrel emergency pill		• Single dose of 1.5 mg up to 72 hours after UPSI • Limited efficacy after 72 hours	Pregnancy	• If woman vomits within 2 hours of taking pills she must repeat the dose • Possible risk of ectopic pregnancy	If used within 72 hours prevents 84% of pregnancies
Emergency copper IUD		• Up to 5 days after UPSI • If ovulation has not occurred can be used up to 5 days post suspected time of ovulation		• PID, consider antibiotic prophylaxis for high risk women • Possible risk of ectopic pregnancy	1%
Ulipristal acetate		• 30 mg as a single dose ASAP, no later than 120 hours after UPSI • Efficacy affected by enzyme inducing drugs	Allergy and pregnancy	• Headache, nausea, abdominal pain • If woman vomits within 3 hours of taking pills she must repeat the dose	Around 1.4% in first 72 hours

General Practice at a Glance, First Edition. Paul Booton, Carol Cooper, Graham Easton, and Margaret Harper.

A request for contraception is a common reason for consultation in general practice. As there are many different contraceptive methods, each with their own limitations, you should know about all of them so you can offer patients an informed choice.

History

Main points to consider:

- Age of patient – if under 16 years, are they Fraser competent? A competent person:
  o Is able to understand and retain the information pertinent to the decision about their care, as well as the consequences of not having treatment.
  o Is able to use this information to consider whether or not they should consent to the intervention offered.
  o Is able to communicate their wishes.
- When a patient asks about contraception, your first question should be what they would like. A patient may have clear ideas or have no knowledge at all, so it is important to ask 'Do you have any thoughts about what you might like to use?'
- Previous contraceptive use can affect their choice due to side effects or they may prefer to 'stay with what they know', but this may not be the best so discuss other options.
- Current circumstances like relationship status, number of children, is the family complete? Establish how pressing it is for the woman not to conceive. A medical student in the middle of her degree may react differently to an unplanned pregnancy compared with a mother of three in a stable relationship.
- Menstrual history including last menstrual period (LMP) to establish whether the patient has regular cycles (irregular, infrequent cycles may point to polycystic ovary syndrome [PCOS] or other pathology) and to exclude pregnancy and to advise when to start using contraception.
- Obstetric and gynaecological history, including history of ectopic pregnancy (some methods can increase the risk of this, e.g. progestogen-only pill [POP], intrauterine device [IUD]), previous pelvic infection (also increases the risk of ectopic pregnancy), fibroids (can distort the uterine cavity and cause problems with coil use).
- Sexual history including any STIs. The coil can introduce infection into the uterus and Fallopian tubes. STIs are more common in the young and if someone is not in a stable relationship (see also Chapter 21).
- Medical history. A history of thrombo-embolic disease, breast cancer or hypertension impacts on the use of oestrogen-containing contraceptives.
- Drug history and OTC medicines. Some interact with combined oral contraceptive pill (COCP).
- Is the partner present and does he or she have any views on contraceptive method?
- Can you exclude pregnancy? You may need to perform a test.
- When to start contraceptive method – the safest time to start most methods of contraception is at the onset of a normal menstrual period to ensure no pregnancy has already occurred.

Examination

Check the woman's blood pressure and weight. This is also a good opportunity to make sure her cervical smear is up to date.

Contraceptive options

Female methods

Hormonal methods

Containing oestrogen and progestogen:
- **COCP**
- **Contraceptive patch**
- **Contraceptive vaginal ring**

Mode of action: acts on the hypothalamic–pituitary–ovarian axis to suppress FSH and LH production therefore blocking ovulation. Thickens cervical mucus and creates hostile endometrial lining.

Containing progestogen alone:
- **Progestogen-only pill.** Mode of action: Thickens cervical mucus. Makes uterine lining thinner and hostile to implantation. Can prevent ovulation. Desogestrel 75 µg (Cerazette®) inhibits ovulation in >9 out of 10 women.
- **Contraceptive injection.** Mode of action: prevents ovulation, thickens cervical mucus, thinning of uterine lining.
- **Contraceptive implant.** Primary mode of action: prevents ovulation.
- **Intrauterine system (IUS).** Mode of action: effect on endometrial lining preventing implantation, and effect on cervical mucus to reduce sperm penetration.

Non-hormonal methods

Intrauterine device (containing copper): Mode of action: effect on endometrial lining preventing implantation, effect on cervical mucus to reduce sperm penetration.

Barrier methods: Female condom, cap and diaphragm. Mode of action: physical barrier to sperm reaching egg.

Permanent methods

Female sterilisation: tubal occlusion is most often with Filshie Clips. It is a laparoscopic procedure, usually performed as a day case, and carries surgical risk. Overall failure rate is about 1 in 200.

Emergency contraception
- **Levonorgestrel.** Mode of action: efficacy is thought to be due primarily to inhibition of ovulation rather than inhibition of implantation.
- **Ulipristal acetate.** Mode of action: ulipristal is a progesterone receptor modulator and is thought to delay or inhibit ovulation and maturation of the endometrium.
- **IUD.**

Male methods

Barrier method

Condoms (not prescribable in general practice although many practices stock them).

Permanent method

Vasectomy involves excision of part of the vas deferens and carries a surgical risk. However, vasectomy is minimally invasive and can usually be carried out under local anaesthetic. The failure rate is 1 in 2000. Sterility is not immediate and the patient should be warned to continue to use contraception. Two negative semen samples, starting 3 months after the operation and taken 1 month apart, are recommended before reassuring the patient that he is sterile.

(a) Algorithm for management of subfertility in general practice

	Male	Male and female	Female

History
 	
Patient presents with infertility
– see both members of couple together
	• Testicular history
	  – torsion/mumps/
	  undescended
	• Occupational history
		• Ask about sex:
		  – frequency?
		  – penetrative?
		  – pain/problems?
		• Contraception history
		• Previous children/pregnancies
		• Previous sexually transmitted infections
		• Smoking
		• Alcohol
		• Caffeine
		• Illicit drugs
		• Body Mass Index
		• Illness – thyroid, diabetes, etc
		• Medications
		• Previous treatments – esp cancer treatment
		• Surgery – pelvic, undescended testes
			• Age
			• Periods regular?

Examination	• Gynaecomastia	• External genitalia	• Pelvic exam • Galactorrhoea? • Acne/hirsutism?

Investigation – after 12 months of trying **or earlier if:**
– history of undescended testes or pelvic inflammatory disease
– irregular periods
– woman >35
	• Semen analysis
	  – abstain 3 days prior
	  – to lab within 1–2 hours
			• Chlamydia
			• Day 3 FSH, LH
			• Day 21 progesterone
			  – or mid luteal
			• Consider prolactin, TSH
			  – only if symptoms of disease
			• **Avoid** ovulation kits

Referral – after 18 months of trying **or earlier if:**
– known cause for infertility or added concern:
  – e.g. history cancer treatment
  – e.g. history chronic infection e.g. HIV, Hep B/C
	• Surgery for varicocele/obstruction
	• Sperm recovery
		• Treat underlying systemic disease
		• In vitro fertilisation and embryo transfer (IVF-ET)
		• Intrauterine insemination (IUI)
		• Gamete intrafallopian transfer (GIFT)
		• Intracytoplasmic sperm injection (ICSI)
			• Hysterosalpingogram/laparoscopy and dye
			  – ?tubal patency
			• Remove endometriosis/fibroid
			• Ovulation stimulation
			  – clomifene
			  – gonadotrophin analogues
			  – ovarian drilling

FSH = follicle-stimulating hormone; LH = luteinising hormone; TSH = thyroid-stimulating hormone

(b) Causes of subfertility

Common and systemic causes of infertility

• Women ≥35
• Over or under weight
• Stress
• Polycystic ovarian syndrome
• Thyroid disorders
• Premature menopause
• Hyperprolactinaemia
• Some cancers and cancer treatments

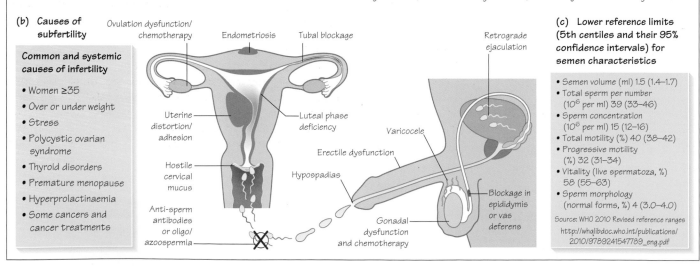

(c) Lower reference limits (5th centiles and their 95% confidence intervals) for semen characteristics

• Semen volume (ml) 1.5 (1.4–1.7)
• Total sperm per number (10⁶ per ml) 39 (33–46)
• Sperm concentration (10⁶ per ml) 15 (12–16)
• Total motility (%) 40 (38–42)
• Progressive motility (%) 32 (31–34)
• Vitality (live spermatoza, %) 58 (55–63)
• Sperm morphology (normal forms, %) 4 (3.0–4.0)

Source: WHO 2010 Revised reference ranges
http://whqlibdoc.who.int/publications/2010/9789241547789_eng.pdf

General Practice at a Glance, First Edition. Paul Booton, Carol Cooper, Graham Easton, and Margaret Harper.

Definition and background

Subfertility is a reduced capacity to conceive. It can lead to considerable psychological distress in those affected. Subfertility is relatively common and seen frequently by the GP – 1 in 6 UK couples are affected. Some 30% of couples will conceive after 1 month of trying; 60% of couples after 6 months; 84% after 12 months and 92% after 24 months. So, in the first 12 months of trying to conceive, simple advice is usually enough. Beyond 12 months, or if there is any special cause for concern, the GP needs to be proactive with investigations, support and understanding.

Aetiology

Female fertility is known to decline with age, especially after 35 years. However, subfertility can commonly be caused by problems in either partner: up to half by female disorders; about one-third by male disorders; about 10% by both partners; and in 10% the cause will remain unexplained.

History

Ideally, you should see both partners. Your history should include the following:
- Lifestyle issues for both partners, especially smoking and alcohol (see management section, below).
- Contraception (fertility can take a while to return after some contraceptive methods – up to 12 months following the Depo injection, for example).
- Ask about the woman's normal menstrual cycle and age, history of undescended testes or varicocele in the man, chronic infection such as HIV, hepatitis B or C and any previous cancer treatment in either partner.
- Previous pregnancies involving either partner (is this primary or secondary infertility?).
- History of sexually transmitted infection.
- Ask both partners about their occupation (do they involve hazards that can affect male or female fertility).
- Full medical, surgical and drug history. Systemic disease such as thyroid, diabetes or inflammatory bowel disease can have an adverse effect on fertility, as can their treatments; pelvic, abdominal or genital surgery is also relevant.

Examination

- Calculate **both** partners' body mass index (BMI), particularly relevant for the woman (see Figure 23a).
- Look for signs of polycystic ovaries in the **woman**: acne, hirsutism, male pattern baldness. Examine the breasts if there is a history of galactorrhoea and perform an abdominal, speculum and pelvic examination – look also for signs of undisclosed sexual difficulties such as vaginismus.
- Examine the **man** for gynaecomastia and also examine his external genitalia – observe the appearance of the penis, the testicular location, size and consistency, any sign of varicocele or inguinal hernia.

Investigations

Start investigations for couples who have not conceived after 1 year of regular unprotected intercourse or before if you suspect a problem (e.g. a woman >35 years or with irregular periods, history of pelvic infection or surgery, or male history of undescended testis). In primary care, blood tests can be arranged for the woman to check her ovulation and semen tests organised for the man.

Management

Couples should be seen together wherever possible. Remember that this can be a very stressful time for both of them. They will need support and assurance that something is being done – even though many will go on to conceive without any intervention. Remember that there may be feelings of guilt (e.g. about previous terminations or delaying start of family) or inadequacy (particularly in some cultures, where pressure to have children is high) that may need exploring for both partners.

GPs should make all couples aware of lifestyle changes to improve their chances of conception. Some of these questions are very personal, but explaining why they are relevant can help put the couple at ease:
1 Frequency and timing of sexual intercourse
2 Smoking
3 Alcohol
4 Medications and recreational drugs
5 Body weight.

Address any identified potential causes for the couple's fertility problems (e.g. treat thyroid disorders or refer for fibroid removal). If a couple still hasn't conceived naturally after 18 months, then refer them to a gynaecologist for further investigations and management (see Figure 23a).

Those who have had a cause for their subfertility identified by your initial investigations should be referred sooner, as should those whose fertility you are more concerned about (e.g. previous cancer treatment or HIV).

Pre-conception counselling

Couples may ask your advice before trying to get pregnant. Key areas to discuss include the following:
- The need for frequent unprotected penetrative sex.
- Smoking, alcohol, weight, drug use and medications including contraception.
- Rubella status testing can be offered to enable vaccination, when needed, before trying to conceive.
- Cervical smear history and a smear offered if appropriate.
- Daily folic acid supplements to reduce the risk of neural tube defects in the developing fetus. Ideally, to be taken from intention to fall pregnant until 12 weeks into pregnancy – 0.4 mg/day for most women, 5 mg/day in those who have previously had an infant with a neural tube defect, are taking anti-epileptic medication or are diabetic.

(a) Methods of termination according to gestational age in weeks

Medical using mifepristone and prostaglandin							Medical using mifepristone and multiple doses of prostaglandin																
Early aspiration technique to strict protocol							Suction termination								Dilatation and evacuation								
1	2	3	4	5	6	**7**	8	**9**	10	11	12	13	14	**15**	16	17	18	19	20	21	22	23	**24**

(b) A comparison of the different methods

	Medical		Surgical		
Method	Anti-progesterone mifepristone followed by prostaglandin 48 hours later	Anti-progesterone mifepristone followed by multiple doses (vaginal or oral) of prostaglandin	Early aspiration technique involving magnification of aspirated material and serum βHCG follow up	Suction termination	Dilatation and evacuation
Timing according to gestational age	Up to 9 weeks	9 – 24 weeks	Up to 7 weeks	7 – 15 weeks	>15 weeks
Anaesthetic	None required	None required	Sedation +/– local anaesthetic	Sedation +/– local anaesthetic/general anaesthetic	General anaesthetic
Efficacy	Risk of failure 1–14/1000 (higher in earlier terminations)		Risk of failure 2.3/1000 (higher in earlier terminations)		

Complications	All risks are lowered in early terminations
	
	• Peri-operative:
	  – haemorrhage during termination 1/1000
	  – uterine perforation at time of termination 1–4/1000
	  – uterine rupture – <1/1000 higher in mid trimester medical termination
	  – cervical trauma – higher in surgical – around 1/100
	
	• Post operative:
	  – infection – up to 10% – risk lower if given prophylactic antibiotics
	  – fertility – no known association with infertility, small increased risk miscarriage/preterm birth
	  – psychological consequences				

General Practice at a Glance, First Edition. Paul Booton, Carol Cooper, Graham Easton, and Margaret Harper.

The definition of termination of pregnancy is the voluntary ending of a pregnancy by removal of the products of conception. Terminations can be carried out using medical or surgical methods.

In England and Wales there are around 195,000 terminations performed annually, and at least one-third of British women will have had a termination before they reach the age of 45. Most women visit their GP as the first step in the referral procedure. Patients requesting your help are often unsure of what they want, are emotionally fragile and are uncertain how the doctor will react to their situation. It is vital therefore that the GP acts sensitively and empathically and provides accurate information, is aware of the legal requirements and provides non-judgemental support and counselling for a women who is facing an often difficult decision that she will have to live with for the rest of her life.

Box 24.1 The law

Terminations in England, Scotland and Wales are regulated under the Abortion Act 1967 and the Human Fertilisation and Embryology Act 1990.

Terminations can be carried out under 24 weeks if there is:

(a) risk to the physical or mental health of the woman
(b) risk to the physical or mental health of her children or family.

There is no upper limit to the time at which a termination can be performed if there is:

(a) risk to the woman's life
(b) risk of grave permanent damage to the woman's physical or mental health or
(c) risk of physical or mental disability if the baby was born.

Terminations are still illegal in Northern Ireland apart from exceptional circumstances where there is immediate risk to the life of the mother or long-term or permanent risk to her physical or mental health.

Under the Acts, two doctors must sign a legal document (HSA1 form) to indicate under which grounds the termination can be performed. Females under the age of 16 can have a termination without parental consent if the two medically responsible professionals deem that she is 'Gillick' competent and the Fraser guidelines are followed.

Key points to address in the GP consultation

• **Confirm pregnancy**, if necessary.
• **Assess dates** – a pregnancy is dated from the first day of the last normal menstrual period. If it is not clear the patient may need bimanual examination or a referral for an urgent ultrasound.
• **Prompt referral to local services.** The risks of complications from a termination are fewer the earlier in the pregnancy it can be carried out so a speedy and a fail safe referral mechanism is paramount. Ideally, she should be seen within 5 days from the point of referral and the termination should be completed in no longer than 2 weeks from the clinic date.
• **Fill out and sign a HSA1 form** for her to take to her clinic appointment along with a referral letter.
• **Provide her with information regarding the process** and what is likely to happen next.
• **Consider contraception following the termination.** She can become pregnant within 1 week of her termination so this is your window of opportunity to discuss her options.

Psycho-social issues to consider in the consultation

• **Counsel the patient to consider all her options.** You may be the first person she has spoken to, and you can offer unbiased advice and support. Questions you may want to ask include: Does her partner/family know? What are their views? Has she considered alternatives? What are the pros and cons of each? How does each option make her feel? What are her future plans?
• **Consider whether she needs additional support to help her make this decision** (e.g. if she is particularly vulnerable because of mental health issues, poor social support or if there is any suggestion of coercion from her partner and/or family). Counselling is available at the clinic.
• **Make sure she knows that she can change her mind** at any time up to the actual termination procedure.
• **Consider the possibility of domestic violence, sexual abuse or even incest as factors in an unwanted pregnancy.** You may have to support your patient through testing for STIs and even criminal proceedings.
• **Offer follow-up and support** – there may well be psychological consequences so be proactive and prepared. Risk factors for post termination distress include lack of social support, preceding mental health issues, ambivalence before termination and being a member of a cultural society that considers termination to be wrong.

What if you feel unable to provide adequate counselling or referral because of religious or personal beliefs?

You are not obliged to refer patients or to take part in terminations if your personal or religious beliefs prevent you. However, you have a duty of care towards your patient, so you should ensure that she is seen the same day by a colleague who can provide her with the help she needs. You must never let your personal feelings or beliefs get in the way of your duty as a doctor to give your patient the care she needs (see GMC guidance *Personal beliefs and medical practice*).

What happens in the specialist clinic?

• The patient will be offered counselling if she or her GP feels it is necessary.
• The doctor will perform an ultrasound to confirm the gestational date as well as check FBC, blood group and Rhesus type (in case the patient needs anti-D immunoglobulin postoperatively) and screen for sexual transmitted infections (e.g. *Chlamydia*).
• All women routinely receive empirical antibiotics to prevent the risk of postoperative infection.
• Contraception will be discussed – she will be encouraged to have the chosen method initiated immediately after the termination (e.g. IUD/IUS or an implant can be inserted immediately afterwards, and oral contraceptives can be started the next day).
• It may also be an opportunistic time to offer cervical screening if she is due a smear test.

Aftercare

• The patient will be provided with information regarding what she can expect to happen (e.g. bleeding patterns, pain).
• She will be seen for follow-up within 2 weeks of the abortion for review. This may include an ultrasound to check the products have all been passed.

Inform the patient to seek help if after the termination she has:
➤ Increased or severe pain
➤ Increased or severe bleeding
➤ Fever.

(a) Woman presenting with heavy menstrual bleeding (HMB)

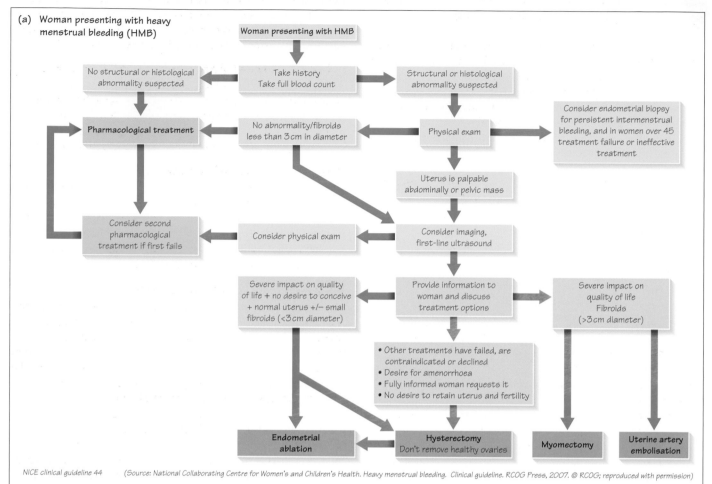

Woman presenting with HMB

↓

Take history
Take full blood count

No structural or histological abnormality suspected ← → Structural or histological abnormality suspected

Pharmacological treatment ← No abnormality/fibroids less than 3cm in diameter → Physical exam → Consider endometrial biopsy for persistent intermenstrual bleeding, and in women over 45 treatment failure or ineffective treatment

Uterus is palpable abdominally or pelvic mass

Consider second pharmacological treatment if first fails ← Consider physical exam ← Consider imaging, first-line ultrasound

Severe impact on quality of life + no desire to conceive + normal uterus +/– small fibroids (<3cm diameter) ← Provide information to woman and discuss treatment options → Severe impact on quality of life Fibroids (>3cm diameter)

• Other treatments have failed, are contraindicated or declined
• Desire for amenorrhoea
• Fully informed woman requests it
• No desire to retain uterus and fertility

Endometrial ablation ← Hysterectomy Don't remove healthy ovaries   Myomectomy   Uterine artery embolisation

NICE clinical guideline 44   (Source: National Collaborating Centre for Women's and Children's Health. Heavy menstrual bleeding. Clinical guideline. RCOG Press, 2007. © RCOG; reproduced with permission)

(b) Polycystic ovarian disease

On examination look for:

• Acne

• Hirsutism
  – distribution often on chin, upper lip, nipples and around umbilicus and a line beneath the umbilicus

• Poor breast development

• Central abdominal obesity

• General examination
  – including BP and weight BMI and waist measurement

Polycystic features of ovaries in ultrasounds are diagnostic

Normal ovary

Polycystic ovary

(c) Investigations for PCOS

• **Blood tests:** Hormone profile ratio of LH, FSH normal ratio of 1 is altered and generally greater than 1:1 (tested third day of cycle). Serum (blood) levels of androgens, including androstenedione and testosterone – elevated
  – best measure – free testosterone level. The free androgenic (ratio of testosterone to sex hormone binding globulin [SHBG]) is also high and thought to be a predictor of free testosterone
  – fasting sugar and lipid profile
  – 2 hour glucose tolerance test (GTT) in patients with obesity
  – fasting insulin level (if available) alone or with GTT helps diagnose insulin resistance and indicates who will respond to the metformin
• **Ultrasound:** May show multiple cysts (>12) in both ovaries with increased stroma, arranged around the periphery (rosary pattern) or scattered throughout with an increased ovarian size. Remember not all patients with polycystic ovarian syndrome have polycystic ovaries
• **Diagnostic criteria:** According to Rotterdam criteria any of two out of three is diagnostic:
  – oilgomenorrohea/anovulation
  – androgen excess
  – polycystic appearance by u/s

Menstrual disorders are common in primary care.

Menorrhagia

Bleeding that is heavier than the patient's normal flow. Blood loss may be a problem but is often less than the patient perceives.

History

• Ask if the cycle is regular or not, the usual cycle interval, bleeding, pain and dyspareunia. A menstrual chart helps establish the pattern. Normal cycles may vary from 22 to 34 days.
• Establish the amount of blood loss. More than 80 ml per cycle is menorrhagia. Ask about the number of pads or tampons used, clots and the number of days of heavy bleeding.
• Exclude any co-morbidity or history of HRT, tamoxifen, irregular pill-taking or any herbal medicine.

Examination

Exclude anaemia and evidence of thyroid disease. Examine the abdomen for any obvious mass or tenderness in the lower abdomen. Vaginal examination is **mandatory** if there is a history of an irregular cycle in perimenopausal or post-menopausal women or if there is menorrhagia with intermenstrual or post-coital bleeding.

Investigations

FBC; FSH, LH, testosterone, prolactin; clotting screen; pelvic scan.

Common causes of menorrhagia

• Functional – hormonal imbalance is a diagnosis by exclusion.
• Fibroid and/or endometriosis – most common above 30 years.
• Pelvic inflammatory disease.
• Carcinoma.
• Systemic disease (e.g. hypothyroidism).

Management

• Treat anaemia, exclude pathology, and beware of **cancer** in patients around menopause with co-morbidity like diabetes.
• If no apparent pathology try mefenamic acid or tranexamic acid, then oral contraceptive pill (OCP) to achieve better cycle control.
• In peri-menopausal women, if contraception is needed and the scan is normal, consider a Mirena®. This has **reduced the number of hysterectomies for menstrual disorders.**
• Refer all cases of post-menopausal bleeding, and patients with an abnormal scan (e.g. submucous fibriods or fibroids larger than 5–6 cm, and endometriosis) for hysteroscopy and/or laparoscopy.

Dysmenorrhoea

Dysmenorrhoea can be primary or secondary. In primary dysmenorrhoea, no cause is detected. It occurs in young women soon after puberty or when regular ovulation is established. Prostaglandin and other inflammatory substances are thought to cause uterine cramps and spasm of blood vessels.

Secondary dysmenorrhoea is associated with an existing condition. The most common is endometriosis. Other causes include fibroids, adenomyosis, ovarian cysts and pelvic congestion and the presence of IUD.

Diagnosis

In primary dysmenorrhoea, typical symptoms are pain, lower abdominal cramps from a few days before menstruation and lasting for the first half of the cycle. Other symptoms include vomiting, diarrhoea, constipation, headache and fainting attacks.

In secondary dysmenorrhoea carry out a full examination and a vaginal examination to detect any tenderness or lumps, a cervical smear, vaginal and cervical swabs.

A pelvic scan and laparoscopy is useful if endometriosis is suspected.

Treatment

For secondary dysmenorrhoea, treatment depends on the cause.

For primary dysmenorrhoea, consider NSAIDs or OCP. Complementary measures like changing posture during cramps, stopping smoking, yoga, omega-3 foods and exercise may all help.

Intermenstrual and post-coital bleeding

The cause is commonly local to the cervix (e.g. a cervical polyp or erosion). Do a speculum and internal examination to exclude the above causes, infection or pregnancy. If no local cause is found, refer for hysteroscopy to exclude an endometrial polyp. Malignancy is uncommon but must be considered in all patients.

Post-menopausal bleeding

Any vaginal bleeding after 1 year after stopping menstruation, whether a normal period or just spotting, must be taken seriously. Take a full history and internal examination. Refer for a pelvic scan and hysteroscopy (2-week pathway to exclude malignancy). The return of normal periods is uncommon but can be confirmed by a normal level of FSH or a normal scan.

Polycystic ovarian syndrome

The incidence is about 5–10% in women in the reproductive period and 20% in patients with subfertility. It may present with amenorrhoea, oligomenorrhoea, hirsutism, acne, subfertility, recurrent miscarriages or obesity in young adults. There is a wide spectrum of symptoms. In mild cases menstruation may be normal, the patient may conceive but then go on to have miscarriages.

Underlying cause and long-term effect

The exact cause is unknown. There is:
• Increased incidence with a family history.
• Imbalance in hypothalamic–pituitary–ovarian axis feedback mechanism. The ovaries secrete more testosterone resulting in symptoms. Ovulation may cease because of changed levels of luteinising hormone (LH) and follicle-stimulating hormone (FSH).
• **PCOS is often associated with insulin resistance** resulting in obesity, hypertension, diabetes and coronary heart disease later.
• Endometrial hyperplasia may occur due to cycle reduction (<3/yr) and without the protection effect of progesterone lead to endometrial cancer.
• An increase in the incidence of ovarian cancer.
• Depression and mood swings because of lack of progesterone.

History

Ask about menstruation (length and amount of bleeding), age of menarche, onset and distribution of excess hair, weight gain, family history of PCOS or diabetes.

Treatment

1 **Lifestyle** – mainstay of treatment. Weight reduction, healthy diet, regular exercise all increase the chance of ovulation, improve insulin resistance and prevent long-term risk.
2 **Metformin** is not licensed for PCOS and studies show no substantial benefit but it may help weight loss and restore ovulation.
3 **Hormonal treatment.** For primary amenorrhoea advise lifestyle changes. Then consider Dianette® or Yasmin®, particularly if there are raised testosterone levels. If the presentation is miscarriages or subfertility, achieving normal BMI is the first step. Clomifene may be the next step but refer to a specialist subfertility clinic.

26 The menopause

Box 26.1   Diseases after the menopause

- Cardiovascular disease (CVD) risk increases
- Osteoporosis increases for women after the menopause
- Breast disease: A woman whose menopause is in her late 50s has approximately twice the risk of developing breast cancer as one whose menopause was in her early 40s

Box 26.2   Causes of premature menopause

- Idiopathic
- Radiotherapy and chemotherapy: bilateral oophorectomy results in instant menopause and hysterectomy without oophorectomy can induce a premature menopause
- Surgery
- Infection (e.g. TB)
- Chromosomal abnormalities (e.g. involving the X chromosome)
- Autoimmune diseases (e.g. diabetes, hypothyroidism, Addison's disease)
- FSH receptor abnormalities
- Disruption of oestrogen production

The experience of the menopause can vary dramatically between women. Some need information and reassurance and others require medical intervention.

The menopause is characterised by a **reduction in oestrogen** production due to primary ovarian failure. There is an increase in LH/FSH levels due to negative feedback. It occurs gradually with the **climacteric** or 'peri-menopausal' phase. The average age of the menopause in the UK is approximately 51–52 years.

Menopause in a woman <45 years is defined as premature (see premature menopause box). Treatment with HRT is usually recommended until the age of 50.

Diagnosis

The menopause is defined as >12 months of amenorrhoea. It can be difficult to establish when the menopause has occurred, especially if HRT is taken in the peri-menopausal phase.

History

Ask the patient about the following:
- **Severity of symptoms.** The impact is probably multi-factorial and may be influenced by culture and psycho-social factors.
- **Menstrual changes.** Periods usually become less regular as there are an increased number of anovulatory cycles.
▶ Post-coital, intermenstrual, post-menopausal or heavy and/or painful bleeding may indicate other pathologies.
- **Flushes/sweats:** experienced by up to 85%. The severity can vary dramatically; they are often associated with palpitations.
- **Psychological:** a complex and controversial area. Symptoms including anxiety and depression, irritability, insomnia, loss of libido and memory loss have been said to be attributable to the menopause. However, these may be multi-factorial and also caused by changes going on in the individual's life at that time. Some symptoms such as hot flushes may have direct impact on sleep.
- **Urogynaecological:** urinary and sexual symptoms are common:
  o As the vagina, urethra and bladder trigone are oestrogen dependent they gradually atrophy
  o Vaginal dryness and atrophy are common and may lead to superficial dyspareunia and vaginal bleeding
  o A reduction in bladder elasticity and pelvic floor support can produce symptoms of stress incontinence.

Investigations

Investigations are usually unnecessary except if the diagnosis is in doubt or premature menopause is suspected.

A serum FSH (>30 IU/L) is usually diagnostic in women not taking hormonal contraception (if in doubt repeat in 6 weeks).

Management

Due to emerging evidence treatment recommendations have changed over the years and it remains a complex area. Consider patient choice, symptom control and the risk–benefit balance for each individual patient when deciding on management:
- **No specific treatment:** symptoms of the menopause usually last 2–5 years and are variable in severity. Increasing physical activity, reducing caffeine and alcohol can be of help with hot flushes.
- **HRT alternatives:**
  o **Clonidine:** may reduce hot flushes although its side effects (e.g. dizziness, dry mouth) often limit its use.
  o **SSRIs:** can help reduce hot flushes.
  o **Complementary treatments:** include ginseng, black cohosh and red clover (oestrogenic properties). There is limited evidence to prove their value and some may have long-term risks.
- **HRT:** aspects to discuss with the patient:
  o **Types:** women without a uterus can use oestrogen-only preparations but women with a uterus must have a preparation containing both oestrogen and progestogen to prevent endometrial proliferation. This can be given as a continuous combined preparation (no bleed) or with cyclical progestogen for the last 10–13 days of the cycle.
  o **Preparations:** tablets, skin patches, gels and nasal sprays. Topical oestrogen preparations can be helpful for vulval symptoms.
  o **Side effects:** weight gain, nausea, breast tenderness, premenstrual syndrome (PMS) type symptoms.
  o **Benefits:** currently HRT is recommended for symptomatic control only and not for primary or secondary prevention of CVD nor as a first line treatment for osteoporosis.
  o **Risks:** this has been an area of concern for many women and clinicians. Therefore the decision to take HRT is taken jointly between the patient and doctor after looking at the risk–benefit profile. Risks are usually greater the older the woman and the longer they have been on HRT. It is important that women regularly review their medication with their GP and ensure that it remains appropriate for them.

27 Common gynaecological cancers

Role of the GP in gynaecological malignancies

For these cancers much of the treatment takes place in secondary care. As a GP your main role is to encourage disease prevention and education (e.g. cervical screening, human papilloma virus [HPV] immunisations) and to refer potential pathology early. Referral is via the current system of cancer networks and the '2-week rule' for seeing and investigating patients with red flags. This aims to improve survival as well as alleviating much of the anxiety around cancer for patients.

The GP, along with the multi-disciplinary team, provides medical, practical, educational and psychological support for patients (and relatives). The GP has a vital role with patients when the treatment is not curative and the patient moves towards the terminal stages of their illness.

Ovarian cancer

- **Incidence:** 5000 new cases per year – 20.3 per 100 000[i]
- **Risk Factors:**
  - age: most in women over the age of 50
  - ovulation: Factors that reduce ovulation, COC/parity/breast-feeding/ sterilisation and hysterectomy, slightly lower the risk. Slightly increased risk – HRT/obesity/late menopause
  - family history: Most NOT genetic. Approximately 1 in 20 cases are genetic – commonest identifiable genes – BRCA1 and BRAC2[ii]
- **History: Often no early or specific symptoms resulting in late diagnosis. Ask about the more common symptoms:**
  - abdominal or pelvic pain
  - frequent of persistent bloating
  - difficulty in eating/feeling full early
  - urinary symptoms (urgency and frequency)

  See NICE guidelines – advise prompt investigation in women over the age of 50 with such symptoms using CA125[iii]
- **Diagnosis: Includes use of USS and CA125**
- **Treatment: Refer urgently**
- **Prognosis:** Often poor due to the late presentation of this cancer – the overall 5-year survival – below 35%[iv]
- **Future Screening for Ovarian Cancer:** Current trials looking at the use of USS and CA125

[i] http://www.gpnotebook.co.uk
[ii] http://www.patient.co.uk/
[iii] NICE guidelines: Ovarian Cancer, April 2011
[iv] NICE guidelines: Ovarian Cancer, April 2011

Endometrial cancer

- **Incidence:** 4500 new cases each year
  - common age of presentation in UK: 50s to 60s
- **Risk Factors:**
  - age,
  - (unopposed) oestrogen exposure
  - nulliparity
  - obesity
  - late menopause
  - endometrial hyperplasia
  - PCOS and tamoxifen
  - diabetes
  - family history: strong family history of breast, ovary or colonic cancers
- **History and examination:** Ask about – ▶ abnormal vaginal bleeding, post-menopausal bleeding, post-coital/inter-menstrual bleeding or other abdominal/pelvic symptoms
- **Diagnosis:** includes ultrasound, endometrial sampling and hysteroscopy
- **Treatment:** urgent referral
- **Prognosis:** good if diagnosed early

Cervical cancer (80% squamous)

- **Incidence:** 16 per 100 000 women
- **Age of presentation in UK:** 40 to 50s
- **Risk Factors:** HPV (Human Papilloma Virus: 16 and 18 subtypes) – can lead to pre-malignant condition of CIN – increased risk with age/lower social class/ smoking, impaired immunity (e.g. HIV infection) and use of COC
- **History and examination:** Abnormal vaginal bleeding – initially post-coital bleeding, also inter-menstrual or even post-menopausal bleeding, offensive vaginal discharge, dyspareunia
- **Examination:** may reveal ulceration/cervical mass that bleeds on contact
- **Diagnosis:** Colposcopy
- **Treatment:** Urgent referral
- **Prognosis:** Depends on stage at presentation – average 5-year survival – 58%

Cervical screening

60% of women who develop cervical cancer have never been screened. In England and Northern Ireland 1st invitation for screening is age 25 years (Scotland and Wales 20 years) – then every 3 years 25–48 years and every 5 years 48–65 years Screening – liquid-based cytology has reduced the number of inadequate tests
- **Smear results:**
  - normal
  - inadequate: smear sample could not be analysed and needs repeating
  - abnormal: includes borderline (repeat at 6 months – often resolves spontaneously), mild dyskaryosis (repeat at 6 months – CIN 1), moderate dyskaryosis (refer for colposcopy – CIN 2), severe dyskaryosis (refer for colposcopy – CIN 3) and ▶ suspected invasive carcinoma (refer urgently)
- **Treatment of abnormal smears:** via a colposcopy service – may include cryotherapy, laser treatment or loop diathermy. HPV immunisation programme (see Chapter 16)

Vulval cancer (90% squamous)

- **Incidence:** Uncommon. 1000 cases diagnosed each year
- **Age of presentation in UK:** usually over the age of 55 yrs
- **Risk Factors:**
  - age
  - VIN (vulval intraepithelial neoplasia): can develop on the vulva. It can cause a persistent itch/skin can look abnormal with thickening and red/white patches. Approximately 1/3 vulval cancers develop in women with VIN
  - HPV (human papilloma virus) subtypes 16, 18 and 31 can lead to VIN
  - lichen sclerosus and lichen planus cause chronic vulval inflammation increasing the risk of cancer
  - smoking
  - genital herpes virus type 2 increases the risk but most women with genital herpes **do not** develop vulval cancer
- **History and examination:** Post-coital bleeding, followed later by an offensive watery discharge, persistent vulval itch, pain in vulva, non-healing vulval lesion e.g. ulcer, thickened/raised/white/red/brown lesion/patch on vulva
- **Diagnosis:** Biopsy
- **Treatment:** Refer suspected cases urgently
- **Prognosis:** The overall prognosis is relatively good if caught early

General Practice at a Glance, First Edition. Paul Booton, Carol Cooper, Graham Easton, and Margaret Harper.

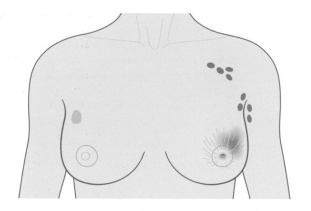

Benign
- Younger patient
- Pain, especially cyclical
- No lump, or well-defined mobile lump
- No skin changes
- Can be generalised nodularity
- Cyst which is no longer palpable after aspiration
- Painful tender lumps especially if breast-feeding (can be blocked duct or abscess)

Malignant
- Absence of pain (usually but not always)
- Ill-defined lump with tethering superficially or deeply
- Blood-stained nipple discharge
- Skin changes e.g. peau d'orange
- Nipple changes e.g. retracted nipple, Paget's disease of nipple
- Lymphadenopathy
- Systemic features e.g. weight loss, bone pain (especially new back pain in woman over 50)

Every year, about 3% of women visit their GP with breast symptoms, and many of them are terrified of having cancer.

The most common breast symptoms are:
- **Pain:** usually means a benign condition, especially if pain is cyclical and is the only symptom
- **Lump:** 9 out of 10 lumps are benign, but you cannot assume that at presentation
- **Nodularity:** can be cyclical and is often benign, but may coexist with cancer.

History
- Ask 'How long have you had the symptoms?'
- Enquire about other symptoms such as discharge, skin changes or any change in the nipple or breast shape.
- Find out if pain or nodularity is related to periods. Are periods regular? Is the woman on HRT or the contraceptive pill?
- Is she breast-feeding now? While it's interesting to know about previous breast-feeding, age at menarche and alcohol intake, these will not aid your diagnosis.
- Family history is important. Apart from being a risk factor, a close family history can also explain a patient's high anxiety.

Examination
- Look first for any contour abnormalities or asymmetry, bearing in mind that size discrepancy between right and left is usual.
- Check for skin changes such as eczema round the nipple (could be Paget's disease of the nipple, a localised cancer) or a pitted surface like the skin of an orange (called *peau d'orange*, a sign of more advanced cancer).
- Check for inverted nipples or discharge from the nipple.
- Palpate both breasts quadrant by quadrant, including each axillary tail, with the flat of your hand.
- Check for regional lymph nodes, even though axillary examination can be misleading.
- You may need to examine other areas (e.g. the spine or the abdomen), depending on your patient's symptoms.

Management
Clinical features (see Figure 28) help discriminate between benign and malignant disease. **Even so, your patient needs referral if there is a lump.** A well-defined mobile lump in a young woman is likely to be benign, but it needs to be confirmed by biopsy.

You should also refer if there is:
► Blood-stained discharge
► Recent nipple inversion
► Nipple eczema – can be Paget's disease of the breast
► Asymmetric nodularity that persists more than 2 weeks.

One-stop breast clinics are ideal, with most investigations including ultrasound, mammography and fine-needle aspiration often performed in one session.

Benign breast disease
Thanks to hormone fluctuations, a woman's breasts undergo many changes, from puberty to the menopause. Men too can develop breast disorders, including gynaecomastia which can be pubertal or drug-induced.

Around 20% of women have some benign breast disease, which includes cysts, fibrocystic disease and fibroadenomas. Once it's established that breast symptoms are benign, reassurance is the main treatment.

Breast abscess is most common during breast-feeding, and is often caused by *Staphylococcus aureus*. If diagnosed early, antibiotics may be enough, but a fluctuant mass or large abscess needs surgical drainage.

Pain is a hallmark of benign breast disease, but try to exclude rib pain by palpation (cervical spondylosis can also cause breast pain). If breast pain is the only symptom then your patient needs reassurance rather than referral. However, pain can merit referral if it's severe and goes on for over 6 months.

With breast cysts, pain can come on suddenly, with a lump that literally appears overnight. Cysts are most common in women in their late thirties and forties, but they also occur in post-menopausal women, especially those on HRT.

General Practice at a Glance, First Edition. Paul Booton, Carol Cooper, Graham Easton, and Margaret Harper.

It can be tempting to aspirate a cystic lump in the surgery but it is better to refer the patient so the cyst can be confirmed by ultrasound and aspirated in the clinic. Cysts are usually benign but can be linked with an increased risk of breast cancer.

Breast cancer

One in eight women can now be expected to develop breast cancer. Every year, the disease also occurs in around 300 men in the UK.

Most breast cancers are survivable. Of the 48,000 women diagnosed with it in the UK annually, over three-quarters survive at least 10 years, and almost two-thirds live 20 years. The GP's job is to diagnose it at an early stage when survival is most likely, to support the woman and her family through often gruelling treatment, and to help her achieve quality of life.

There are several kinds of breast cancer:
- **Invasive breast cancer:** may or may not have receptors for oestrogen, progesterone and the protein HER2.
- **Ductal carcinoma *in situ*** (DCIS): most women with DCIS have no signs or symptoms, and only discover they have DCIS after a routine mammogram. As a result of the national breast screening programme, DCIS is diagnosed much more often than it once was. Treatment depends on the extent of the condition.
- **Lobular carcinoma *in situ*** (LCIS): it is usually enough to monitor LCIS.

Treatment is now highly specialised. It may include surgery (either mastectomy or breast-conserving), radiotherapy, chemotherapy, hormone treatment (e.g. the anti-oestrogen tamoxifen and the aromatase inhibitor anastrozole), biological treatment with trastuzumab (Herceptin®) or a combination of several options. The management depends on the stage of the disease and the type of tumour as well as on patient preference. Breast reconstruction can sometimes be performed, either at mastectomy or later.

Should you mention 'cancer'?

Students worry about how to broach the possibility of cancer without scaring patients unnecessarily, when referring for instance. The chances are that your patient is already thinking about cancer and it's usually best to be honest if cancer is in your differential diagnosis. You can explain that 9 out of 10 lumps are benign, but you need to rule out the 1 in 10 chance to be safe. Remember there can be serious consequences of **not** mentioning the word 'cancer': your patient may not come back if things worsen, may fail to attend their appointment or could be scared when someone mentions cancer at hospital.

NHS breast screening

The NHS breast screening programme offers free screening every 3 years for all women aged 47 to 74.

Every year, around 2 million women are screened. The cancer detection rate is around 8 per 1000 women screened. Most of the invasive cancers detected are under 1.5 cm in diameter, and are more likely to be treated without mastectomy. Nowadays over one-quarter of all breast cancers are picked up by screening but mammography also finds benign lesions and less invasive cancers. Investigating and treating these can cause much anxiety. This is one of the reasons some experts doubt the value of breast screening.

Approach to antenatal care is woman-centred, with primary purpose to pre-empt serious complications and ensure (so far as possible) a healthy baby is born to a healthy woman

In an uncomplicated pregnancy, nulliparous women ('nullips') usually have 10 antenatal appointments, while parous women have 7. This is based on the fact that nullips can have a higher incidence of pre-eclampsia and other complications. They also need more information and emotional support

NHS maternity records are standardised. They are held by the woman herself, and updated every time she is seen during pregnancy. At every appointment, blood pressure should be taken, and urine checked for proteinuria

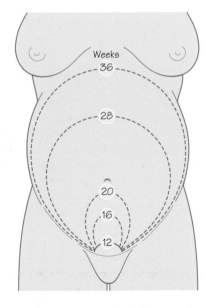

Timing	Type of contact	What happens
Before 10 weeks ideally	Booking appointment for all pregnant women – long consultation with midwife	• Identify women in need of extra care • Woman gets information on screening for Down's, breast-feeding, healthy eating and other lifestyle matters • Early ultrasound scan offered. Also blood tests: blood group, rhesus status, anaemia, haemoglobino-pathies, HIV, rubella status, syphilis • Identify women who have had female genital mutilation (FGM)
16 weeks	Appointment for all	• Review and discuss results of tests • Offer information on routine anomaly scan
18-20 weeks	Ultrasound scan ('anomaly scan')	• Detects major structural anomalies • Women with placenta praevia are offered another scan at 32 weeks
25 weeks	Appointment for nullips	• Blood pressure and urine • Plot symphysis-fundal height
28 weeks	Appointment for all	• Second screening for anaemia and red cell autoantibodies • Investigate Hb below 10.5 g/100 ml • Offer anti-D prophylaxis to rhesus-negative women • Plot symphysis-fundal height
31 weeks	Appointment for nullips	• Review results of tests done at 28 weeks • Blood pressure and urine • Plot symphysis-fundal height
34 weeks	Appointment for all	• Review results of tests done at 28 weeks • Offer 2nd dose of anti-D to rhesus-negative women • Blood pressure and urine • Plot symphysis-fundal height • Give information on labour and birth, including birth plan and pain relief • Breast-feeding discussed if not already done earlier
36 weeks	Appointment for all	• Blood pressure and urine • Plot symphysis-fundal height
38 weeks	Appointment for all	• Blood pressure and urine • Plot symphysis-fundal height • Discuss management of prolonged pregnancy
40 weeks	Appointment for nullips	• Blood pressure and urine • Plot symphysis-fundal height
41 weeks	Appointment for women who have not given birth	• Blood pressure and urine • Plot symphysis-fundal height • Offer a membrane sweep and induction of labour

General Practice at a Glance, First Edition. Paul Booton, Carol Cooper, Graham Easton, and Margaret Harper.

66 © 2013 Paul Booton, Carol Cooper, Graham Easton, and Margaret Harper. Published 2013 by Blackwell Publishing Ltd.

The pregnant woman

Pregnancy is not an illness. By and large it is a normal healthy life-affirming process. Pregnant women are therefore not necessarily 'patients'. Understandably, many dislike being treated as if they were. Many also hold strong views about pregnancy and birth, and about how they want to experience it.

All the same, pregnancy can bring problems for both mother and baby. In the UK, the maternal death rate is 6.7 per 100,000 live births, and every year there are thousands of stillbirths and perinatal deaths (deaths around birth and the first week of life).

Substandard care is a major factor in many of these deaths. Antenatal care needs to deliver woman-centred care that doesn't neglect the medical risks.

Antenatal care

Most antenatal care is shared between the hospital antenatal clinic and the practice. Midwives, whether hospital-based or in the community, are the lead professionals involved in normal pregnancy. But GPs too care for pregnant women, and are often the first health professional the woman consults at a pivotal moment in her life. As the lynchpin of continuity of care, a GP is well-placed to reassure the woman at a time of physical and emotional change.

Equally importantly, the GP has a key role in recognising and managing any complications, and may also see the pregnant woman for unrelated illness, such as flu. You therefore need to know about pregnancy in general, and the antenatal routine, screening tests and medical problems that can affect pregnancy or arise from it.

History

At the first consultation, ask the woman about her last period, whether it was normal and what her usual cycle is. The expected date of delivery (EDD) is 9 months and 7 days, which you can calculate by subtracting 3 months and adding 7 days to the first day of her LMP. Make allowances if her cycle is unusually long or short and remember that the due date is not set in stone. The first scan may suggest a different date. Besides, few babies arrive exactly on time.

By now you will have a good idea of whether the pregnancy is wanted or not. If you're unsure, ask how she is feeling about the pregnancy, and read her face as well. Throughout the consultation be alert to any hints of domestic violence or rape.

Ask about alcohol, smoking and drugs (prescribed, over-the-counter and recreational). The dangers of smoking in pregnancy include miscarriage, premature labour and small-for-gestational age babies. Women who want to stop smoking may need nicotine replacement therapy as well as support. The Department of Health advises women to abstain from alcohol from before conception to the end of the first trimester, but there is no hard evidence that small amounts of alcohol, such as 2–3 units a week, harm the fetus. Many women also feel needlessly guilty for having had a few drinks before they knew they were pregnant.

Always enquire about previous pregnancies. These affect expectations and can flag up an increased risk of complications.

Pre-eclampsia, premature labour, ante-partum or post-partum haemorrhage and small-for-gestational-age-babies can all recur. Miscarriage is common and is usually a one-off but a woman may be very concerned about a recurrence (see Chapter 30). Women who have had a termination are often anxious about their current pregnancy too.

Family history is important. 'Did any of your family have problems during pregnancy, or with their babies?' and 'Are there any twins in the family?' Ask specifically about diabetes and pre-eclampsia (or 'toxaemia') as these have a strong familial element.

Is she already taking folic acid? A daily dose of 400 μg is recommended from before conception to 13 weeks' gestation to reduce the risk of spina bifida, neural tube defects and cleft lip and palate.

Examination

- Take the blood pressure and check heart and lungs.
- Examine the abdomen. In a singleton pregnancy, the fundus should not be palpable above the pelvic brim before 13 weeks.
- You need not examine the pelvis or breasts routinely.
- Routine weighing is no longer recommended during antenatal care, but check weight and height and calculate BMI early on in the pregnancy.

Women with a BMI over 30 kg/m^2 need extra care: they are at increased risk of miscarriage, gestational diabetes, pre-eclampsia, thrombo-embolic disease, caesarean section and wound infections. They are also less likely to breast-feed. Their babies are at higher risk of prematurity, stillbirth and congenital abnormalities and neonatal death.

Management

- Give out information on pregnancy and on screening tests, and provide information and support for the woman and her partner if she has one.
- Remember to be sensitive to cultural and religious values, especially when discussing tests and procedures.
- The woman may have questions about work, diet, weight, medication, alternative therapies, exercise and common infections. Pregnant women are often concerned about toxoplasmosis. As long as the litter tray is kept clean and she practises good hygiene, the threat from the family cat is almost non-existent. However, gardening, visiting petting farms and eating undercooked meat or unwashed produce do carry a risk of toxoplasmosis.
- Give her a prescription for folic acid if she isn't already taking 400 μg/day, and assess whether she needs anything else.
- There is a good case for all pregnant women to take vitamin D supplements. These are not yet a routine part of antenatal care, but they are vital for many women, for instance vegans, those with darker skins and those who have had short gaps between babies.
- Iron supplements are no longer routine and are best kept for those with iron deficiency.

Finally, refer her promptly to the antenatal clinic of her choice, as long as her choice seems compatible with her obstetric history. It's appropriate to be upbeat, but remember that normal labour is a retrospective diagnosis.

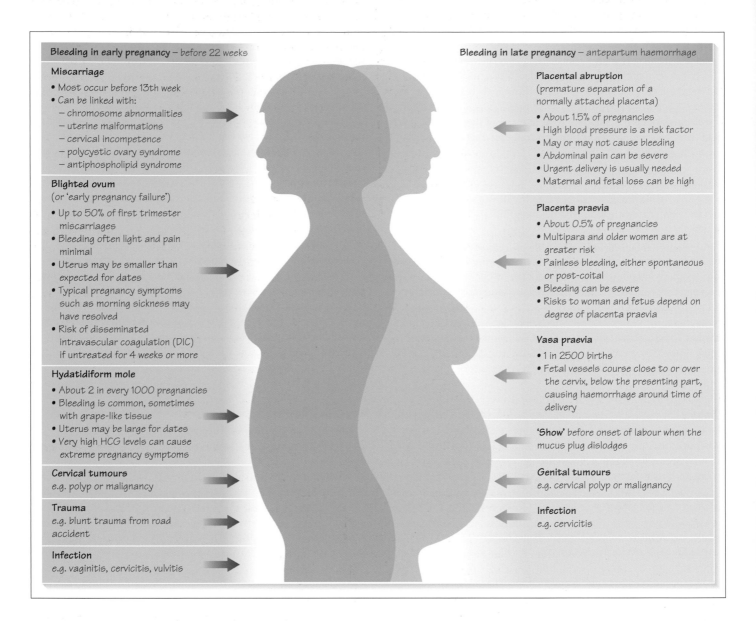

Bleeding in early pregnancy – before 22 weeks

Miscarriage
- Most occur before 13th week
- Can be linked with:
  – chromosome abnormalities
  – uterine malformations
  – cervical incompetence
  – polycystic ovary syndrome
  – antiphospholipid syndrome

Blighted ovum
(or 'early pregnancy failure')
- Up to 50% of first trimester miscarriages
- Bleeding often light and pain minimal
- Uterus may be smaller than expected for dates
- Typical pregnancy symptoms such as morning sickness may have resolved
- Risk of disseminated intravascular coagulation (DIC) if untreated for 4 weeks or more

Hydatidiform mole
- About 2 in every 1000 pregnancies
- Bleeding is common, sometimes with grape-like tissue
- Uterus may be large for dates
- Very high HCG levels can cause extreme pregnancy symptoms

Cervical tumours
e.g. polyp or malignancy

Trauma
e.g. blunt trauma from road accident

Infection
e.g. vaginitis, cervicitis, vulvitis

Bleeding in late pregnancy – antepartum haemorrhage

Placental abruption
(premature separation of a normally attached placenta)
- About 1.5% of pregnancies
- High blood pressure is a risk factor
- May or may not cause bleeding
- Abdominal pain can be severe
- Urgent delivery is usually needed
- Maternal and fetal loss can be high

Placenta praevia
- About 0.5% of pregnancies
- Multipara and older women are at greater risk
- Painless bleeding, either spontaneous or post-coital
- Bleeding can be severe
- Risks to woman and fetus depend on degree of placenta praevia

Vasa praevia
- 1 in 2500 births
- Fetal vessels course close to or over the cervix, below the presenting part, causing haemorrhage around time of delivery

'Show' before onset of labour when the mucus plug dislodges

Genital tumours
e.g. cervical polyp or malignancy

Infection
e.g. cervicitis

While bleeding can occur with or without pain, and pain can occur with or without bleeding, either symptom is significant in pregnancy. Bleeding is especially alarming for a pregnant woman and her family.

Some women go straight to hospital, but many consult their GP so it is important to know how to manage these common symptoms.

Bleeding in early pregnancy

This means before 22 weeks, the time at which the fetus is considered viable.

Any blood comes from the woman, not her fetus, and not every cause is related to her pregnancy (see Figure 30). However, in many cases bleeding is indeed pregnancy-related and can lead to fetal or even maternal death, so always take it seriously.

Miscarriage

This is often a woman's greatest fear. It's said that 20% of all pregnancies end in miscarriage, but ultrasound studies show that the real proportion is much higher because many occur early on, before the woman even knows she is expecting.

Miscarriage can be:
- **Threatened:** bleeding can be light, and pain minimal. The cervical os is shut.
- **Inevitable:** pain may or may not be severe. The os is open and there may be products of conception in the cervical canal.
- **Incomplete:** the woman continues to bleed after passing some products of conception. There may be also be products of conception visible in the canal.
- **Complete:** bleeding and pain stop, and the os closes.
- **Recurrent:** this is defined as three or more miscarriages.

General Practice at a Glance, First Edition. Paul Booton, Carol Cooper, Graham Easton, and Margaret Harper.

History

• Establish how many weeks pregnant she is.
• Miscarriage usually causes both pain and bleeding, with bleeding often preceding pain. Ask if she has pain (like contractions or a bad period) and whether she has passed anything other than liquid blood ('Did you pass clots or see anything in the blood?').
• Did anything trigger the symptoms, for instance sex or injury?
• Find out whether she has had previous bleeds in this pregnancy, or any previous miscarriages.

Examination

• Check her pulse and blood pressure.
• Examine the abdomen, but not the pelvis as this can make things worse. However, a gentle speculum examination may help as it will tell you if the os is open and whether there are visible products of conception.

Management

If bleeding is severe, send the woman urgently to A&E. If it is mild, same-day referral to the Early Pregnancy Unit (EPU) is more appropriate.

The GP also has an important role in supporting a woman after miscarriage. You can usually reassure her that a first-trimester miscarriage is most often a one-off. However, do not underestimate recurrent miscarriage. **It can be an important – even the only – sign of antiphospholipid syndrome, a major and often preventable cause of fetal and maternal loss.**

Bleeding in late pregnancy

This is known as antepartum haemorrhage (APH) and occurs in up to 5% of pregnancies.

Even though there are many possible minor causes, you cannot afford to give false reassurance. Light bleeding is not necessarily less serious than heavy bleeding. **Send every woman with APH to hospital urgently.** She may need transfusion and/or emergency caesarean section, and her baby may need resuscitation and neonatal intensive care.

Before referring, quickly gain some idea of the woman's condition:
• Ascertain the gestational age and her rhesus status.
• Is she known to have placenta praevia?
• Is she in shock? Check her pulse and blood pressure as well as her general state.
• Examine her abdomen. Is it irritable or tender (early abruption) or hard and board-like (late abruption)?

Antiphospholipid syndrome

As it has so many possible manifestations, every doctor should know about antiphospholipid syndrome (APS) and how to test for it. Also called Hughes' syndrome and 'sticky blood', APS is linked with hypercoagulability. Deep vein thrombosis (DVT) is perhaps the most common problem. APS also causes 20% of strokes and MIs in under-45-year-olds, and about 20% of cases of recurrent miscarriage. It is also linked with pre-eclampsia, placental abruption, intrauterine growth restriction and stillbirth, so it has a role across the whole spectrum of fetal compromise and loss.

Women who suffer late pregnancy loss or recurrent miscarriage should have a blood test for antiphospholipid antibodies. With treatment (typically aspirin or heparin under specialist supervision), the successful pregnancy rate can rise to 80%.

Abdominal pain

Pain is not always linked with the pregnancy, but it may be. **If there is bleeding as well, it probably is pregnancy-related, but remember that in ectopic pregnancy pain often precedes bleeding and there may be no bleeding at all.**

As the pregnancy progresses and the uterus enlarges, non-pregnancy pain becomes harder to diagnose as well as more serious in outlook.

Some of the pregnancy-related causes to consider include:
• Ectopic pregnancy (early pregnancy)
• Heartburn/reflux (both early and late pregnancy)
• Hyperemesis (early pregnancy)
• Constipation (anytime)
• Urinary tract infection (anytime)
• Pain from uterine fibroids (anytime)
• Acute fatty liver (late pregnancy)
• Severe pre-eclampsia (HELLP – also late pregnancy, see Chapter 31).

Some of the unrelated causes include:
• Appendicitis
• Gall bladder pain (see Chapter 44)
• Ureteric colic
• Accidents to ovarian cysts (e.g. bleeding, torsion)
• Gastroenteritis
• IBS
• Intestinal obstruction
• Sickle cell crisis.

If pain is mild and there are no worrying signs, it can be appropriate to perform an MSU and review the woman. However, if you have any doubts, refer her to hospital without delay.

Other pregnancy problems

Headache
- Common in early pregnancy and usually benign
- Occasional paracetamol is safe

Heartburn
- In early pregnancy, caused by progesterone which relaxes the gastro-oesophageal sphincter and allows reflux
- Later the growing uterus exerts pressure effects
- Milk, simple antacids and Gaviscon all help
- Raising the head of the bed can be useful

Bleeding gums
- Gums become hyperaemic in early pregnancy because of hormone changes
- Good dental hygiene is important

Breast tenderness or pain
- Can occur before the first missed period
- Is due to rising oestrogen levels

Nausea – 'morning sickness' is thought to be due to high HCG levels, and can last all day
- Small regular meals and carb snacks help
- Some women swear by nibbling on root ginger
- Usually resolves by 2nd trimester but may need treatment if vomiting is frequent ('hyperemesis gravidarum')

Back pain
- Usually worse in late pregnancy
- Minor injuries common as relaxin loosens ligaments
- Good posture, low heels and keeping active all help
- Swimming useful

Constipation (a progesterone effect)
- Fibre, fruit, vegetables, more water and regular exercise all help
- Strong laxatives are contra-indicated in pregnancy

Carpal tunnel syndrome
- Fluid retention puts pressure on median nerve
- Resting or shaking hand can help
- Wrist splint is useful

Haemorrhoids ('piles')
- Results from constipation and pressure in the pelvis
- Prevent constipation
- Avoid straining

Vaginal discharge
- Clear discharge often due to oestrogen rise and increased vascularity
- No treatment needed unless itch, smell or discharge is coloured

Varicose veins
- Due to progesterone and pressure in the pelvis
- Tend to run in families
- Walking and resting (not standing) help
- Support tights are useful

Mild ankle swelling
- Due to fluid retention and pressure in the pelvis
- Is normal if mild
- Check for proteinuria
- Otherwise manage as for varicose veins

In addition, **tiredness** is common especially early in pregnancy, and **insomnia** especially in late pregnancy

Remember that these symptoms can be severe with multiple pregnancy as well as hydatidiform mole. You should also be aware that some 'minor' symptoms can have serious significance when they occur later in pregnancy especially: ▶Headache, ▶Oedema

General Practice at a Glance, First Edition. Paul Booton, Carol Cooper, Graham Easton, and Margaret Harper.

70 © 2013 Paul Booton, Carol Cooper, Graham Easton, and Margaret Harper. Published 2013 by Blackwell Publishing Ltd.

Common minor symptoms

Pregnancy can cause a variety of complaints. A woman may feel frustrated when these are dismissed as 'minor'. Reassurance and self-help are key to dealing with many of these symptoms (see Figure 31). Many women find it useful to hear that symptoms such as morning sickness and breast tenderness are worse when the pregnancy is doing well.

More serious problems

Hypertensive disorders of pregnancy include **gestational hypertension** and **pre-eclampsia**. Gestational hypertension complicates up to 15% of pregnancies. Pre-eclampsia is a multi-system disorder that comes on after 20 weeks (usually 3rd trimester). It affects 5–10% of pregnancies and is severe in around 2%. **In the UK, pre-eclampsia kills around 1000 babies a year, and about 10 women.**

Some women are more prone to it: those over 40, in their first pregnancy, expecting twins or more, or with a previous/family history of pre-eclampsia.

Assessment early in pregnancy aims to spot women at higher risk so they can have more frequent fetal monitoring. **Even so, it is impossible to predict who will develop it, so you should have a high level of awareness and know what to do.**

Refer her to hospital without delay for any of these:
- Diastolic BP is ≥90 mmHg, or systolic BP is ≥160 mmHg
- Urine shows 2+ protein or more.

While there are usually no symptoms, these are very significant and should also trigger immediate referral:
- Severe headache with or without vomiting
- Visual problems such as blurred vision or flashing lights
- Epigastric pain (usually severe pain just below the ribs, not heartburn)
- Sudden swelling of the face, hands or feet
- Signs of fetal compromise such as reduced fetal movements or a small-for-gestational-age fetus. You may have a local protocol.

Never delay action for suspected pre-eclampsia. It can develop quickly, becoming lethal to mother and baby within 2 weeks.

Gestational diabetes

Gestational diabetes (GDM) occurs in 2–5% pregnancies. It is often asymptomatic but can increase perinatal mortality. Some women should be offered screening in pregnancy:
- Those with BMI >30
- Previous baby weighing 4.5 kg or more
- Previous GDM
- A first degree relative with diabetes
- Family origin with a high prevalence of diabetes (South Asian, black Caribbean, Middle Eastern).

GDM can often be treated by diet and exercise, but up to 20% need insulin or glibenclamide (avoid other sulfonylureas).

Multiple pregnancy

While twins are common at 1 per 65 maternities, most receive specialist care. But you should know that minor symptoms are often worse, and serious complications more common, especially:
- Pre-eclampsia
- Bleeding (including post-partum haemorrhage)
- Premature labour
- Malpresentation
- Cord prolapse
- Fetal distress
- Twin-to-twin transfusion syndrome.

Over half of all twins are delivered by caesarean. The women you see in primary care may need help to appreciate the hazards of carrying multiples.

Medical disorders in pregnancy

Pre-existing conditions are common as the average age of first pregnancy is rising. Always mention these in your antenatal referral.

Thyroid disease

Both oestrogen and human chorionic gonadotrophin (hCG) affect thyroid hormones. **Hyperthyroidism** can present or relapse in the first trimester. Treating it is important for a woman and her baby.

In **hypothyroidism**, thyroxine needs can soar. Women with an underactive thyroid should have thyroid function tests as soon as they know they are pregnant, and every 6–8 weeks thereafter.

Hypertension

Chronic hypertension affects 1–5% of pregnancies and these women should have specialist care. ACE inhibitors and angiotensin-receptor blockers (ARBs) have been linked with intrauterine death, so they should be stopped within 2 days of diagnosing the pregnancy and other treatments used. Target BP in pregnancy for those with existing (not pregnancy-related) hypertension is under 150/100 mmHg (or 140/90 mmHg if target organ damage).

Asthma

Asthma can be serious for the developing fetus if it is poorly controlled. However, most pregnant women with asthma have few problems (although their condition may worsen after delivery). Preventing attacks is important, and inhaled bronchodilatators and steroids appear safe to use throughout pregnancy.

Epilepsy

While many women have fewer fits in pregnancy, about one-third have more. Every year, about four women die in the UK.

Most babies are fortunately unaffected but it's still desirable to minimise fits. If the woman already attends a neurology clinic, bring forward her appointment, especially if her fits are poorly controlled.

Pre-existing diabetes

Refer the woman as early as you can to the joint diabetes and antenatal clinic. If possible, the aim is a fasting blood glucose below 5.9 mmol/L and 1-hour post-prandial blood glucose below 7.8 mmol/L.

Pregnant women can take metformin, but ideally all other oral hypoglycaemic agents should be stopped before she conceives, and if necessary she should go on to insulin.

Remember that hypo awareness can be poor in pregnancy, especially in the first trimester.

(a) Some of the differences between dementia and acute confusional state

Remember, the patient who has dementia can develop an acute confusional state

Features	Dementia	Acute confusional state (delirium)
Aetiology	• Alzheimer's (60)%, vascular (20%) • Dementia with Lewy bodies, fronto-temporal dementia, rarer causes like Huntington's, Creutzfeldt–Jakob disease (CJD), Parkinson's • Mixed pattern e.g. Alzheimer's plus vascular dementia	• Infection: Urinary tract infection, chest infection, meningitis • Anoxia-CCF, respiratory failure, carbon monoxide poisoning • Toxic: Medication – (tranquillisers, antidepressants, analgesia), alcohol and drug misuse. Alcohol withdrawal • Metabolic: Electrolyte imbalance, uraemia, glycaemia • Intracranial: subdural, vascular, tumour • Other causes: surgery, nutritional e.g. B12 deficiency, thyroid
Onset	• Gradual over months or years	• Acute or sub-acute
Consciousness	• Normal	• Altered, typically fluctuating and associated with poor attention and sleep disturbance
Thought content	• Impoverished	• Disorganised – flights of ideas, may be frightened, agitated or aggressive
Speech	• Normal with a good social conversation until later stages when deteriorates. Maybe language problems such as aphasia	• Confused, rambling and incoherent
Memory	• Impaired	• Impaired
Neurological signs	• Usually none unless vascular dementia, Parkinson's/Lewy body dementia	• Common e.g. unsteady gait or tremor
Attention	• Normal until late stage	• Poor attention
Perception	• Normal until late stage	• May have hallucinations and delusions
Motor	• Normal until late	• Hyper or hypoactive
Autonomic features	• Only in later stages	• May be present with agitation , sweating, tachycardia
Physical features	• None but look for risk factors – see below	• May be signs of acute medical cause
Differential diagnosis	• Normal ageing, depression, acute confusional state or a sub-acute presentation of any of the organic causes of delirium e.g. subdural or anoxia	• Depression, dementia, bipolar disorder, psychosis
Risk factors	• Non-modifiable – age, sex, genetic • Modifiable – smoking, alcohol, social stimulation and physical activity. Vascular dementia – hypertension, cardiovascular disease, diabetes, obesity	• Dementia, age, male, surgery or major illness
Prognosis	• Progressive deterioration with premature death	• Depends on underlying cause. May be full recovery but carries a high mortality

(b) Management in General Practice

Dementia

- **Early referral** to psychogeriatric unit. Discuss the diagnosis and management plan with the patient and carer. Give support and information
- **Treat factors** that may improve or slow the progression e.g. vascular dementia – smoking, diabetes, hypertension and cardiovascular disease
- **Look after** the physical health – health promotion, immunisations, smoking and alcohol advice. Monitor hypertension and lipids in vascular dementia
- **Look for** and treat physical illness
- **Management of complex behaviour** like aggression, wandering, restlessness, incontinence and poor mobility – liaise with community team
- **Shared care** with the community team ensuring there is a good pathway in place for communication between the professionals (the patient may not be able to remember or to pass on information)
- **Day centre** attendance stimulates the patient in a safe environment and gives carers a break
- **Regular review** if there is significant deterioration and the patient is at risk residential care may become necessary
- **Drug treatment** (secondary care) – cholinesterase inhibitor in some cases. Use of anti-psychotic drugs to treat aggression carries a potential high risk of strokes and is not recommended (NICE) in most cases

Acute Confusional State

- **Management** depends on the cause
- **Treat** underlying cause e.g. UTI – if no response, the diagnosis is in doubt, you suspect serious illness or the patient is too difficult to manage at home refer to secondary care
- **Assess safety** of the patient to remain at home – any doubts admit to hospital
- **Assess social situation** – do they live alone?
- **Give advice** to the carer on how to manage – e.g. clear communication with the patient, to try and avoid conflict, help with orientation, time and place. Distract if they tend to wander. Look after nutrition. Try and anticipate physical needs – cold/too warm or need the toilet

General Practice at a Glance, First Edition. Paul Booton, Carol Cooper, Graham Easton, and Margaret Harper.

72 © 2013 Paul Booton, Carol Cooper, Graham Easton, and Margaret Harper. Published 2013 by Blackwell Publishing Ltd.

The elderly population is increasing and with it the incidence of dementia, posing an enormous challenge to primary care, psychiatry and social services. At 75 years 5.9% of elderly people have dementia, rising to 20.3% at 85 years.

Dementia. A patient with dementia has a progressive irreversible global deterioration in cognitive ability, including memory loss, personality changes, deterioration in language, problem-solving and social and personal functioning. The most common dementias are Alzheimer's disease and vascular dementia.

Acute confusional state can be difficult to distinguish from dementia, and the two can coexist. Acute confusional state is caused by an underlying medical cause which is usually reversible. Typical features are an acute or semi-acute onset and fluctuating course.

Your key aims are to:
• Make a diagnosis and differentiate between treatable and non-treatable cognitive decline
• Refer promptly to secondary care when appropriate
• Make sure that patients who have mental capacity are given the same rights of determining their management plan as anyone else
• Look after the patient's physical problems
• Take part in shared care.

Patients may refer themselves to the GP or be brought by a partner or carer. Always take a presentation of dementia seriously **especially in the early stages as these are patients who benefit most from intervention.**

Clinical presentation of dementia
• Memory loss – short or long term
• Language problems (e.g. aphasia)
• Deterioration in problem-solving, orientation, concentration and judgement
• Gradual loss of daily living skills
• Behaviour problems (e.g. aggression). **Depression is common in dementia** but remember that depression alone can present with features of dementia.

Clinical presentation of acute confusional state
• Acute or subacute onset
• Fluctuating course
• Disordered thought, memory impairment, agitation
• Maybe hallucinations and delusions
• Underlying medical cause.

History
You need to take a careful history which, along with the examination, will help you distinguish between the progressive dementias and acute confusional states.

You may have to rely on a carer for the history, **but always involve the patient as well,** giving them time and building a rapport.
• Ask about the onset. Has it been gradual or relatively quick?
• What was the patient like before? In a patient with previous high level of functioning it may be difficult to spot early signs of dementia.
• Ask about any drugs or medications – including OTC drugs, alcohol and recreational drugs.
• Enquire about any recent head injury, signs of infection (e.g. chest infection or UTI). Infections may be asymptomatic in the elderly, presenting only with confusion, or they may be responsible for increasing confusion in a patient who already has dementia.
• Are there any mood changes? **Remember depression.**
• Establish whether the confusion fluctuates from day to day, is worse at night or if there is any alteration in level of consciousness.
• Ask specific questions about short and long-term memory, understanding, grasp of language and judgement. Has their personality changed? If so how?
• In suspected dementia ask about everyday tasks. Are they able to dress, manage their hygiene, go shopping and cook? Have these altered? Ask about safety issues. Typically, they start a task and forget it (e.g. burning food because they forget to turn the gas off, wandering and find it difficult to get home). Ask about medication. Are they able to manage it themselves, if not who does?
• Take a careful medical history, particularly of any previous episode of confusion, or any deterioration in vision or hearing. Ask about family history of dementia.
• Ask about the social situation and any support for the patient or family.

Examination
To rule out a treatable cause, carry out a careful physical examination looking for any undiagnosed infection, thyroid disease, neurological abnormality or signs of vascular disease or injury.

Investigations
It is important to eliminate any treatable causes. Send an MSU. Request FBC, ESR or CRP, TFTs, LFTs, calcium, U&E, B12, folate and glucose. Consider chest X-ray.

There are a number of tests for cognitive ability. The most used one in primary care is the Mini Mental State Examination (MMSE). This accesses short and long-term memory loss, language ability and visuo-spacial and construction abilities. As a guide, 25/30 or more is considered a normal score (depending on their previous ability). The tests are useful if performed early as they provide a base to compare progress.

When administering these tests make sure that the patient feels comfortable and you establish a good rapport. Avoid interruptions. Make sure that the patient can hear and let them have enough time. If the patient wishes the partner or carer can stay, but tell them not to give any clues as to the answers.

Management
If you diagnose dementia, refer the patient to secondary care to a memory clinic or psychogeriatric department to confirm the diagnosis, for further investigations (MRI/CT scan to establish the diagnosis, type of dementia and exclude other pathology) and to form a management plan.

If you suspect acute confusional state, treat any obvious cause. Refer to secondary care if the diagnosis is more complex or the patient does not respond to treatment.

Long-term management of dementia
The aim is to keep the patient at home if possible. This involves balancing any risks between the patient's safety and quality of life.

The psychogeriatric team initiate community care plans, tailoring them to the patient's needs. The team includes a psychogeriatrician, a community psychiatric nurse (CPN), an occupational therapist and a social worker, plus the carers.

Fits, faints, falls and funny turns

Table 33.1 Key differences between fits and faints

Fits	Faints
In the (uncommon) temporal lobe seizures an aura (often a smell or a memory) may precede a seizure	There is no aura, but there may be preceding light headedness, nausea and sweating
Unconsciousness normally of several minutes or longer	Unconsciousness is brief usually less than 20 secs (and often only a few seconds)
Patient initially goes stiff (tonic seizure) then after short period relaxes and develops rhythmic jerking (clonic seizure). Often one happens without the other	Tonic and clonic features absent, though children in particular may have erratic twitching and jerking during syncope
Incontinence is common	Incontinence may occur if patient faints whilst bladder full
Tongue biting may happen as part of clonic phase of fit	Patients may injure themselves in fainting so tongue biting could occasionally occur
Often confused on recovery, headache common, may take an hour or more to get back to normal, often feel very tired and may sleep following fit	Usually feels back to normal within 10 minutes of recovering consciousness

Assessing falls in the elderly

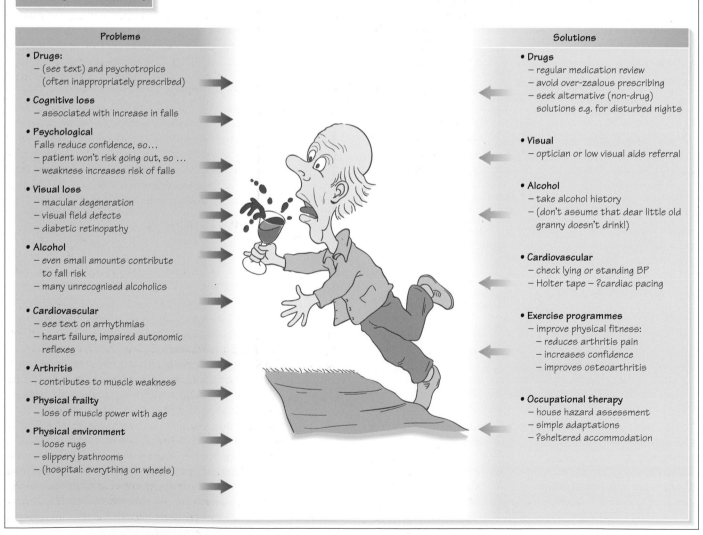

Problems

- **Drugs:**
  - (see text) and psychotropics (often inappropriately prescribed)
- **Cognitive loss**
  - associated with increase in falls
- **Psychological**
  Falls reduce confidence, so…
  - patient won't risk going out, so …
  - weakness increases risk of falls
- **Visual loss**
  - macular degeneration
  - visual field defects
  - diabetic retinopathy
- **Alcohol**
  - even small amounts contribute to fall risk
  - many unrecognised alcoholics
- **Cardiovascular**
  - see text on arrhythmias
  - heart failure, impaired autonomic reflexes
- **Arthritis**
  - contributes to muscle weakness
- **Physical frailty**
  - loss of muscle power with age
- **Physical environment**
  - loose rugs
  - slippery bathrooms
  - (hospital: everything on wheels)

Solutions

- **Drugs**
  - regular medication review
  - avoid over-zealous prescribing
  - seek alternative (non-drug) solutions e.g. for disturbed nights
- **Visual**
  - optician or low visual aids referral
- **Alcohol**
  - take alcohol history
  - (don't assume that dear little old granny doesn't drink!)
- **Cardiovascular**
  - check lying or standing BP
  - Holter tape – ?cardiac pacing
- **Exercise programmes**
  - improve physical fitness:
    - reduces arthritis pain
    - increases confidence
    - improves osteoarthritis
- **Occupational therapy**
  - house hazard assessment
  - simple adaptations
  - ?sheltered accommodation

General Practice at a Glance, First Edition. Paul Booton, Carol Cooper, Graham Easton, and Margaret Harper.

Blackouts and 'funny turns' present very commonly to general practice and can be confusing to sort out. This chapter is an overview of common presentations which will help you make sense of them. They are common and serious in the elderly, but all ages are considered in this chapter.

It is useful to think of these problems in three categories:
1 Blackouts, where there is loss of consciousness
2 True vertigo
3 Non-vertiginous dizziness.

Blackouts

Blackouts can mainly be subdivided into syncope and seizures, of which the former are common and the latter unusual in practice. The diagnosis relies on the history which is usually straightforward with a careful history from both patient and any witnesses. Table 33.1 compares the key features of each; differentiating fit from faint is an important first step in management.

Syncope

Syncope has a multitude of causes which may be difficult to disentangle. In children and young people it is common and usually vasovagal in origin, provoked by intercurrent infection, standing up suddenly and emotions (the first visit to the operating theatre for some medics). An accurate diagnosis needs to be made, particularly for those children who twitch when they faint and who are at risk of a misdiagnosis of epilepsy. In elderly people blackouts are common and have a multitude of causes. Although benign in themselves, the injuries they cause can be fatal (e.g. fractured hip, head injuries). A good history from both patient and witnesses is crucial. It is important, particularly in elderly people, to find out whether there was a blackout (unconsciousness) or a conscious fall – this can be surprisingly hard to tease out.

The more common causes can be grouped together as:
• **Drug causes:** a huge problem in the elderly, antihypertensives, alpha-blockers (for prostatic hypertrophy), diuretics, drugs causing arrhythmias or significant bradycardia (e.g. digoxin, beta-blockers), sulfonylureas and other hypoglycaemic agents – this is a small selection. Always ask yourself 'Could this be drug related?' Review the medication list and avoid overzealous treatment.
• **Cardiac causes:** e.g. paroxysmal arrhythmias (both fast and slow), sick sinus syndrome, episodic heart block. These can be difficult to pin down as patients can go for long periods without symptoms. A Holter (24-hour ECG) tape is useful – 12-lead ECGs generally aren't. Valvular disease such as aortic stenosis is rare.
• **Vascular causes:** postural hypotension is important in the elderly – drugs are again a major cause but also carotid hypersensitivity is common, autonomic neuropathies in diabetics and hypovolaemia acutely from illness and chronically from sodium-wasting renal lesions and diuretics. Postural hypotension can be also be induced by exercise and eating.

Seizures

Most epilepsy starts in childhood and is idiopathic. It is common in people with learning difficulties. A second peak occurs in patients over 60 years when a structural lesion is more likely. Causes of epilepsy in adults include cerebrovascular disease (e.g. infarction or haemorrhage), degenerative disease (e.g. Alzheimer's), head injury (e.g. road traffic accidents), metabolic causes (e.g. hypoglycaemia, uraemia, hypocalcaemia and hypercalcaemia), drugs (e.g. phenothiazines, but most importantly alcohol and in

particular alcohol withdrawal which precipitates seizures). Brain tumours, most of which will be secondary, are also an important cause.

Diagnosis of seizure can only be made from the history: carefully interview the patient and any witnesses. Table 33.1 indicates the key features that differentiate it from other blackouts. EEGs provide confirmation in some childhood epilepsies and scans can show structural lesions, but diagnosis rests on the history.

A patient with a first seizure should be referred for neurological assessment as the diagnosis has significant implications for life. The patient should be advised not to drive while investigations are pending and to be careful in situations that could put them at risk (e.g. swimming, using machinery). A formal diagnosis of epilepsy is not made until two episodes have occurred. Therapy is usually initiated by the specialist, but the GP should be aware that some anti-epileptic drugs induce liver enzymes that reduce contraceptive pill efficacy, the dose of which will need to be increased to maintain effectiveness. In pregnancy, anti-epileptic medication is associated with teratogenicity so try to simplify and reduce medication, but not at expense of seizure control.

Vertigo

True vertigo is uncommon: many patients use the term for dizziness of one sort or another so it is important to clarify that it is a true rotational sensation. Ask about falls (or having to hold on to something to stop falling) and nausea and vomiting. The most common cause in practice is **acute vestibular neuronitis**, which starts with a sudden vertigo and then settles over about 3 or 4 days. It is presumed of viral origin. Advise your patient not to drive or use machinery until symptoms settle. Vestibular sedatives may be useful in severe attacks. **Benign positional vertigo,** common in women and in middle age and over, presents with intermittent episodes of vertigo, usually worse on rising from bed in the mornings, and with changes in position during the day. Attacks last a few minutes, patients often having a bad spell over several weeks then a period of remission. Other causes: **migraine** can produce vertigo (and vaguer dizziness); **Ménière's disease** (uncommon and over-diagnosed) is associated with tinnitus and deafness.

Non-vertiginous dizziness

This is a problem area for GPs. Many patients complain of poorly described muzziness or dizziness. A large proportion of these will be psychosomatic (see Chapter 63) although remember that psychosomatic illness produces real physical symptoms (e.g. hyperventilation causing dizziness via respiratory alkalosis). The key to the diagnosis is a careful history that relates physical symptoms to psychological stressors. In elderly patients, any of the items listed under syncope can cause dizziness instead of or in addition to syncope. Other common causes include acute viral illness and migraine. Serious physical illnesses such as pneumonia and heart attacks sometimes present with non-specific 'dizziness' symptoms – in the latter, diabetic patients (with autonomic damage) may develop 'silent' MIs, without pain, but with a general feeling of wretchedness. Intermittent vertebrobasilar ischaemia, where the vertebral arterial flow is compromised as a result of atheroma and/or vertebral spondylosis (and precipitated by movements like bending down to look into a cupboard) can cause dizziness, blackouts, vertigo and drop attacks. Diagnosis relies on careful history-taking and examination, sometimes repeated after a few weeks when symptoms may have progressed.

Table 34.1 Features suggesting cardiac ischaemia (SOCRATES)

	Possible questions to ask	Patient history which may suggest ischaemic heart disease
Site	Where is the pain?	Often central, retrosternal (If continually moving site, less likely to be cardiac)
Onset	When did the pain start, and was it sudden or gradual?	Often starts slowly and gets worse with time
Character	What is the pain like? How would you describe it?	Often described as tight, squeezing, crushing or constricting
Radiation	Does the pain go anywhere else?	May radiate to left arm and/or throat or jaw
Associations	Any other signs or symptoms associated with the pain?	Nausea/vomiting, sweating, dizziness, palpitations breathlessness, syncope
Time course	Does the pain follow any pattern?	Often lasts >15 minutes (Less than 30 seconds duration suggests non-cardiac cause)
Exacerbating/ relieving factors	Does anything make the pain better or worse?	Worsened by exertion (and sometimes emotion) Relieved by rest or GTN (glyceryl trinitrate) within a few minutes
Severity	How bad is the pain? (Scale of 1–10)	Often severe (8–10)

Table 34.2 Examples of features suggesting non-ischaemic cause of chest pain

Pericarditis	Sharp, stabbing. Worse lying down, better when sitting up or leaning forwards. Tends to be worse on inspiration or coughing
Oesophageal reflux	Tends to be a burning sensation, rising up from stomach or lower chest. May be related to food, lying down, stooping or straining. Relieved by antacids
Tietze's syndrome (or costochondritis)	Pain aggravated by physical activity or movement, coughing or sneezing. Tender on palpation. Swelling of costochondral joint in Tietze's syndrome
Aortic dissection	Chest or back pain, often starts suddenly, and described as severe and 'sharp', 'ripping' or 'tearing' in nature
Pleuritic pain (e.g. viral respiratory tract infection, pneumonia, pulmonary embolus, pneumothorax)	Usually sharp, stabbing pain worse on inspiration or coughing. Breathlessness, cough, or haemoptysis
Panic attack	Over-breathing, numbness/tingling in fingers or round mouth. Can also include palpitations, nausea, sweating, dizziness. (NB similarity with ischaemic pain associated symptoms)

(a) Causes of chest pain

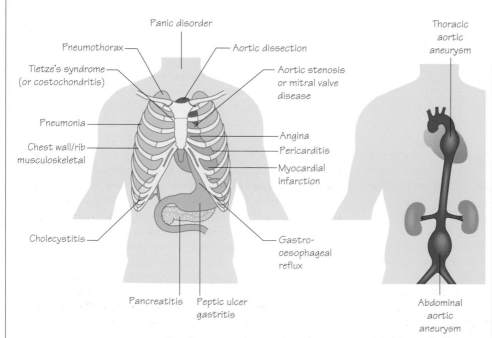

Panic disorder
Pneumothorax
Aortic dissection
Tietze's syndrome (or costochondritis)
Aortic stenosis or mitral valve disease
Pneumonia
Chest wall/rib musculoskeletal
Angina
Pericarditis
Myocardial infarction
Cholecystitis
Gastro-oesophageal reflux
Pancreatitis
Peptic ulcer gastritis

(b) Aortic aneurysm

Thoracic aortic aneurysm

Abdominal aortic aneurysm

- Dilatation of the aorta
- 6% men and 2% women over 65 have abdominal aortic aneurysm (AAA)
- 8000 die every year of ruptured aortic aneurysm in UK
- Risk factors: men and women >60 years old; smoking, diabetes, hyperlipidaemia, obesity, hypertension
- Close family history
- Unruptured: often no symptoms, possibly mild abdominal, back or chest pain
- Ruptured: usually fatal. Sudden, severe chest, abdominal back or groin pain, and collapse
- Screening programme for AAA introduced in 2009 in England, offering ultrasound scans to all men over 64 years old
- An abdominal aortic aneurysm <50 mm wide has a low chance of rupture
- Operation to repair the aneurysm may be advised if >50 mm as above this size the risk of rupture increases
- Open repair with graft is a major operation, carries significant risk of mortality
- Newer approach, endovascular repair, considered safer

Chest pain is common in general practice (about 1.5% of all presentations), and can make both patients and doctors feel anxious. The priority for the GP is not to miss any life-threatening causes, such as MI. Only about 8% of all the chest pain that a GP sees is caused by cardiac disease. Most chest pain in general practice has a more benign origin, such as musculoskeletal problems, gastro-oesophageal reflux or panic disorder (see Figure 34a). The key to managing chest pain lies in taking a careful history. So, unless the patient is acutely unwell, take your time getting the story straight.

Taking a history

• Start with open questions to let the patient describe the pain in their own words ('Tell me more about this chest pain you've been getting').
• Encourage the patient to open up more ('And was there anything else about it . . .?').
• Find out if they have any particular ideas or worries about the pain.
• Use more direct questioning later, to establish whether the patient has any features of cardiac ischaemia. You could use a mnemonic such as SOCRATES to remember what to ask (see Table 34.1).
• Does the patient have a **past history** of a heart attack or a stroke or any clotting disorders?
• Is there any **family history** of cardiovascular disease?
• Any patient with chest pain should also be asked about the **risk factors for cardiovascular disease**: smoking, diabetes, hypertension, hyperlipidaemia, obesity, lack of exercise and stress.
• The patient's **medication** may give you a clue as to their medical problems. Patients often forget to mention they have hypertension, but may be able to tell you that they take a daily ACE inhibitor.
• Differentiate stable from unstable angina. Stable angina is reliably provoked by (for instance) climbing two flights of stairs. Unstable angina comes without apparent provocation and requires urgent hospital assessment.

Examination

The history alone should give you a clear idea about what is causing the patient's pain but however confident you feel (and however rushed), a careful cardiovascular examination is essential. You don't want to miss, for example, aortic stenosis (which can cause angina) or the signs of heart failure. In particular, check:
• Pulse (rate and rhythm) and blood pressure (ideally both arms)
• Auscultate the heart and examine the lungs
• Check for peripheral oedema and a raised jugular venous pulse (JVP).

The examination is also helpful for pinpointing non-cardiac causes of chest pain. In Tietze's syndrome or costochondritis you may find localised tenderness of the chest wall. In peptic ulcer disease there may be epigastric tenderness and, if the pain is pleuritic, you may pick up a pleural rub or other focal lung signs.

Investigations

The following investigations may be helpful in general practice:

ECG: may show ischaemia, pericarditis or pulmonary embolism. (But remember; a normal resting ECG doesn't rule out ischaemia or even an infarct: they are normal in more than 90% of patients with recent angina. If you think the patient needs an urgent ECG, consider sending them to hospital.)

Blood tests: FBC (exclude anaemia, and high white cell count possible in pneumonia); fasting lipids and glucose.

Chest X-ray: to pick up, for example, chest infection, pneumothorax, enlarged heart, fractured rib or aortic aneurysm.

Other tests: these may be required to exclude non-cardiac causes: ultrasound abdomen (gallstones); upper gastrointestinal endoscopy (peptic ulcer or oesophagitis); serum amylase (pancreatitis).

Further tests (in hospital): troponin I or T; exercise ECG (to confirm cardiac ischaemia); coronary angiography; ventilation/perfusion scan (to exclude pulmonary infarction); echocardiography.

Management

Most patients presenting with chest pains in primary care do not have serious pathology. However, they are often very frightened that they do. Eliciting the patient's ideas and concerns (fears) about what this pain represents will allow you to reassure them about their specific fears in most cases. For many patients this is all they will require of their doctor. Others will need a plan to investigate their symptoms further before offering treatment.

Patients in whom ischaemic chest pain is high on the list of differential diagnoses are often referred to the local **rapid access chest pain clinic** for further assessment. For the minority who are **acutely unwell or are currently having chest pain**, get help from surgery staff and arrange for a 999 ambulance for rapid admission to hospital. The patient may need oxygen via a face mask, pain relief (usually opioids) and an anti-emetic. Give any specific treatments according to diagnosis (e.g. 300 mg aspirin chewed or dispersed in water for MI if no contraindications).

Acute attacks of stable angina are managed with glyceryl trinitrate (as spray or sublingual tablets). Patients having more than two attacks a week need regular drug therapy, usually with a beta-blocker. If beta-blockers are not tolerated or are contraindicated, a long-acting nitrate or suitable calcium-channel blocker can be used.

In patients who do not have cardiac chest pain, but are given no clear diagnosis, the GP's job can be challenging. Gastro-oesophageal reflux is a common cause of non-cardiac chest pain; some suggest trying a course of a proton pump inhibitor (PPI) or arranging endoscopy. A chest X-ray is important if you suspect a chest infection or pneumothorax for example, and management will depend on the findings. Psychological therapies can be very helpful for panic disorder, but discussions with patients need to be handled sensitively. Costochondritis or other musculoskeletal causes tend to resolve with time and possibly anti-inflammatory medication.

GPs often have to deal with the uncertainty of caring for patients with undiagnosed chest pain while investigations are underway. For both doctor and patient, safety netting (telling the patient when to return to the surgery or to seek urgent help) is a crucial part of dealing with this uncertainty.

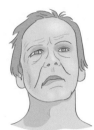

The Face, Arm, Speech Test (FAST)

Face: has the face fallen on one side?

Arms: can they raise both arms and keep them up?

Speech: is speech slurred?

Time to call 999 if you see any one of these signs

(Source: ABC of Stroke, Edited by Jonathan Mant and Marion F Walker. 2011. Wiley-Blackwell)

Every 5 minutes someone in the UK has a stroke. It's the biggest cause of adult neurological disability in industrialised countries, and it accounts for about 11% of all deaths.

Role of the GP

The GP must make a rapid diagnosis and assessment of the patient who may have had a stroke or transient ischaemic attack (TIA) (features similar to stroke but lasting less than 24 hours), and make sure they receive timely referral and treatment. The GP also has a crucial role in **preventing** strokes, and in supporting the patient and coordinating care during **rehabilitation**. GP activity in preventing strokes focuses on smoking cessation advice, screening for atrial fibrillation, BP checks and monitoring, cholesterol control, weight loss and encouraging physical activity, and monitoring co-morbidities (e.g. diabetes) (for more details on preventing cardio-vascular problems see Chapter 37).

History

As well as the familiar symptoms of rapid onset of unilateral weakness, speech or vision problems, patients may also present with severe headache, confusion, loss of consciousness or vomiting. Ask about:
• **Risk factors** for stroke, including previous strokes or TIAs, atrial fibrillation, ischaemic heart disease, diabetes, hypertension and smoking.
• **Medications**, including whether the patient is on aspirin or warfarin.
• There are many conditions that mimic strokes; bear in mind for example CNS tumours, facial palsies, hypoglycaemia.

Examination

The examination should pay particular attention to:
• Level of consciousness
• Neurological signs (including incontinence and dysphagia)
• Blood pressure, heart rate and rhythm
• Carotid bruits and heart murmurs
• Other systemic signs of infection or neoplasm.
 In people with sudden onset of neurological symptoms outside hospital, a validated tool such as FAST (Face, Arm, Speech Test) can be used as a quick screen to diagnose stroke (Figure 35).

Acute management of stroke and TIA

If a **stroke** is suspected the patient should be referred immediately by ambulance to a hospital with an acute stroke unit. Early thrombolysis in a specialist unit reduces mortality and morbidity.

 If a **TIA** is suspected, assess carefully the risk of the patient going on to have a stroke. The ABCD2 risk scoring system can be used which assesses the patient's age, BP, clinical features, duration and whether or not they have diabetes. High risk patients should be assessed at a TIA clinic within 24 hours of first presentation to a healthcare professional. Low risk patients should be assessed at a TIA clinic within 7 days. Patients are usually started on aspirin (unless already on warfarin).

After a stroke

The GP has an important role in supporting the patient and their family and carers after a stroke. Secondary prevention involves lifestyle advice including smoking, monitoring risk factors such as BP and diabetes, atrial fibrillation (should the patient be on warfarin?), use of antiplatelet medication for secondary prevention and considering carotid endarterectomy for significant carotid stenosis. GPs provide information and support, help with psychosocial issues (screen for depression in both patients and carers) and help with disabilities.

Rehabilitation

Up to half of people who have a stroke are left with some sort of disability. Rehabilitation starts in hospital but outside hospital many different types of health professionals may be involved, and the GP can help to coordinate care:
• **Physiotherapist:** helps to regain mobility and muscle control.
• **Occupational therapist:** can use range of techniques to help with basic everyday living tasks such as washing, dressing, eating or going up stairs. Helps with physical and mental skills.
• **Speech and language therapist:** helps with swallowing, speech, reading, writing and understanding words.
• **Continence adviser:** helps with bowel or bladder problems.
• **Clinical psychologist:** helps with anxiety, depression, memory problems or cognition.
• **Stroke clubs:** social support from other stroke patients.

(a) **Leg ulcers** are very common, particularly in older patients. Try to distinguish between venous and arterial ulcers as management is different (although they may coexist in the same patient).

	Arterial	Venous
History	• Cardiovascular disease, diabetes, obesity, immobility	• Varicose veins, DVT, phlebitis
Appearance	• 'Punched out', deeper	• Shallow, large, oozing
Position	• More distal, dorsum of foot, heel or toes • Sometimes shin	• Anywhere between mid-calf and malleoli
Pain	• Painful, worse at night, relieved by hanging leg over edge of bed	• Usually mild
Associated features	• Ischaemia features: pale, cold, hairless, nail dystrophy, absent pulses	• Varicose eczema, hyperpigmentation of surrounding skin
Investigation	• Ankle-Brachial Pressure Index (ABPI) duplex scan • Exclude diabetes • Angiography if revascularisation considered • Wound swabs only if suspect active infection	• Ankle-Brachial Pressure Index (ABPI) duplex scan • Exclude diabetes • Wound swabs only if suspect active infection
Management	• As for peripheral vascular disease	• Graduated compression bandaging (once established ABPIs) • Debridement • Antibiotics only if infection • Topical steroids for varicose eczema

(b) **The most common sites for venous ulceration** are above the medial or lateral malleolus

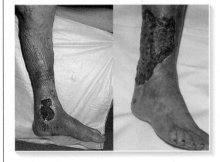

(c) **A hand-held Doppler** being used to measure the ankle-brachial pressure index

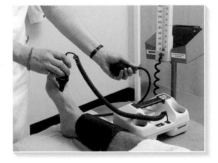

(d) **Multilayer elastic compression bandaging**

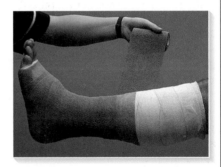

People with **peripheral vascular disease** have increased risk of MI, stroke and mortality. So, although a patient may present with an acute problem such as lower limb pain, leg ulcers or gangrene, the GP must also address the patient's overall cardiovascular risk.

History

Typically:

1 Intermittent claudication: leg or buttock pain on walking, disappears when still, often worse in one leg

2 Ischaemic rest pain: severe, constant pain in foot, usually worse at night, sometimes relieved by hanging leg over side of bed.

Ask about medications (e.g. beta-blockers), cardiovascular risk factors (e.g. smoking, diabetes) and history of cardiovascular disease or erectile dysfunction.

Consider other causes of leg pain, including sciatica, spinal stenosis or musculoskeletal injury.

Examination

Full cardiovascular examination including pulses and abdomen for aortic aneurysm is essential. Key findings:

• Weak or absent pulses in lower limb
• Leg pale, cold and there is often loss of hair
• In severe disease ulcers or gangrene on leg or foot.

Investigations

Full cardiovascular risk assessment including blood pressure, FBC (anaemia), fasting glucose and lipids, ESR (exclude inflammatory vasculitis), ECG and Doppler ultrasound (duplex scan) to measure Ankle–Brachial Pressure Index (ABPI). (This is the ratio of systolic BP at ankle and arm and gives a measure of blood flow at the ankle.)

Management

Most patients' symptoms improve with medical treatment and by modification of lifestyle factors, such as stopping smoking, regular exercise (even if some pain as improves collateral circulation), weight loss, control of diabetes, hypertension and cholesterol, antiplatelet therapy, and possible use of peripheral vasodilators (e.g. naftidrofuryl). Refer to secondary care if severe or diagnosis unclear.

General Practice at a Glance, First Edition. Paul Booton, Carol Cooper, Graham Easton, and Margaret Harper.
© 2013 Paul Booton, Carol Cooper, Graham Easton, and Margaret Harper. Published 2013 by Blackwell Publishing Ltd.

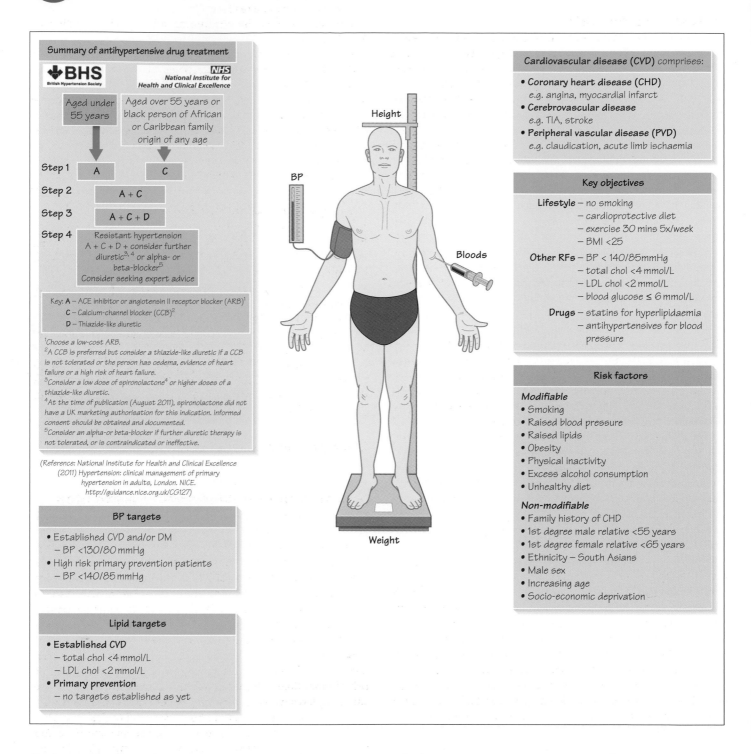

Summary of antihypertensive drug treatment

BHS British Hypertension Society

NHS National Institute for Health and Clinical Excellence

Aged under 55 years

Aged over 55 years or black person of African or Caribbean family origin of any age

Step 1   A   C

Step 2   A + C

Step 3   A + C + D

Step 4   Resistant hypertension A + C + D + consider further diuretic[3, 4] or alpha- or beta-blocker[5] Consider seeking expert advice

Key: **A** – ACE inhibitor or angiotensin II receptor blocker (ARB)[1]
C – Calcium-channel blocker (CCB)[2]
D – Thiazide-like diuretic

[1]Choose a low-cost ARB.
[2]A CCB is preferred but consider a thiazide-like diuretic if a CCB is not tolerated or the person has oedema, evidence of heart failure or a high risk of heart failure.
[3]Consider a low dose of spironolactone[4] or higher doses of a thiazide-like diuretic.
[4]At the time of publication (August 2011), spironolactone did not have a UK marketing authorisation for this indication. Informed consent should be obtained and documented.
[5]Consider an alpha-or beta-blocker if further diuretic therapy is not tolerated, or is contraindicated or ineffective.

(Reference: National Institute for Health and Clinical Excellence (2011) Hypertension: clinical management of primary hypertension in adults, London. NICE. http://guidance.nice.org.uk/CG127)

BP targets

- Established CVD and/or DM
  – BP <130/80 mmHg
- High risk primary prevention patients
  – BP <140/85 mmHg

Lipid targets

- **Established CVD**
  – total chol <4 mmol/L
  – LDL chol <2 mmol/L
- **Primary prevention**
  – no targets established as yet

Height

BP

Bloods

Weight

Cardiovascular disease (CVD) comprises:

- **Coronary heart disease (CHD)**
  e.g. angina, myocardial infarct
- **Cerebrovascular disease**
  e.g. TIA, stroke
- **Peripheral vascular disease (PVD)**
  e.g. claudication, acute limb ischaemia

Key objectives

Lifestyle – no smoking
– cardioprotective diet
– exercise 30 mins 5x/week
– BMI <25

Other RFs – BP < 140/85mmHg
– total chol <4 mmol/L
– LDL chol <2 mmol/L
– blood glucose ≤ 6 mmol/L

Drugs – statins for hyperlipidaemia
– antihypertensives for blood pressure

Risk factors

Modifiable
- Smoking
- Raised blood pressure
- Raised lipids
- Obesity
- Physical inactivity
- Excess alcohol consumption
- Unhealthy diet

Non-modifiable
- Family history of CHD
- 1st degree male relative <55 years
- 1st degree female relative <65 years
- Ethnicity – South Asians
- Male sex
- Increasing age
- Socio-economic deprivation

Cardiovascular disease (CVD) is the main cause of death in the UK, accounting for more than one in three deaths. It places a huge burden on the NHS, yet much of CVD is preventable. Patients rarely consult specifically on how to prevent heart disease and stroke, but promotion makes up a large part of a GP's work. Consultations for primary prevention of cardiovascular disease can be very rewarding. Done well, they offer a holistic approach to patient care, and make a real difference to patients.

An important part of this work is the **NHS Health Check**. This aims to prevent heart disease, stroke, diabetes and kidney disease by inviting people aged 40–74 for an assessment of their risk. The GP then calculates a 10-year cardiovascular risk, expressed as a percentage chance of developing disease in the next 10 years.

The consultation must balance the doctor's agenda and the patient's, especially if the patient is really there for something else. Consider how to approach the subject, for example: 'Did you

General Practice at a Glance, First Edition. Paul Booton, Carol Cooper, Graham Easton, and Margaret Harper.

know that we're offering a health check? Have you heard about this?'

Risk factors for CVD

Some risk factors matter more than others. Smoking far outweighs the other modifiable factors. If a patient has two or more risk factors, their total risk increases by more than the sum of each risk. Some coexisting conditions also increase the risk of CVD, such as diabetes type 1 or 2, chronic kidney disease, hypertension, hyperlipidaemia, rheumatoid arthritis and other autoimmune diseases.

In the surgery, primary prevention of CVD can be done by GPs, practice nurses or suitably trained healthcare assistants. Patients may also attend after health checks elsewhere such as a pharmacy, gym or the dentist. Even some supermarkets now offer health checks.

You need the following information for a full CVD risk assessment:
- **Lifestyle factors:** smoking, diet, physical activity, alcohol
- **Examination findings:** BP, BMI, waist circumference
- **Blood tests:** random or fasting glucose, fasting lipids (cholesterol, cholesterol:high density lipoprotein ratio).

Risk calculators

These rely on these data to calculate an individual's 10-year risk of developing CVD. Two of the most common risk calculators in use are QRISK2 and JBS2. The Joint British Societies have also produced risk prediction charts which are at the back of the British National Formulary (BNF). These are an easy-to-understand pictorial method for patients to visualise their risk. Having calculated the risk, you need to understand the implications for the patient, and be able to explain what a particular risk score means for that patient.
- 10-year CVD risk ≥20% is high risk and warrants active management of all risk factors, including drug therapies for hypertension and hyperlipidaemia
- 10-year CVD risk <20% involves encouraging patients to make healthy lifestyle choices.

Reducing risk

Some people can make huge reductions in their CVD risk with lifestyle changes such as stopping smoking, losing excess weight, doing regular exercise and taking up a heart-healthy diet (at least five portions per day of fresh fruit and vegetables, reduced intake of total and saturated fat, alcohol consumption up to ≤3 units/day for men and ≤2 units/day for women; see Figure 37).

Dietitians, exercise on referral and smoking cessation groups can all help. Discussing lifestyle changes and taking on board patients' preferences can be a great way of motivating people to make changes.

Management of hypertension

The latest recommendations from NICE advise carrying out 24-hour BP monitoring to make the diagnosis of hypertension. This is thought to overcome the effects of 'white coat' hypertension, where BP readings taken in the surgery are higher than the usual readings at home or elsewhere.

Consider 24-hour BP monitoring after a clinic reading of ≥140/90 mmHg.

Based on results from this, consider the following management:
- BP ≥ 150/95 mmHg → start treatment
- BP ≥ 135/85 mmHg:
  ○ Total CVD risk ≥20% or target organ damage or diabetes → start treatment
  ○ Total CVD risk <20% and no target organ damage and no diabetes → lifestyle advice and annual review
- BP <135/85 mmHg → normotensive

Note: if clinic reading ≥180/110 mmHg → start treatment

Management of hyperlipidaemia

Hyperlipidaemia means either raised total cholesterol, low density lipoprotein (LDL-C), triglycerides (TG) or combination of total cholesterol and TG. Exclude and treat secondary causes of hyperlipidaemia.
- If the patient already has established CVD or familial hyperlipidaemia → start treatment (usually statins)
- If total CVD risk ≥20% → start treatment
- If total CVD risk <20% → lifestyle advice, repeat CVD risk assessment within 5 years.

For both hypertension and hyperlipidaemia there are easy to follow guidelines from NICE. The GP surgery may have also produced local guidance for best practice including specific medications and doses.

Management of raised glucose

See Chapter 41.

How to talk to patients about prevention

It can be hard to persuade patients to take medications (which may have side effects) in order to treat high blood pressure or cholesterol which are not causing them any symptoms at all. Ultimately, it is the patient's choice, but you have a duty to explain the pros and cons clearly. Make it clear that high blood pressure or high cholesterol are risk factors for disease, but are not strictly diseases in themselves. You need to talk about CVD in terms the patient is used to (e.g. 'heart attacks, strokes and blood circulation problems'). It is also worth finding out what the patient's experience of these conditions is: they may have a relative or friend who has been affected. Explain the patient's level of risk in clear terms (e.g. 'A risk of more than 20% means you have a greater than one in five chance of having a heart attack or a stroke in the next 10 years'). Check that the patient is clear about their level of risk, and what options are open to them to reduce it. Invite any questions and try, between you, to arrive at a shared management plan that the patient is happy with.

Assessing psychosomatic breathlessness

This can be clinically difficult to disentangle. The breathlessness is often ill-defined and may be perceived as a blockage in the throat or something pressing on the windpipe ('globus hystericus'). Look for possible stressors and try to relate attacks to these. Physical breathlessness is usually worse with exertion, psychosomatic breathlessness is often worse at rest and better on exertion (but so can asthma be). Try to relate the symptoms to anxiety-provoking situations. Palpitations are often part of anxiety – find out what the patient means and tap out the rhythm – a normal speed pounding in the chest suggests psychosomatic causes. Fast regular palpitations coming on out of the blue are more suggestive of a true arrhythmia, most commonly supraventricular tachycardia (SVT).

Managing psychosomatic breathlessness

- Some patients respond to simple explanation of the link between stress and physical symptoms. Others may refuse to accept their diagnosis is other than physical which can be a block to treatment and produce a difficult relationship between patient and physician. Try using the 'reattribution model' as a way of moving patients towards accepting a diagnosis and treatment (bottom right)
  - investigations have only a limited effect in reassuring the patient (one study showed a CT scan reassured headache patients for only 4 months), and may paradoxically confirm the patient's suspicion something serious is wrong ('the doctor wouldn't have done it unless he was worried')
  - referrals (like investigations) have little to offer unless for clear medical reasons. They complicate management, often result in an excess of investigations and confirm the patient's fears that something serious is going on
  - combined psychotherapy, relaxation therapy and physical therapy has the best results. If the patient will accept it, CBT may also be used

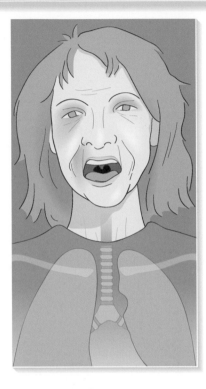

Panic attacks/panic disorder

- A very common problem in general practice
  - explain physiological basis of patient's symptoms 'fight and flight' hormone response etc 'vicious circle' of anxiety panic producing physical symptoms, producing more anxiety, worsening symptoms etc
  - CBT is the best long term approach to panic disorder, but patients may require short term support whilst new coping mechanisms are developing
  - support groups – such as Anxiety UK help patients come to terms with their symptoms and gain support from fellow sufferers
  - SSRIs (and as a second line tricyclics) are recognised as helping sufferers
  - beta blockers work by reducing the physical (adrenergic) symptoms of panic and can be useful, but are contraindicated in diabetes and asthma, and hypotension or other side effects may be problematic

The 'Reattribution Model'

- Make the patient feel understood
  - explore history thoroughly
  - explore emotional cues
  - explore social and family factors
  - explore health beliefs
  - focused physical examination (mainly to reassure patient)

- Broaden the agenda to include psychosocial explanations
  - feed back the results of the examination
  - acknowledge reality of symptoms
  - reframe the complaints in social and psychological terms
  - be realistic about therapeutic goals

- Make the link between psyche and soma
  - keep explanations simple
  - link to life events
  - focus on the 'here and now'
  - NB remember depression lowers the pain threshold
  - patient may only be able to accept depression caused **by** the physical problems – but this is a starting place to work from

Frequent attenders

- Patients with psychosomatic disorders are often frequent attenders in general practice and make considerable demands on practice staff. Managing demand is difficult but it helps to:
  - see the same doctor – coordinates care, avoids 'divide and rule' tactics
  - arrange to meet the patient regularly (more effective at controlling demand than patient making appointments)
  - avoid secondary referral – raises unrealistic expectations of a physical cure

General Practice at a Glance, First Edition. Paul Booton, Carol Cooper, Graham Easton, and Margaret Harper.

The sensation of breathlessness is common and causes range from physiological to psychological and physical pathology. It is frequently regarded with grave foreboding by patients but is also a vital symptom for doctors.

Sudden acute causes of breathlessness

While these are usually the most serious, they are the most straightforward to disentangle. They can be broken down into those more likely to present in younger or older ages.

Acute breathing difficulties at younger ages

• **Pneumothorax:** sharp unilateral pain and no history of respiratory problems (except in those with previous pneumothorax who will probably recognise their problem), typically tall thin young men (including the rare Marfan's syndrome).
• **Asthma:** usually a history of episodic breathlessness and/or nocturnal cough and waking, and past history of childhood 'chest troubles' (frequently wrongly or vaguely diagnosed as: 'wheezy bronchitis' or similar colloquialism) (see Chapter 40).
• **Pulmonary embolism:** actually more common in older patients but is one of relatively few common acute causes of breathlessness in younger people. History of immobilisation (e.g. inpatient, long haul flight, plaster cast), smoking and combined oral contraceptive pill users (risk from both increases with age). Associated with pain and haemoptysis.
• **Panic attacks:** common and debilitating. Unlike the above where urgent admission is essential, avoiding admission and de-medicalising are more helpful here. First episodes are more likely to be associated with psychological stressors, later episodes less so. Episodes often come out of a background of emotional stress with acute provocation (e.g. an argument, or agoraphobic or claustrophobic situations). Symptoms and anxiety are disproportionate to physical findings, which may be of erratic or deep sighing breathing. Oxygen saturation levels will be normal, peak flow is usually unrecordable (due to inability to cooperate). A past history of panic attacks is helpful in diagnosing the current episode, but do not assume the current attack is panic just because of the past history.

Acute breathing difficulties at older ages

All the above continue to present. Pneumothorax is more likely in those with emphysema. The pill and smoking dramatically raise the risk of pulmonary embolism with age.
• **Pneumonia:** the classic acute pneumococcal lobar pneumonia is relatively unusual nowadays, but pneumonia is common, often complicating an acute viral illness. Patients with pre-existing respiratory or other co-morbidities (e.g. diabetes, chronic obstructive pulmonary disease [COPD]) are more at risk (hence the winter flu vaccination strategy). Careful chest examination is often revealing but remember atypical organisms often give few respiratory signs. A pulse oximeter (most practices have them now) will show decreased O2 saturations and add to your diagnostic certainty.
• **Acute left heart failure:** may present as a complication of MI (and so usually with cardiac pain, although may be silent in diabetes) or by itself in those with pre-existing ischaemic heart disease. Thus, past medical history (and drug history as a proxy for PMH) are helpful, smoking and other risks indicative. Examination may show basal crepitations (you need lots for a diagnosis – scattered crepitations are common in older people and frequently without significance). Because biventricular failure is common, look for right heart failure signs too.

• **Arrhythmias:** cause breathlessness but usually the palpitations form part of the presenting symptoms, although older people may often not notice the palpitations of fast atrial fibrillation. Paroxysmal atrial tachycardias are common, particularly in younger women.

Slowly progressive causes of breathlessness

• **Chronic obstructive pulmonary disease (COPD)**, a term now preferred to the older chronic bronchitis, and emphysema are much the most common in primary care. It is estimated that only one-third of patients are diagnosed, so many are not receiving optimal care. On the other hand, the assumption that all older people with such presentations have COPD leaves other potentially treatable conditions (particularly asthma) unrecognised (see Chapter 40).
• **Tuberculosis** is increasing in frequency in particular risk groups, the destitute, immigrants and debilitated patients (especially HIV). Symptoms and signs may be subtle. A history of weight loss, night sweats, cough with or without haemoptysis, especially in at risk groups, requires assessment with at least a chest X-ray. A patient presenting with breathlessness is likely to have advanced disease.
• **Pneumoconiosis and fibrosis** are uncommon in primary care, but locally problematic depending on where you practise. Remember it's not just the asbestos worker who is at risk, but his wife who did the laundry too. Poor industrial practices may expose the whole surrounding population – large quantities of asbestos dust were released around East London's Barking asbestos factory. Diagnosis is suggested by history and crackles, particularly in the upper lobes, and characteristic X-ray appearances. The picture is often complicated by coexisting COPD.
• **Pulmonary oedema** produces characteristic orthopnoea (and sometimes paroxysmal nocturnal dyspnoea). Causes are legion, but ischaemic and alcoholic dilated cardiomyopathy are common in primary care. Mitral stenosis, still beloved of clinical examinations, is relatively uncommon nowadays. Mitral incompetence is common, usually caused by cardiomyopathy (see above) producing valve ring dilatation. Aortic stenosis (now the most common primary valve lesion due to congenital bicuspid aortic valve) can give acute pulmonary oedema at a late stage.
• **Obese** patients may present with breathlessness: the GP needs to sort out whether it is the obesity itself or one of the many causes associated with it that is causing the symptoms.

Vague breathlessness

Vague breathlessness is a common presenting symptom in general practice. It could be an early form of any of the above, or numerous other physical causes for which breathlessness may be a symptom, such as **anaemia, acute viral illness** or a **developing pleural effusion**. Perhaps most commonly it is a psychosomatic symptom of underlying psychological malaise. These present considerable management problems for the GP. One needs to be sure it is not due to an underlying physical problem while at the same time investigation and secondary referral (even if negative) all tend to confirm to the patient that there is a physical problem. Fastidious history-taking and precisely targeted investigation is crucial. Many doctors believe a negative investigation reassures: it often achieves the exact opposite ('He wouldn't have done the test if he wasn't worried'), so only use investigations if they are likely to contribute to your diagnosis.

39 Cough, smoking and lung cancer

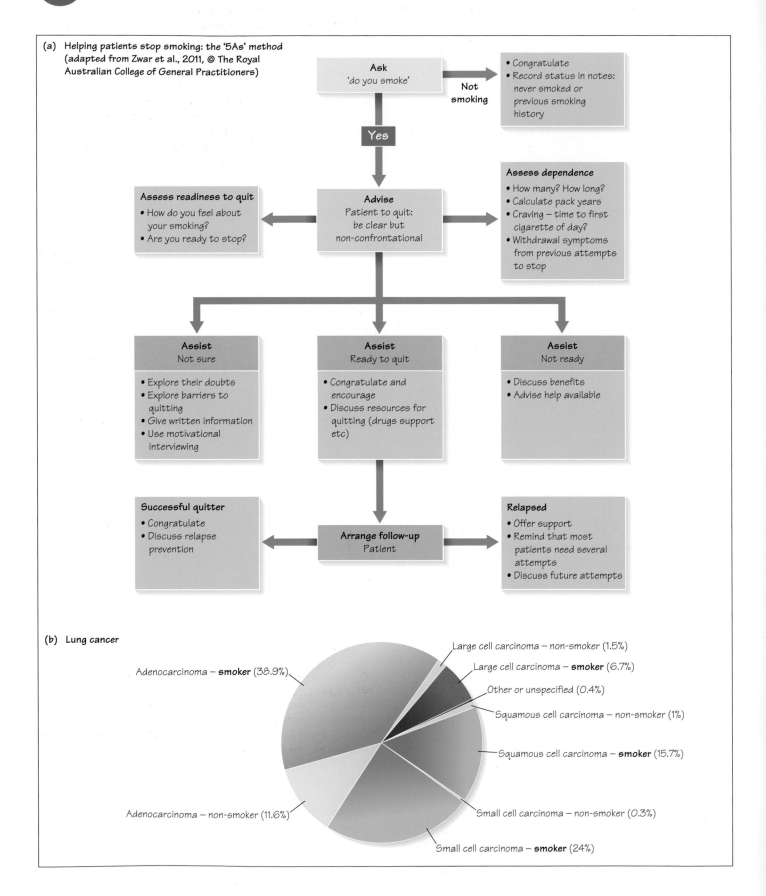

(a) Helping patients stop smoking: the '5As' method (adapted from Zwar et al., 2011, © The Royal Australian College of General Practitioners)

Ask
'do you smoke'

Not smoking
- Congratulate
- Record status in notes: never smoked or previous smoking history

Yes

Advise
Patient to quit: be clear but non-confrontational

Assess readiness to quit
- How do you feel about your smoking?
- Are you ready to stop?

Assess dependence
- How many? How long?
- Calculate pack years
- Craving – time to first cigarette of day?
- Withdrawal symptoms from previous attempts to stop

Assist
Not sure
- Explore their doubts
- Explore barriers to quitting
- Give written information
- Use motivational interviewing

Assist
Ready to quit
- Congratulate and encourage
- Discuss resources for quitting (drugs support etc)

Assist
Not ready
- Discuss benefits
- Advise help available

Successful quitter
- Congratulate
- Discuss relapse prevention

Arrange follow-up
Patient

Relapsed
- Offer support
- Remind that most patients need several attempts
- Discuss future attempts

(b) Lung cancer

- Large cell carcinoma – non-smoker (1.5%)
- Large cell carcinoma – **smoker** (6.7%)
- Other or unspecified (0.4%)
- Squamous cell carcinoma – non-smoker (1%)
- Squamous cell carcinoma – **smoker** (15.7%)
- Small cell carcinoma – non-smoker (0.3%)
- Small cell carcinoma – **smoker** (24%)
- Adenocarcinoma – **smoker** (38.9%)
- Adenocarcinoma – non-smoker (11.6%)

General Practice at a Glance, First Edition. Paul Booton, Carol Cooper, Graham Easton, and Margaret Harper.

Cough is one of the most common symptoms to present in general practice. It may be the presenting symptom of many serious disorders, but also of a vast range of self-limiting or minor conditions. It is a great cause of concern to patients who may interpret it as a 'chest infection' requiring antibiotics, cancer or pretty much anything else. Understanding the patient's ideas and concerns is vital in unpicking symptoms and giving patients tailored advice.

Cough

More or less any respiratory condition may produce cough, together with a fair number of non-respiratory ones. Most adults presenting with a cough of short duration will have an URTI. Look for confirmatory coryzal symptoms and manage symptomatically. Exploring the patients' concerns is important if you are to educate them to manage their own symptoms and be less reliant on medical services in future. However, in patients with pre-existing respiratory disease a URTI may precipitate an exacerbation and this risk should be factored into your management.

► Persistent coughs of more than 3 weeks' duration should be explored in more detail. Most of these will turn out to be either **serial URTIs** (the presence of a young family makes this almost inevitable) or a relatively long-lasting infection. Related to this, **post infectious coughs** can follow mycoplasma (primary atypical) pneumonia and whooping cough, which often presents atypically in adulthood. Campaigns encouraging patients with a cough of longer than 3 weeks to see the doctor aim at early identification of lung cancer. It remains to be seen if this will be effective, but protracted cough is a very common symptom in general practice with many causes.

Of the more serious causes of cough the two huge contributors are COPD and asthma. **Asthma** is common and under-diagnosed. Mild asthma presents with a cough rather than wheeze and there is often nothing to find when the patient appears in surgery. Sputum production is part of the pathology of asthma and eosinophils colour it bright green. Coloured sputum is therefore not synonymous with infection or need for antibiotics. **COPD** is under-diagnosed even more than asthma, particularly when mild. It should always be considered in those aged above 40 years especially if the patient is or was a smoker. A **'smoker's cough'** is quite likely to represent mild COPD (see Chapter 40).

Other respiratory causes of cough include **bronchiectasis,** a long history of recurrent cough and often foul sputum are charactreristic; a childhood history of whooping cough or inhaled foreign body may be found. Listen for the characteristic patches of treacly crepitations. In **lung fibrosis,** with its characteristic dry cough, an occupational history may be helpful and consider rheumatological causes.

► Haemoptysis (although common in COPD) should always make you consider **tuberculosis** (ask about ► weight loss, night sweats and more common in immigrants, homeless and the immunocompromised) and **lung cancer** (see Figure 39b). Consider **lung**

irritants: apart from smoking look for occupational causes – working in dusty or polluted atmospheres, which includes exposure to pollution from road traffic.

Mild degrees of **heart failure** frequently produce cough (usually dry and almost never the classic pink-tinged frothy sputum). Outside the chest consider **oesophageal reflux** (worse when lying down at night and more common in obese patients).

Remember certain **drugs** produce cough, particularly the ACE inhibitors. Patients may not associate starting the drug with the onset of their symptoms, which may in turn take weeks to settle when the drug is discontinued. The problem does not usually occur with ARB drugs, so it is worth switching on suspicion and monitoring to ensure the cough does settle (and if not investigating further).

Lung cancer

Background
- Most common cancer worldwide.
- Most common cause of cancer death in the UK. Around 39,000 new cases per year; rate stable for men, rising for women following smoking habits.
- Secondary cancers in lung from kidney, prostate, breast, bone, gastrointestinal tract, cervix and ovary are all very common – they are not covered further here.
- Most (90%) patients are smokers: risk rises with amount smoked. Other aetiological factors include asbestos, occupational exposure (e.g. nickel, arsenic, chromium, uranium).
- 80% aged over 60 years at diagnosis, rare below 40 years.
- Much lung cancer is silent until a late stage.
- UK 5-year survival rates (9%) are below Europe (12%) and USA (15%), probably as a result of late presentation.

Symptoms
Symptoms are non-specific. Have a low threshold of suspicion in patients:
- Progressively above age 40
- With risk factors – smoking, COPD, asbestos, previous history of cancer.

Consider in patients with unexplained cough (longer than 3 weeks):
► Haemoptysis
► Breathlessness
► Chest and/or shoulder pain
► Chest signs
► Hoarseness (involvement of recurrent laryngeal nerves)
► Clubbing
► Cervical or supraclavicular lymphadenopathy
► Weight loss.

Management in primary care
Chest X-ray will identify most patients with lung cancer, but if there is a high index of suspicion despite normal chest X-ray refer for urgent assessment.

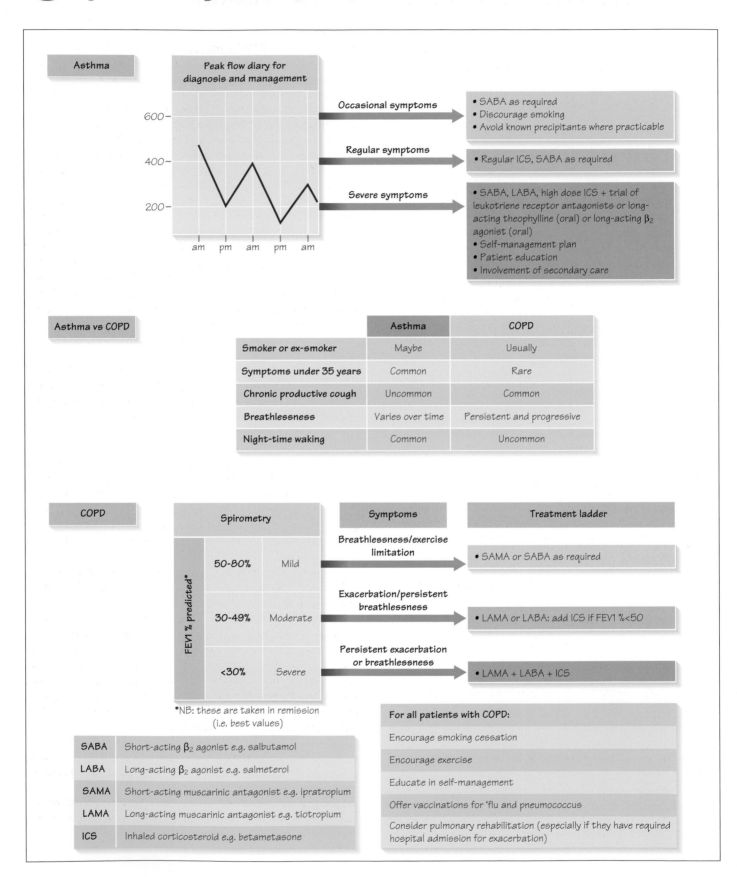

Asthma

Peak flow diary for diagnosis and management

Occasional symptoms
- SABA as required
- Discourage smoking
- Avoid known precipitants where practicable

Regular symptoms
- Regular ICS, SABA as required

Severe symptoms
- SABA, LABA, high dose ICS + trial of leukotriene receptor antagonists or long-acting theophylline (oral) or long-acting β_2 agonist (oral)
- Self-management plan
- Patient education
- Involvement of secondary care

Asthma vs COPD

	Asthma	COPD
Smoker or ex-smoker	Maybe	Usually
Symptoms under 35 years	Common	Rare
Chronic productive cough	Uncommon	Common
Breathlessness	Varies over time	Persistent and progressive
Night-time waking	Common	Uncommon

COPD

Spirometry			Symptoms	Treatment ladder
FEV1 % predicted*	50-80%	Mild	Breathlessness/exercise limitation	• SAMA or SABA as required
	30-49%	Moderate	Exacerbation/persistent breathlessness	• LAMA or LABA: add ICS if FEV1 %<50
	<30%	Severe	Persistent exacerbation or breathlessness	• LAMA + LABA + ICS

*NB: these are taken in remission (i.e. best values)

SABA	Short-acting β_2 agonist e.g. salbutamol
LABA	Long-acting β_2 agonist e.g. salmeterol
SAMA	Short-acting muscarinic antagonist e.g. ipratropium
LAMA	Long-acting muscarinic antagonist e.g. tiotropium
ICS	Inhaled corticosteroid e.g. betametasone

For all patients with COPD:

Encourage smoking cessation

Encourage exercise

Educate in self-management

Offer vaccinations for 'flu and pneumococcus

Consider pulmonary rehabilitation (especially if they have required hospital admission for exacerbation)

General Practice at a Glance, First Edition. Paul Booton, Carol Cooper, Graham Easton, and Margaret Harper.

Asthma and chronic obstructive pulmonary disease (COPD) are overwhelmingly the most common respiratory problems in primary care. They pose significant diagnostic and management problems for GPs.

Asthma

Asthma is common at all ages, is increasing in incidence and occurring in younger age groups.

Diagnosis

Diagnosis may be challenging, particularly in children (see Chapter 14). Diagnosis of moderate or severe asthma is generally straightforward, especially as many patients will have a long past history of asthma or other atopic symptoms. Explore the past history for 'weak chests' and 'wheezy bronchitis' as children and 'bronchitis' and 'everything goes onto my chest' as an adult – there are many undiagnosed asthmatics in the community. Asthma can arise *de novo* in adults, most commonly in their twenties. It is often wrongly diagnosed as COPD in older age groups. In some patients airflow obstruction appears irreversible on spirometry but a course of corticosteroids may unveil reversibility. Mild asthma may present with nocturnal cough only, a patient who describes always taking a long time to recover from everyday colds and URTIs, or someone in whom physical exertion (e.g. running, swimming) is limited by breathlessness or cough often has undiagnosed asthma. A history of cough in the small hours, of coughing on exercise and when allergens are around (hay fever season, changing the beds, brushing the cat) should all alert you to the possibility of asthma. By the time a patient reaches the surgery there are frequently no expiratory wheezes or anything else abnormal to hear in the chest. Diagnosis relies on a careful history, peak flow diaries and spirometry with bronchodilator challenge (which many surgeries now undertake).

Management

While effective treatment for asthma exists for all but the most severe, compliance is often poor and so symptoms are often poorly controlled. Helping patients to:
• Understand the role of their different inhalers
• Ensure they have an inhaler they can physically cope with
• Learn to use their inhaler correctly
• Agreeing a management plan that the patient can understand are key tasks for general practice teams. Much routine asthma monitoring devolves to practice nurses, so it is essential they are well equipped for the task. The stepped use of medication is well described in the excellent guideline *On The Management Of Asthma* (revised 2011; available at http://www.sign.ac.uk/guidelines/fulltext/101/index.html). Allergen avoidance is only useful where it is practicable, whereas smoking cessation is a vital goal.

Chronic obstructive pulmonary disease

COPD is a major cause of death in the UK, at around 5% of all deaths (about 30,000 per year, just behind lung cancer). Around 85% is attributable to smoking. A typical general practice will have about 200 patients with COPD, but the condition is considerably under-diagnosed (perhaps only one-third of cases are known).

Morbidity is considerable, comprising 1 in 8 of all hospital admissions, mainly in the winter months and causing the loss of over 20 million working days each year.

Diagnosis

The diagnosis of COPD, particularly in the early mild stages, is problematic. There are several definitions – functional, pathological and spirometric – none of which are entirely satisfactory.

Diagnosis is made on the basis of risk (increasing age and usually smoking or, less commonly, other inhaled irritants, mainly occupational), a history of exertional breathlessness, cough and sputum, winter 'bronchitis' and wheeze. The real challenge is to identify mildly affected patients, in whom the natural history can be changed (principally by stopping smoking). A history of protracted cough especially in winter, complicating recovery from URTIs and breathlessness on exertion in at-risk patients are always worth exploring. Never accept the explanation of 'only a smoker's cough, doctor'. On examination look for a plethoric sometimes cyanosed patient, a hyperinflated chest, pursed lips on exhalation and use of accessory muscles (although these signs are usually absent in mildly affected patients). Auscultation is non-specific; wheezes, scattered crackles and non-specific 'moist' noises may be heard. Breath sounds are reduced because of lung destruction in emphysema. Severely affected patients may go on to develop cor pulmonale and right heart failure. Chest X-ray is usually unhelpful diagnostically (except to exclude other pathologies).

Spirometry showing a FEV1/FEV <70% and an FEV1 <80% predicted indicate airflow obstruction. This is suggestive of COPD, but not pathognomonic. It may under-diagnose the elderly and normal values are unreliable for ethnic groups.

Management

As in other chronic diseases, the aim of treatment is to prevent progression and exacerbations. Closely related to this is prevention of hospital admissions which are economically expensive and at least in part represent a failure of community care. The NICE guideline on COPD (http://guidance.nice.org.uk/CG101) is an excellent summary of management. The key issues in primary care are as follows:
• Prevention of progression by encouraging smoking cessation.
• Reducing infective exacerbations through vaccination for flu and pneumococcus.
• Prompt treatment of exacerbations through patient self-management, advice and swift and appropriate GP intervention.

The mainstays of drug treatment are bronchodilators (beta-agonists and antimuscarinics), adding inhaled or, in the most severe disease, oral corticosteroids as the disease progresses (see Figure 40). Prompt antibiotic use with appropriate increases in bronchodilators and steroids may prevent exacerbations and hospital admission. See NICE guideline.

Oxygen therapy for patients with significant hypoxia may prevent complications such as cor pulmonale, but to be effective it needs to be used for at least 15 hours per day and is dangerous for patients who persist in smoking.

Specialist nurses and hospital outreach teams enable community management of more severe disease. The GP often has to coordinate care to manage co-morbidities (such as diabetes).

(a) Differences in T1D and T2D

	T1D	T2D
Symptoms at onset	Polyuria, polydipsia, weight loss of short duration often precipitated by a viral illness or stress	Polyuria, polydipsia, obesity, genital and skin infection
Age of onset	Typically <40	Typically >40
% of diabetic population	5–15%	85–95%
Ketosis	Prone	Rare
Insulin	Absolute deficiency	Relative lack of insulin

(b) Risk factors for T2D

- Family history
- Females (all ethnicities) – waist >80 cm (>31.5")
- Asian males – waist >90 cm (>35")
- White/black males – waist >94 cm (>37.5")
- History of hypertension, stroke or heart attack
- Females – obesity and polycystic ovary syndrome
- Impaired glucose tolerance and impaired fasting glycaemia
- History of gestational diabetes
- Long-standing mental health problems, especially if on anti-psychotic medication

(c) Diagnosis of diabetes

- Fasting glucose of >7.0 mmol/L on more than one occasion, **or**
- 2 hour (plus one other) glucose >11.1 mmol/L in a formal 75 g oral glucose tolerance test (GTT)
- HBA1c ≥6.5% (48 mmol/mol) has been proposed but not gained wide acceptance

(d) Investigations and targets at diabetic reviews

Parameter	Ideal target	Auditable target
Glycosylated haemoglobin (HbAlc)	7% (53 mmol/mol)	<7.5% (58 mmol/mol)
Blood pressure	140/80	145/85 (150/90)
Cholesterol	4.0 mmol/L	5.0 mmol/L

Primary care has progressively embraced the management of diabetic patients over the past two decades. Almost all type 2 diabetes (T2D) and increasingly type 1 diabetes (T1D) are managed in primary care. This has in part been driven by obligations on GPs to produce registers and work towards clinical targets for this group of patients. The surveillance culture of primary care and its role in assessment of risk for cardiovascular morbidity and mortality has led to increasing numbers of diabetic patients being identified and therefore managed. It is estimated that there are over 2.6 million diabetics in the UK, and a further 500,000 who may be undiagnosed.

General Practice at a Glance, First Edition. Paul Booton, Carol Cooper, Graham Easton, and Margaret Harper.

Diagnosis

T1D where there is an absolute lack of insulin and T2D where there is a relative deficiency may present with similar symptoms. Typically, these are polyuria, polydipsia and weight loss. However, onset in T1D is usually acute, with patients becoming seriously ill over a few days, whereas T2D may be almost silent allowing significant end organ damage by the time of presentation. Both conditions have a genetic component. In both conditions insulin resistance and obesity have a vital role in the development of the microvascular and macrovascular complications.

Management

Management involves identifying and assessing new patients followed by regular review of patients, patient education, and lifestyle and pharmacological interventions.

Screening for diabetes in practice is part systematic – newly registered patients have a urine test as part of a health screen (although this has a significant false negative), and the new NHS health check offers a check every 5 years (assessing blood sugar in those judged at risk). GPs have a low threshold of suspicion for testing for diabetes so patients with tiredness and opportunistic infections (boils, *Candida*) as well as more typical symptoms are likely to have opportunistic screening. Because diabetes is so common something like 1 in 10 such tests will be positive.

Regular review is made possible with IT based recall systems allowing UK primary care to be very successful in reaching pragmatic targets to monitor diabetic patients. Almost all T2D and increasingly T1D patients are managed in primary care as expertise in initiating and managing patients on insulin is developed. Recall systems allow patients to be reviewed 3–6 monthly or as required. The holistic nature of primary care allows the healthcare professional to make sensible management decisions with the patient, balancing the risks and benefits of treatment and taking into account the patient's personal, social and psychological needs. In elderly patients this will particularly mean addressing polypharmacy issues (see Chapter 9).

Regular monitoring involves the following:
- Assessing risk factors:
  - obesity BMI and waist circumference
  - lifestyle factors – enquire about diet, smoking, exercise, mood.
- Managing the primary problem of hyperglycaemia:
  - glycosylated haemoglobin, home blood glucose monitoring.
- Reducing secondary complications:
  - ophthalmic complications (retinal photography and screening)
  - nephropathy (renal function tests including estimated glomerular filtration rate [eGFR], albumin : creatinine ratios)
  - cardiovascular disease and hypertension (e.g. blood pressure monitoring, lipid measurements)
  - neuropathy (assessment of peripheral sensation)
  - foot complications (observation of skin, assessment of blood supply and neurological assessment).
- Medication review: to assess patient concordance, review drug effectiveness and for interactions and side effects.

Educating diabetic patients to understand and take care of their condition is vital. Practice based nurses and increasingly patients themselves are key players in the education of newly diagnosed and established patients to enhance their understanding of diet, exercise and management aims. Practice nurses have developed a major role in monitoring diabetic patients. Dietitians have a vital role, particularly in newly diagnosed patients. Lifestyle management is the first stage of diabetes management unless pharmacological intervention is urgent.

Drug management is of both the diabetes itself, but also of the other often coexisting pathologies that are at increased risk in diabetes.
- **First line therapy for T2D** (if HbAIc >7.5% [58 mmol/mol]) is metformin. If not tolerated consider sulfonylurea (although not if overweight, as appetite is increased).
- **Second line therapy** (if HbAIc >7.5% [58 mmol/mol]): add sulfonylurea, if not overweight. Gliptins are better for overweight patients.
- **Third line therapy** (if HbAIc >7.5% [58 mmol/mol]) remains controversial. More conservative clinicians move on to insulin, while others favour the use of glucagon-like peptide (GLP-1) agonists as early use may preserve pancreatic beta cell function.
- **Insulin.** Modern injectable pen devices and the use of insulin pumps have greatly enhanced options for patients. Initiation is usually with a long-acting drug, with the addition of shorter acting insulins to achieve tighter control in more brittle diabetics.

Other interventions

Lipids are commonly elevated in T2D, but even where apparently normal increase the already high risk of cardiovascular disease. All diabetics receive statins as part of aggressive cholesterol management.

Blood pressure again adds to cardiovascular risks. ACE inhibitors and ARBs are drugs of choice in view of their additional renal protective effects.

Anti-thrombotics: there is an increased risk of thrombosis (MI, stroke) so all patients over 50 and those under 50 with additional risk factors should be on 75 mg/day aspirin.

Future directions for hyperglycaemic control in T2D

The therapeutic options available to clinicians have increased in recent years with the introduction of newer agents – especially gliptins and GLP-1 agonists. Unfortunately, research findings in diabetes have focused more on reductions in proxy markers of good control such as HbAIc rather than true reductions in morbidity and mortality. It is to be hoped that lessons learned from the use of the glitazones (rosiglitazone was withdrawn when it became apparent that cardiovascular mortality was increased despite impressive reductions in HbA1c) will allow the research community to focus more on clinically relevant end points. While the newer agents are now licensed for use and are included in NICE guidance, their use by clinicians remains cautious as long-term evidence from studies of safety and efficacy is lacking. As the market for the newer agents is continually changing clinicians are advised to check licensed indications in mono and in combination therapy. Emerging evidence that bariatric surgery improves glucose homeostasis (even before weight loss is achieved) may have implications for future diabetes management.

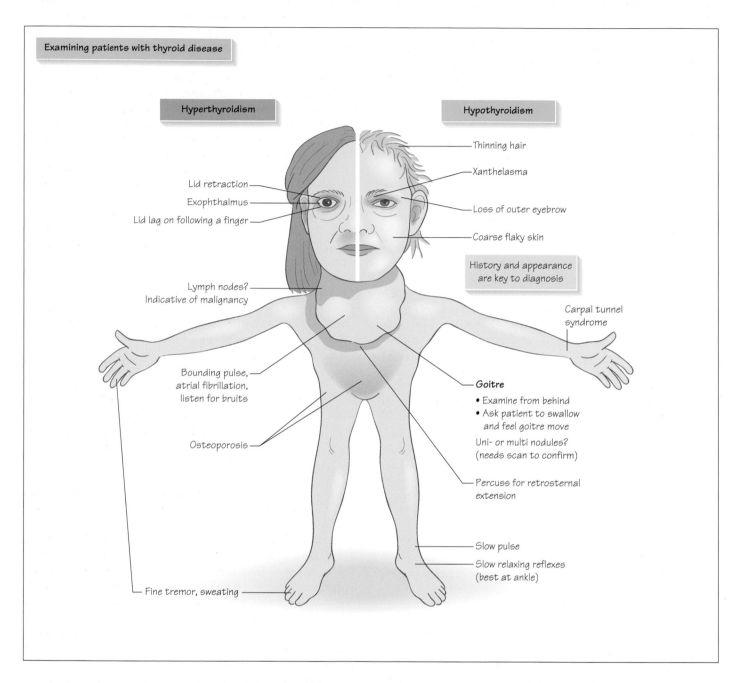

Examining patients with thyroid disease

Hyperthyroidism

Hypothyroidism

Lid retraction

Exophthalmus

Lid lag on following a finger

Thinning hair

Xanthelasma

Loss of outer eyebrow

Coarse flaky skin

History and appearance are key to diagnosis

Lymph nodes? Indicative of malignancy

Carpal tunnel syndrome

Bounding pulse, atrial fibrillation, listen for bruits

Osteoporosis

Goitre

• Examine from behind
• Ask patient to swallow and feel goitre move

Uni- or multi nodules? (needs scan to confirm)

Percuss for retrosternal extension

Slow pulse

Slow relaxing reflexes (best at ankle)

Fine tremor, sweating

Next to diabetes, thyroid disease is the most common endocrine condition. GPs manage most patients with hypothyroidism; other thyroid conditions usually require joint working with specialists.

Pathology

Thyroid disease can essentially be broken down into physiological change, autoimmune disease, presenting as hyperthyroidism or hypothyroidism, and benign or malignant lumps in the neck. Malignancy is rare.

A lump in the neck

Physiological goitre is common and caused by 'puberty, pregancy and poverty', the former from increased demand, the last from decreased supply in those parts of the world where dietary iodine is low and supplements not available. This may be worsened by diets containing goitrogens (e.g. cabbage which has a thiouracil-like action). In Japan, seaweed eating produces goitre from iodine excess. Be aware that kelp (seaweed) found in many health tonics contains large amounts of iodine and may produce goitre or transiently interfere with thyroid function. Patients with physiological goitre are normally euthyroid and asymptomatic.

Autoimmune goitre: both thyroid stimulation and destruction by autoantibodies can both lead to goitre and often the two processes coexist (although known as Graves' and Hashimoto's diseases). The soft diffuse swelling in Graves' disease is the most common autoimmune goitre.

Thyroid nodules are common but only occasionally toxic. The main issue is to differentiate the rare malignancy from the rest. Benign nodules might appear single but scanning often reveals them to be multiple.

Thyroid tumours are rare. Warning signs are single, sometimes painful nodules, growing rapidly and fixed to deep structures or skin. Check for local lymph nodes.

Thyroid function tests reveal the minority of toxic goitres. Ultrasound scans reveal the size, extent and nodularity of the goitre. Any suspicion of malignancy requires urgent secondary assessment, usually by ultrasound guided needle biopsy.

Goitres occasionally put pressure on underlying structures and may require surgical removal; more commonly, surgical treatment is for cosmetic reasons.

The overactive thyroid

Most commonly due to autoimmune Graves' disease, but less commonly from transient (viral) thyroiditis or caused by excess iodine consumption (usually kelp as above).

The typical case is a woman in her twenties presenting with hyperactivity (or sometimes tiredness) weight loss, palpitations, sweating and tremor. Amenorrhoea is common, as are irritability and anxiety. Patients feel the heat and may dress inappropriately for the weather. It can happen at all ages and in the elderly may present with atrial fibrillation as the sole symptom. A goitre is often present and frequently a bruit from the greatly increased blood flow. Exophthalmos and other signs of thyroid eye disease are common.

Free thyroxine and T3 are high and thyroid stimulating hormone (TSH) suppressed. Autoantibodies, particulary peroxidase, are usually positive.

Treatment is with an anti-thyroid drug (most commonly carbimazole). This takes several weeks to work and meanwhile beta-blockers give good symptom control. Check the thyroid at weekly or 2-weekly intervals as patients move swiftly from overactivity to underactivity due to the drug. Carbimazole can cause agranulocytosis – check the white cell count (WCC) at the outset and insist the patient immediately reports symptoms suggestive of infection (e.g. sore throat). The purpose of the drugs is to control thyroid activity until the hyperactive episode remits (typically 3–9 months). Further episodes may occur over time after which the gland often becomes inactive and treatment becomes that of hypothyroidism. Large goitres, or difficulties gaining adequate control may require surgical excision (usually leaving a remnant of gland to maintain endocrine activity) or in older patients the use of radioactive iodine, which generally produces hypothyroidism sooner or later. Thyroid eye disease can be exacerbated by treatment and requires specialist advice.

The underactive thyroid

This presents insidiously, usually in older age groups. This is one of the times when continuity of care may present problems as the GP (and the patient's family) may not notice the slow but characteristic changes in appearance.

Patients gain weight, skin becomes thickened and hair lost (in particular the outer one-third of the eyebrows); menorrhagia may be a presenting symptom. Patients feel the cold and complain of slowness of thought and action. Constipation is common. In extreme and rare cases patients may become comatose or an apparently psychotic condition 'myxoedema madness' occurs.

Thyroid hormones are usually reduced but an elevated TSH is of most significance. An unexplained macrocytosis may be due to hypothyroidism. Asymptomatic patients with a slightly raised TSH are common and there is no agreement whether they require treatment.

Treatment is straightforward: progressively increase the dosage of thyroxine until the TSH falls within the physiological range. Pitfalls are provoking cardiac ischaemia in vulnerable patients (hypothyroidism exacerbates the development of atherosclerosis). The most vulnerable may require hospital admission and starting treatment with T3, which has a shorter half-life, until the patient has been stabilised. Goitre size may temporarily increase in response to treatment and rarely this may put pressure on the airway and require surgical treatment.

Regular TSH checks are necessary as the gland usually fails progressively over a period of 12–18 months and the dosage of thyroxine replacement needs to keep pace with the decline. Once all gland activity has failed, the dose of thyroxine remains more or less constant and only occasional check-ups are required (usually annually to coincide with the patient's medication review).

Some important causes of adult gastroenteritis in UK

		Symptoms	Transmission	Management
VIRUSES	**Norovirus** Commonest cause of viral infectious gastroenteritis in England and Wales – also known as 'winter vomiting disease' due to its seasonality and typical symptoms	• Vomiting, diarrhoea, fever • Generally mild, usually recover in 2–3 days	• Person to person by the faecal oral route; contaminated food and water, especially bivalve molluscs **Incubation period:** usually 24–48 hours	• Supportive • Rehydration
BACTERIA	**Salmonella**	• Diarrhoea, vomiting and fever	• Predominantly from food-stuffs (most commonly red and white meats, raw eggs, milk and dairy products) following contamination of cooked food by raw food or failing to achieve adequate cooking temperatures **Incubation period:** 12–72 hours	• Supportive – antibiotics not routinely recommended
	Escherichia coli O157	• Mild to severe bloody diarrhoea • Can cause haemolytic uraemic syndrome and thrombotic thrombocytopaenic purpura which affect blood, kidneys and occasionally central nervous system • Relatively rare cause in UK but can be fatal in infants, young children or elderly	• Consuming food or water contaminated with faeces of infected animals • Also through contact with infected animals or with environment contaminated with faeces of infected animals, e.g. farms • Also human–human	• Entirely supportive – no specific treatment
	Campylobacter The commonest cause of food poisoning in Britain	• Abdominal pain, profuse diarrhoea, malaise • Vomiting is uncommon	• Raw or undercooked meat (especially poultry), unpasteurised milk, bird-pecked milk on doorsteps, untreated water, and domestic pets with diarrhoea • Person to person if personal hygiene is poor **Incubation period:** 1–11 days (usually 2–5 days)	• Usually no specific treatment – if needed (e.g. severe or enduring symptoms or in immuno-compromised), a macrolide antibiotic or ciprofloxacin
PROTOZOA	**Giardia**	• Diarrhoea, abdominal cramps	• Person to person • Foodborne transmission is rare • Faecal oral in young children • Waterborne • Spread within families is common **Incubation period:** 5–25 days	• Antibiotics: metronidazole
	Cryptosporidium	• Watery or mucoid diarrhoea	• Contact with infected animals • Outbreaks have been associated with public water supplies and contaminated food • Seasonal outbreaks are associated with farm visits to feed and handle lambs • Person to person spread, particularly in households and nurseries **Incubation period:** average 7–10 days; range 1–28 days	• Supportive – no effective antibiotics available

(Reproduced with permission of Health Protection Agency)

Acute diarrhoea

Acute diarrhoea can be defined as passing three or more loose or watery stools a day, lasting for fewer than 14 days. It is very common, affecting almost every adult in the UK every year (although most people won't see a doctor about it). Most cases are caused by **infective gastroenteritis**, which is often accompanied by vomiting and resolves on its own within 2–4 days (see Figure 43). But the GP also needs to be alert to the rarer but more serious causes of diarrhoea, such as inflammatory bowel disease, coeliac disease or bowel cancer, and infective diarrhoea needing investigation and treatment. More persistent diarrhoea may point to irritable bowel syndrome or lactose intolerance. Look out for systemic complications of diarrhoea such as dehydration, sepsis or abdominal disease.

History

• Clarify what the patient means by diarrhoea – people often use the term to mean passing normal stools frequently, or any minor change in their normal bowel habit.
• How long has the patient had diarrhoea? If more than a week this should prompt investigations to identify persistent infectious and non-infectious causes.
• Does the patient have any ideas about what has caused their diarrhoea? Have they eaten anything unusual recently, or are they in touch with people who have similar symptoms (this could suggest an infective cause)?
• Ask about recent foreign travel (raises the possibility of 'traveller's diarrhoea').

General Practice at a Glance, First Edition. Paul Booton, Carol Cooper, Graham Easton, and Margaret Harper.

- Ask about past medical history (e.g. thyroid disorders, diabetes, HIV or existing gastrointestinal conditions).
- Ask about medications, including recent treatment with antibiotics (risk of *Clostridium difficile* infection). Many medications (not only laxatives) have diarrhoea listed as a possible side effect.
- Ask about associated symptoms, such as abdominal pain, vomiting or blood in stools. Mild colicky abdominal cramps often accompany acute gastroenteritis, but more severe or constant abdominal pain could point to irritable bowel syndrome, diverticulitis or even an acute abdomen. **Diarrhoea with vomiting** is a common presentation of infective gastroenteritis, but could have another cause such as systemic illness, medication side effects or diverticulitis.
- Bear in mind the following red flags to guide further investigations or treatment:
▶ Change in bowel habit for >6 weeks (must exclude bowel cancer)
▶ Rectal bleeding: inflammatory bowel disease (IBD; e.g. ulcerative colitis or Crohn's disease), colorectal cancer, some infectious causes (e.g. *Campylobacter, Salmonella, Shigella, Yersinia,* toxogenic *Escherichia coli*)
▶ Weight loss: significant weight loss may indicate malignancy
▶ Dehydration
▶ Sepsis
▶ Systemic illness.

Examination
In the acutely unwell, check vital signs and temperature. About half of patients with infective diarrhoea have a raised temperature, compared with 10% in non-infective diarrhoea. Assess hydration.

Examine the abdomen, noting any masses, tenderness or guarding (mild tenderness is not unusual in gastroenteritis, but bear in mind diverticulitis or acute abdomen; see Chapter 46). Gastroenteritis often causes increased bowel sounds. Consider a rectal examination if there are any red flag signs or if there is any possibility of 'overflow' diarrhoea caused by constipation (particularly in the elderly).

Investigations
Investigations are rarely needed for most cases of acute diarrhoea lasting less than a week. After a week, or if particular concerns, the following tests may be considered in general practice:
- **Stool samples** for ova, cysts and parasites and/or for faecal blood
- **Urinalysis:** specific gravity may be high if dehydrated
- **FBC:** lower haemoglobin (Hb) or raised ESR and/or CRP may suggest IBD or colorectal cancer: white cell count (WCC) may indicate infection or inflammation
- **Urea and electrolytes:** severe diarrhoea may cause electrolyte imbalance
- **Coeliac screen**
- **Thyroid function tests**
- **In hospital:** colonoscopy or tests for malabsorption (e.g. lactose intolerance).

Management
In most cases of acute diarrhoea in general practice, management consists of reassurance and advice (see advice below) after careful assessment. **Safety netting** is important in acute diarrhoea: explain what you expect to happen if your working diagnosis is right, and then what the patient should do if symptoms worsen or persist. Severe dehydration requires immediate admission to hospital for urgent rehydration.

The management of acute diarrhoea is a good example of how GPs often use the **test of time** as a diagnostic approach. There may be one or more planned reviews, depending on the natural history of the condition and how the patient's symptoms develop.

Advice for patients with diarrhoea and/or vomiting
- **Drink plenty of fluids.** This is to avoid becoming dehydrated, a particular danger if you are vomiting as well. Take frequent small sips of water or diluted fruit juice. Avoid milk or dairy products as this can worsen symptoms. Soup can help replace lost salts and fluid.
- **Rehydration salts.** You may be advised to use rehydration salts which you can buy in sachets at a pharmacy. They contain the right balance of sugar, salt and water that your body needs to prevent dehydration.
- **Eat only when you begin to feel like it.** If you don't feel like eating you must continue to take fluids frequently. The latest advice is to eat carbohydrates (plain pasta, rice, bread, potatoes) as soon as you feel like it.
- **Anti-diarrhoea medication.** Medications such as loperamide can relieve the symptoms of uncomplicated diarrhoea in adults. They shouldn't be used if there is blood in the stools or any suggestion of bowel obstruction or colitis, and are not recommended for children.
- **Antibiotics** are generally unnecessary in simple gastroenteritis because the condition usually resolves without them, and in the UK the cause is usually viral. But antibiotics are often needed to treat bacterial infections such as *Campylobacter* enteritis, severe salmonellosis, shigellosis or protozoal infection such as *Giardia lamblia* (see Figure 43).

Vomiting
- Most cases are caused by **gastroenteritis** or food poisoning, and are self-limiting. But there are many possible causes to bear in mind such as gastroenteritis **(often with diarrhoea)**, acute viral labyrinthitis, pregnancy, acute abdomen (e.g. appendicitis), hyperglycaemia and hypoglycaemia, pyelonephritis, migraine, medication (e.g. cytotoxics, some antibiotics), intestinal obstruction, meningitis, bulimia, raised intracranial pressure (e.g. brain tumour), renal failure and acute glaucoma..
- As with diarrhoea, **dehydration** is the big danger.
- Ask about **medication**. Vomiting can be caused by medications, but it can also affect the efficacy of medications people take (e.g. contraception, anti-epileptics, steroids).
▶ Vomiting with **headache** should ring alarm bells: migraine can do this, but don't miss more serious causes such as meningitis or raised intracranial pressure.
- Anti-emetics can be helpful in some circumstances, but watch out for side effects or hiding the real diagnosis.

Box 44.1 Biliary disease

- 10–15% of adults in western world
- Often asymptomatic
- Most common presentations: biliary pain and acute cholecystitis
- Associations: include family history, sudden weight loss, increasing age, oral contraception, diabetes
- **Biliary pain:** Caused by gallstone in cystic duct or ampulla of Vater
  - *Symptoms:* pain often intense, starts suddenly in epigastrium or RUQ (may radiate to scapula); lasts from a few minutes to several hours; often relieved by painkillers. Nausea or vomiting common. Episodic, brought on by fatty foods, can wake patient at night
  - *Investigations:* urinalysis, and possibly CXR, ECG to exclude other serious causes. Ultrasound to visualise gallstones. Liver function tests +/– amylase. Hospital: ERCP (Endoscopic Retrograde Cholangiopancreatogram) best for duct stones. CT scan sometimes used
- **Cholecystitis:** Caused by stretching of the gallbladder with inflammation and subsequent necrosis
  - *Symptoms:* continuous epigastric or RUQ pain (may radiate to scapula) with vomiting, fever, local peritonism. Sometimes jaundice if stone moves to common bile duct
  - *Investigations:* FBC (WCC likely to be raised), LFTs often mildly abnormal. Ultrasound may show thickened gallbladder wall

Box 44.2 Pancreatic disease

- **Acute pancreatitis**
  - *Uncommon:* 5–80/100 000, men>women
  - *Causes:* alcohol, gallstones (less common: infections [e.g. mumps, Hep B, salmonella], autoimmune conditions, injury), 15% no clear cause
  - *Symptoms:* epigastric pain, gradually worsening, often radiates through to back. Also sometimes vomiting, diarrhoea, fever, abdominal tenderness, or jaundice. ? shocked/dehydration
  - *Investigations:* blood tests: amylase, lipase, LFTs. Ultrasound scan. CT scan or ERCP in hospital
  - *Management:* if suspect acute pancreatitis, refer to hospital
- **Chronic pancreatitis**
  - *Uncommon:* prevalence 3/100 000, men>women
  - *Causes:* Underlying aetiology unclear but 70% associated with alcohol misuse
  - *Symptoms:* abdo pain radiating to back (severe). Nausea/vomiting/diarrhoea. Decreased appetite. Malabsorption, steatorrhoea, diabetes mellitus. Abdominal tenderness sometimes. Bear in mind red flags for malignant disease such as wt loss or bowel changes
  - *Management:* assess and counsel re alcohol intake (e.g. with FAST questionnaire). Manage pain (sliding scale from paracetamol to opiates) and malabsorption (may need pancreatic enzyme replacements)
  - *Lifestyle advice/support re:* diet (high protein, low carb) and alcohol and/or illicit drug use

Box 44.3 Dyspepsia (NICE guidance on referral for endoscopy)

- Review medications for possible causes of dyspepsia (for example, calcium antagonists, nitrates, theophyllines, bisphosphonates, corticosteroids and non-steroidal antiinflammatory drugs [NSAIDs]). In patients requiring referral, suspend NSAID use.
- Urgent specialist referral for endoscopic investigation* is indicated for patients of any age with dyspepsia when presenting with any of the following: chronic gastrointestinal bleeding, progressive unintentional weight loss, progressive difficulty swallowing, persistent vomiting, iron deficiency anaemia, epigastric mass or suspicious barium meal.
- Routine endoscopic investigation of patients of any age, presenting with dyspepsia and without alarm signs, is not necessary. However, in patients aged 55 years and older with unexplained** and persistent** recent onset dyspepsia alone, an urgent referral for endoscopy should be made. [June 2005 update]

  * The Guideline Development Group considered that 'urgent' meant being seen within 2 weeks.

  ** In the referral guidelines for suspected cancer (NICE Clinical Guideline no. 27), 'unexplained' is defined as 'a symptom(s) and/or sign(s) that has not led to a diagnosis being made by the primary care professional after initial assessment of the history, examination and primary care investigations (if any)'. In the context of this recommendation, the primary care professional should confirm that the dyspepsia is new rather than a recurrent episode and exclude common precipitants of dyspepsia such as ingestion of NSAIDs. 'Persistent' as used in the recommendations in the referral guidelines refers to the continuation of specified symptoms and/or signs beyond a period that would normally be associated with self-limiting problems. The precise period will vary depending on the severity of symptoms and associated features, as assessed by the healthcare professional. In many cases, the upper limit the professional will permit symptoms and/or signs to persist before initiating referral will be 4–6 weeks.

(From: National Institute for Health and Clinical Excellence (2004) Dyspepsia: Managing dyspepsia in adults in primary care. London: NICE http://www.nice.org.uk/CG017 reflecting updated guidelines of June 2005.)

Figure 44 Causes of epigastric pain

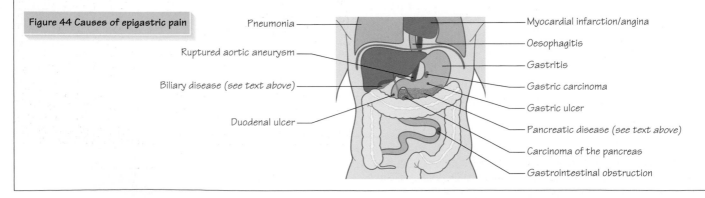

Pneumonia — Myocardial infarction/angina — Oesophagitis — Gastritis — Gastric carcinoma — Gastric ulcer — Pancreatic disease (see text above) — Carcinoma of the pancreas — Gastrointestinal obstruction — Ruptured aortic aneurysm — Biliary disease (see text above) — Duodenal ulcer

General Practice at a Glance, First Edition. Paul Booton, Carol Cooper, Graham Easton, and Margaret Harper.

94 © 2013 Paul Booton, Carol Cooper, Graham Easton, and Margaret Harper. Published 2013 by Blackwell Publishing Ltd.

Dyspepsia

Dyspepsia covers a range of symptoms of the upper gastrointestinal tract including upper abdominal pain or discomfort, heartburn, acid reflux and nausea or vomiting. They are all important and common symptoms in primary care. Up to 40% of adults have symptoms of dyspepsia; 5% of the population consults their GP about it, and 1% of the population is referred for endoscopy each year. Of those who do have an endoscopy, 40% have non-ulcer (functional) dyspepsia, 40% have gastro-oesophageal reflux disease (GORD) and 13% have some form of **ulcer** detected. Gastric and oesophageal cancers only account for 3% of patients who have endoscopy.

History

- Find out exactly what symptoms the patient has. Patients often say they have 'indigestion' or 'heartburn', but the terms can mean different things to different people.
- Ask the usual questions about the nature of any pain, including site, onset and character. Establish whether the symptoms are intermittent or persistent.
- Ask about any worries or ideas the patient has (those who seek medical help for dyspepsia are often worried about significant disease such as cancer).
- Bear in mind other common causes of upper abdominal pain or discomfort such as gallstones or cardiac pain (see Figure 44).
- Ask about **influencing factors** too: the gnawing pain of a peptic ulcer may be improved by food if it's a duodenal ulcer, or worsened if it is a gastric ulcer. Typically, ulcer pain is worse at night. Gastritis or GORD will often be relieved by antacids bought over the counter. GORD is often worse on bending or lying down.
- Ask about the patient's **diet and other lifestyle factors**. Spicy or fatty foods can make dyspepsia worse. Smoking, obesity, alcohol, coffee and chocolate can all worsen symptoms of reflux by lowering lower oesophageal sphincter pressure. Don't forget pregnancy.
- Find out what **medications** the patient is taking: NSAIDs, corticosteroids, aspirin, calcium channel blockers, nitrates, theophyllines, bisphosphonates and SSRIs can all precipitate dyspepsia symptoms.

Alarm features

Enquire specifically about alarm features, which should prompt an urgent referral for further investigations to exclude malignant disease:
► Chronic gastrointestinal bleeding (e.g. vomiting small amounts of blood, blood in stools including melaena)
► Progressive dysphagia (difficulty swallowing)
► Progressive unintentional weight loss
► Persistent vomiting
► Iron deficiency anaemia
► Epigastric mass
► Suspicious barium meal result
► Age 55 years or over if recent, unexplained or persistent dyspepsia.

Examination

Carefully examine the patient's gastrointestinal system, looking particularly for anaemia, jaundice, weight loss, epigastric tenderness or masses (see also Chapter 46).

Investigations

The following investigations may be considered in general practice:

Helicobacter pylori testing (see Box 44.1): carbon-13 urea breath test, stool antigen test or, when validated, laboratory-based serology.

FBC: Hb may be low in underlying malignancy or bleeding peptic ulcer. WCC could be raised in cholecystitis or pancreatitis.

LFT: may be abnormal with gallstones or malignancy or alcohol abuse.

Serum amylase: raised in acute pancreatitis.

Upper gastrointestinal endoscopy: to examine upper gastrointestinal tract, and exclude malignancy (see NICE guidelines on when to refer; Box 44.3).

Ultrasound: to exclude gallstones or other pathology (e.g. pancreatic disease).

Management

Review medications and, if possible, consider stopping any that are known to provoke dyspepsia symptoms. Offer lifestyle advice tailored to the patient, particularly in relation to weight loss, smoking, spicy or fatty foods. Raising the head of the bed may help some patients who have reflux symptoms when lying flat. For many patients, self-medicating with antacids or alginate therapy may give adequate symptom relief. Provide appropriate explanation and reassurance.

If further treatment is needed, there is debate about whether to treat straight away with a month's trial of a proton pump inhibitor (PPI), or to test and treat for infection with *H. pylori* first. The current NICE guidance is to try either treatment first, with the other being offered if symptoms persist or return.

If symptoms continue despite these steps, NICE advises stepping down to the lowest effective dose of PPI that keeps symptoms under control. The patient should be encouraged to use the treatment as needed to manage their own symptoms. If symptoms still return then the patient may need referral for further investigation.

Box 44.1 Helicobacter pylori

About 40% of the UK population is infected with *H. pylori*, and it probably causes no harm in the majority of people. But it is associated with up to 95% of duodenal ulcers and more than 70% of gastric ulcers and is a risk factor for gastric cancer. Eradicating *H. pylori* can cure peptic ulcers and this is the main reason for establishing *H. pylori* status. Eradication only occasionally improves dyspepsia symptoms not caused by peptic ulcer disease.

The main tests for *H. pylori* infection are the carbon-13 urea breath test and a stool antigen test. Patients should stop taking any PPI at least 2 weeks before testing and antibacterials at least 4 weeks before testing as they can cause false negative results. If *H. pylori* positive, the treatment is usually a 1-week eradication regime such as a PPI + amoxicillin + clarithromycin.

Table 45 Typical features and investigations of common lower gastrointestinal conditions

	Rectal bleeding	Change in bowel habit	Abdominal pain	Bloating/ wind	Weight loss	Other possible symptoms	Investigations possible in primary care
Colorectal cancer NB – often asymptomatic	✓ Especially left sided and rectal tumours	✓ Especially to looser and more frequent stools in left sided and rectal tumours	Not usually (though right sided tumours can cause pain)	Not usually	✓ Often	• Anaemia (iron deficiency) • Tenesmus (feeling of incomplete defaecation)	• FBC (anaemia) • Faecal occult blood • Refer for lower GI endoscopy
Crohn's disease	Possibly, mixed with mucous	✓ Diarrhoea, chronic or nocturnal	✓ May mimic appendicitis	Sometimes	✓ Often	• Fatigue • Malaise • Fever • Mouth ulcers • Strictures, fistulae or abscesses	• Systemic features (e.g. skin rashes, arthritis, uveitis) • FBC (iron deficiency common, rarely B12 or folate) • CRP and ESR often raised, U&E, LFT, stool culture and microscopy (exclude infective causes) • Barium enema • Refer for upper and lower GI endoscopy
Ulcerative colitis	✓ Bloody diarrhoea (visible blood in stools in >90% of cases of UC)	✓ Typically bloody diarrhoea	✓ • Crampy ache or pain, left iliac fossa • Pre-defecation pain relieved by passing stools	Sometimes (abdo tenderness and distension suggest toxic megacolon)	✓ Sometimes	• Tenesmus • Urgency • Mucous • Systemic features (e.g. uveitis, arthritis, skin rashes, mouth ulcers)	• FBC, U&E, LFT, ESR, CRP ANCA – found in HLA-DR2 associated form of UC • Plain abdo X-ray (excludes toxic dilatation) • Barium enema • Refer for lower GI endoscopy
Irritable bowel syndrome	No	✓ Constipation or diarrhoea or both	✓ Pain or discomfort, often relieved by defecation	✓ Often abdominal distension or bloating	No	• Symptoms worse on eating • Mucus rectally • Lethargy • Nausea	NB: tests restricted to those that exclude serious pathology • FBC, ESR, CRP, LFT, TFT • Coeliac screen • Faecal occult blood
Diverticular disease (NB: often asymptomatic)	✓ Sometimes	✓ Often constipation with hard stools	✓ • Pain or indigestion, mild or severe • Persistent ache with colicky exacerbations	✓ Distension, flatulence or belching possible	Appetite and weight usually normal	Fever suggests diverticulitis	• Usually diagnosis of exclusion • FBC (leucocytosis in acute inflammation) • Barium meal/enema
Coeliac disease (NB: often mild symptoms)	Not usually	✓ Diarrhoea and steatorrhoea (80%)	✓ Possibly	✓ Abdominal distension and pain (30%)	✓ Possible	• Malaise • Weakness • Iron, folate, vit K and vit D deficiencies • Aphthous ulcers • Nausea/vomiting	• Coeliac screen (antibody tests for coeliac disease – either endomysial antibodies or tissue transglutaminase) • FBC and film (may show iron deficiency) • Ferritin, vit D, calcium may be reduced • Refer for jejunal biopsy (characteristic histology shows partial or subtotal villous atrophy)
Haemorrhoids (NB: often asymptomatic)	✓ Bright red, typically on paper or streaking faeces	Not usually but may cause mucous discharge or faecal soiling	No	No	No	• Itching (pruritus ani) • Anal pain, especially if thrombosed piles	• Proctoscopy • Sigmoidoscopy

From rectal bleeding to a change in bowel habit, GPs encounter the whole range of lower gastrointestinal symptoms, sometimes in the same patient. This chapter gives an overview of the more common conditions GPs have to consider, particularly those that can present with rather vague, intermittent or long-standing symptoms and pose a diagnostic challenge. (For more acute problems, see also Chapters 29–31, 43 and 46.)

History

Using open questions at the start of the consultation is the most efficient way to gather important clinical information. Patients are often understandably uncomfortable talking about lower gastrointestinal complaints (many avoid coming to the doctor at all), and may be anxious about any impending examinations you may need to do. So your empathic listening skills are especially important here.

More specific, closed questions should cover the symptom areas outlined in Table 45, in particular red flag features to exclude serious pathology such as malignancy:
▶ Weight loss (clarify how much, and whether intentional or not)
▶ Change in bowel habit (clarify exactly what patient means, and for how long)
▶ Rectal bleeding (ask about volume, colour and frequency)
▶ Fatigue and/or malaise or symptoms suggesting anaemia (e.g. breathlessness)
▶ Family history of colon cancer or other serious bowel conditions.

Examination

Your examination should be guided by the patient's history, but will usually include a full examination of the gastrointestinal system. Don't forget to check for systemic signs such as anaemia, mouth ulcers or skin conditions. A rectal examination (with consent and chaperone if requested) is a routine part of the abdominal examination. It is not only designed to pick up rectal masses: it may also reveal blood, prostate conditions, abscesses or fistulae, thrombosed piles, faecal impaction and perianal rashes. Also consider urinalysis.

See Table 45 for main features and investigations of key conditions.

Management

Colorectal cancer

If you suspect colorectal cancer then the patient should be referred urgently for further investigations such as lower gastrointestinal endoscopy under specialist care. NICE guidelines recommend (adapted from NICE Guideline 27. London: NICE, 2005. http://www.nice.org.uk/CG27):
▶ Refer urgently patients:
  • Aged 40 years and older, reporting **rectal bleeding** with a **change of bowel habit** towards looser stools and/or increased stool frequency persisting 6 weeks or more.
  • Aged 60 years and older, with **rectal bleeding** persisting for 6 weeks or more without a **change in bowel habit** and without anal symptoms.
  • Aged 60 years and older, with a **change in bowel habit** to looser stools and/or more frequent stools persisting for 6 weeks or more without rectal bleeding.

  • Of any age with a **right lower abdominal mass** consistent with involvement of the large bowel.
  • Of any age with a **palpable rectal mass** (intraluminal and not pelvic; a pelvic mass outside the bowel would warrant an urgent referral to a urologist or gynaecologist).
  • Who are men of any age with **unexplained iron deficiency anaemia** and a haemoglobin of 11 g/100 ml or below.
  • Who are non-menstruating women with **unexplained iron deficiency anaemia** and a haemoglobin of 10 g/100 ml or below.

Crohn's disease and ulcerative colitis

• Specific nutrition advice from dietitian. Contact details for patient support groups.
• Stop smoking – the most effective way to prevent relapse in Crohn's disease.
• Aminosalicylates (more useful in ulcerative colitis than Crohn's), corticosteroids and drugs that affect the immune response (e.g. azathioprine or infliximab) are the mainstays of drug treatment.

Irritable bowel syndrome

Most patients benefit from a clear explanation of the condition and symptom relief.
• Increase fibre content of diet, particularly soluble fibre.
• Anti-spasmodics such as mebeverine can help with pain of smooth muscle contractions. Peppermint oil taken before meals can help colonic spasms and bloating.
• Bulk-forming laxatives for constipation-dominant IBS.
• Anti-diarrhoea medication such as loperamide can help in diarrhoea-predominant IBS.
• Tricyclic antidepressants, cognitive behavioural therapy and hypnotherapy may be effective.

Diverticular disease

• High fibre diet and laxatives are the mainstay of treatment for chronic disease. Anti-spasmodics may provide relief if colic is a problem.
• Antibiotics sometimes prescribed under specialist care if diverticula become infected. Acute diverticulitis usually requires hospital treatment.

Coeliac disease

• Advise on gluten-free diet as well as implications of the condition and importance of follow-up (e.g. for growth in children, or risk of malignancy).
• Recommend contact with dietitian and Coeliac Society for advice and support about living with the condition.

Haemorrhoids

• Advise patients to avoid constipation and reduce time straining at stool by increasing fluid intake and fibre in diet.
• Pharmacological bulking laxatives such as methycellulose or ispaghula husk can decrease abdominal pain and improve stool consistency.
• Local anaesthetic and/or steroid ointments and suppositories can help with pain and itching.
• Washing and drying the perineum after defaecation can also help prevent pruritus ani. Consider surgical approaches such as sclerotherapy, rubber band ligation or haemorrhoidectomy if conservative measures aren't helping.

The site of the pain can be important

R. hypochondrium
- Biliary pain
- Hepatitis
- Trauma to liver
- Subphrenic abscess

Epigastrium
(see also Chapter 44)
- Peptic ulcer
- Pancreatitis
- Duodenitis
- Oesophagitis

L. hypochondrium
- Splenic enlargement or infarct
- Subphrenic abscess

R. loin
- Ureteric colic (e.g. from stone)
- UTI
- Trauma to kidney

Central or peri-umbilical
- Intestinal obstruction
- Early appendicitis
- Meckel's diverticulitis
- Acute pancreatitis
- Ruptured or leaking aortic aneurysm
- Mesenteric infarction

L. loin
- Ureteric colic (e.g. from stone)
- UTI
- Trauma to kidney

R. iliac fossa
- Acute appendicitis
- Appendix mass (abscess)
- Crohn's disease
- Carcinoma of caecum
- Ovarian cyst (e.g. torsion or rupture)
- Pelvic inflammatory disease
- Ectopic pregnancy
- Endometriosis
- UTI
- Ureteric colic
- Rejection of transplanted kidney

Suprapubic area
- Acute retention of urine
- UTI
- Pelvic inflammatory disease
- Ectopic pregnancy
- Dysmenorrhoea
- Endometriosis
- Prostatitis

L. iliac fossa
- Constipation
- IBS
- Diverticulitis
- Ulcerative or ischaemic colitis
- Carcinoma of colon
- Volvulus of the sigmoid
- Ovarian cyst
- Pelvic inflammatory disease
- Ectopic pregnancy
- Endometriosis
- UTI
- Ureteric colic

- **Generalised pain** can occur in many conditions, including
  - early obstruction
  - generalised peritonitis (including acute pancreatitis)
  - gastroenteritis
  - lactose intolerance or food allergy
  - IBS
  - excess flatus

- **Referred pain** can originate in the spine, intercostal nerves or the pleura
- **Medical (i.e. non-surgical) causes** include:
  - diabetic ketosis
  - sickle cell disease
  - acute intermittent porphyria

General Practice at a Glance, First Edition. Paul Booton, Carol Cooper, Graham Easton, and Margaret Harper.

98 © 2013 Paul Booton, Carol Cooper, Graham Easton, and Margaret Harper. Published 2013 by Blackwell Publishing Ltd.

Acute abdominal pain

Most patients with abdominal pain do not have acute pathology, let alone a need for urgent surgery, but it's vital to spot the ones who do. Primary care is often the first or only port of call for the patient, so there's no margin for mistakes.

Take your time. You will regret it if you rush your assessment and get it wrong. You do not need to make an exact diagnosis. You only need a **working diagnosis** to guide your management.

Safety netting can be the difference between life and death.

► Peritoneal irritation (localised or generalised peritonitis, which can be infective, chemical or traumatic in origin) is very important. Always look for it in patients with abdominal pain.

► Children or pregnant women with abdominal pain can worsen rapidly. They may have different pathology too. In children, mesenteric lymph nodes can enlarge and become painful when there is tonsillitis. In late pregnancy, upper abdominal pain can be a warning sign of eclampsia (see Chapter 30).

History

Let the patient tell you about the pain, but be sure to fill in the gaps, noting especially when the pain started and what it is like (using SOCRATES or similar).

► If the pain is worse on movement, it's more likely to be peritonitis. The opposite is true of ureteric colic.

'Have you ever had this pain before?' Previous episodes (and what helped) can guide you this time, especially with biliary pain.

Ask about vomiting and bowel movements.

► Classic symptoms of obstruction are colicky pain, vomiting and constipation (no flatus or stools).

Does the patient feel bloated or distended? Any weight loss?

Are there genito-urinary symptoms? Think UTI and pelvic inflammatory disease. When was the last menstrual period (LMP)? Ask 'Was it a completely normal period for you?'

Take the previous medical history. Ischaemic heart disease is linked with ischaemic colitis and with aortic aneurysm. Is the patient on medication? What about alcohol? Excess intake can lead to pancreatitis or acute alcoholic hepatitis. Don't forget travel (malaria, parasitic infections) and trauma (splenic rupture).

Family history can be important in sickle cell disease, pancreatitis and irritable bowel syndrome, amongst other conditions.

Examination

► Is your patient shocked or dehydrated? Check the colour and feel of the skin, pulse, blood pressure and oxygen saturation (if you have a pulse oximeter). Is there fever? This suggests inflammation but isn't specific to sepsis. The elderly often have little fever and no tachycardia even in advanced sepsis.

Can you smell a foetor? This is more likely in appendicitis and other forms of sepsis within the gut.

When you start examining the abdomen itself, make your patient comfortable, with their hands by their side to help relax the abdominal muscles. One pillow under the head can help.

► Look for any masses, visible peristalsis and signs of trauma. Site can be important (see Figure 46), or it may be misleading.

Check for any signs of peritoneal irritation including:

► Pain on coughing
► Pain on percussion
► Rebound tenderness.

Guarding is a sign too, but it can be absent.

Peritoneal irritation tends to be more serious if it is generalised rather than local, but it is always significant.

Check the hernial orifices and palpate the scrotum (testicular torsion can start with abdominal pain).

Listen for bowel sounds.

► They are usually absent in generalised peritonitis, and may be increased in obstruction.

Does your patient need an intimate examination?

Never omit a rectal examination because it's too much bother. If it could possibly affect your management, you should do one. PR can be helpful if for instance your patient has severe pain and few signs (as can happen with retro-caecal appendicitis).

However, if you are already sure of the diagnosis, a PR is unlikely to change anything.

A vaginal examination can reveal a discharge in pelvic inflammatory disease. However, pelvic tenderness and pain on rocking the cervix can also be diagnosed by rectal examination.

Investigations

You may find urine dipstick useful (nitrites, WBCs or RBCs suggest UTI) and pregnancy test. Check glucose in diabetic patients.

Most tests take place in secondary care, e.g. FBC, CRP, amylase, abdominal X-ray, erect chest X-ray and ultrasound scans.

Management

By now you should have a good idea of how ill your patient is, and what with. Obstruction, peritoneal irritation and hypovolaemia all need hospital assessment or treatment urgently. Patients may need an ambulance, for instance for leaking aortic aneurysm, perforated peptic ulcer and acute pancreatitis.

If you are not sure what is wrong, ask yourself if it could possibly be serious. If so, get help from secondary care without delay. Tell the patient not to eat or drink anything more until seen in hospital.

You will be left with the possibility of a less acute condition. Your choice now lies between reviewing the patient again, sending the patient to hospital or starting treatment empirically. Use this last option only rarely, although it can be reasonable in UTI, for instance.

Referring to hospital

The surgeon on call wants to hear a concise history and salient points from the examination (see Chapter 7). If you think it's really urgent, always say so, even if you're not sure what is wrong.

Should you give analgesia?

The traditional view is that patients with abdominal pain should not have analgesia until seen in hospital, for fear of masking important signs. However, this is now being revised, especially as analgesia sometimes makes assessment easier. But discuss with the surgeon on call before prescribing for someone with an acute abdomen.

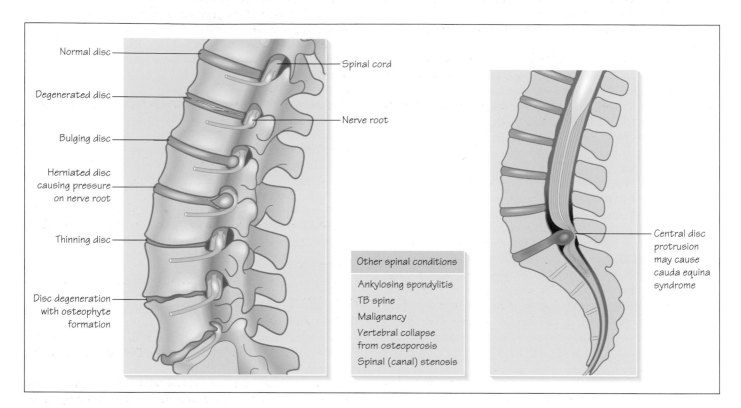

Normal disc
Degenerated disc
Bulging disc
Herniated disc causing pressure on nerve root
Thinning disc
Disc degeneration with osteophyte formation

Spinal cord
Nerve root

Central disc protrusion may cause cauda equina syndrome

Other spinal conditions

Ankylosing spondylitis
TB spine
Malignancy
Vertebral collapse from osteoporosis
Spinal (canal) stenosis

Musculoskeletal symptoms straddle several specialities: orthopaedics, rheumatology and general medicine. To unravel the problem, you need an understanding of anatomy and normal joint function, as well as information about your patient's medical history, lifestyle, daily activities – and their expectations of treatment.

Back pain

Some 60–80% of us will get back pain, so it's a common symptom. Every year around 2.6 million people in the UK see their GP for back pain. It's also the single biggest cause of time off work.

Most back pain is 'mechanical' – linked with posture or the way the back is used – rather than with fracture, inflammation, neoplasia or other pathology. Attacks are often self-limiting, although around 20% develop long-term pain or disability.

The challenge is to spot the 1% who have a serious cause and to treat them promptly.

History

► Onset of new back pain before the age of 20 or after 55 years – more likely to be malignancy (primary or secondary).

Where is the pain?

► Thoracic pain is usually more serious. It may be a disc, TB, osteoporosis, osteomalacia or malignancy.

Radiation of pain to the knee is common with mechanical pain, but involvement of the foot suggests nerve root irritation, for instance from a herniated disc.

► Weight loss or other systemic symptoms – think TB or malignancy.

► Morning stiffness – suggests an inflammatory cause like ankylosing spondylitis.

► Severe night pain – linked with malignancy.

► Pain on walking a certain distance – may be neurogenic claudication from spinal stenosis.

► Loss of bladder or bowel control – important symptoms of cauda equina syndrome.

► Saddle anaesthesia (ask about numbness of the buttocks or the area around the back passage) – also a cauda equina symptom.

• Ask about occupation. It may involve heavy lifting, prolonged driving or work at a visual display unit (VDU) at the wrong height. Workplace factors may also reveal a desire for compensation.

• Family history is important with ankylosing spondylitis and TB.

• Ask about medication (e.g. steroids). You may also be surprised how many patients see their doctor about back pain before even trying paracetamol.

• Cigarette smoking is a risk factor because it affects blood flow to the spine.

• Finally ask 'How are things generally?' Depression can present as back pain.

Examination

Physical examination is informative, and reassures you and your patient.

• If your patient sits happily on the chair with legs crossed, it's unlikely to be severe.

• Look for deformity or asymmetry.

General Practice at a Glance, First Edition. Paul Booton, Carol Cooper, Graham Easton, and Margaret Harper.

- Check for tenderness of the spine.
- Assess spinal movements.
- Test straight leg raising. Pain at less than 80 degrees of hip flexion suggests nerve root irritation.
- Lower limb reflexes are usually normal, but may be reduced with disc prolapse.
- Test muscle power in the legs. It's quicker and more informative than testing sensation, but check sensation in the perianal area for cauda equina.
- With first onset of back pain over 55 years, examine the breasts or perform a digital rectal examination (DRE) to assess the prostate. These carcinomas commonly spread to bone.

Investigations

FBC, ESR, CRP for inflammatory back pain, TB or malignancy. Protein electrophoresis for myeloma. Calcium and vitamin D levels if you suspect osteomalacia.

Patients often want the reassurance of an X-ray but imaging is unlikely to help unless you suspect TB, malignancy, ankylosing spondylitis or fracture (e.g. osteoporotic). You can explain that X-rays only show bones, not muscles or ligaments, the usual cause of back pain. Spinal X-rays also deliver around 50 times the amount of radiation given by a chest X-ray. MRI scans, where available, are far more helpful than X-rays, but even MRI has its limitations.

Management

- Rest for up to 24 hours helps acute back pain, but longer can weaken muscles and worsen the problem.
- Suggest heating pad or hot water bottle.
- Prescribe analgesics such as paracetamol (with or without codeine or dihydrocodeine) or ibuprofen.
- Address lifestyle and work factors. Advise a good bending and lifting technique, using the knees. PC users should adjust their workstation and take frequent breaks. Long-distance drivers also need breaks.
- Consider time off work.
- Advise simple exercises and swimming. Physiotherapy is very useful, especially for recurrent pain.
- Treat nerve root irritation the same way unless severe or worsening, in which case refer. **Always refer suspected cauda equina syndrome urgently to orthopaedics or neurosurgery.**

Cauda equina syndrome

The cause is usually a central disc protrusion at L4–5, but any space-occupying lesion below L2 can produce these symptoms:
▶ Urinary and faecal incontinence
▶ Numbness of the buttocks and the backs of the thighs ('saddle anaesthesia')
▶ Bilateral lower motor neurone weakness, usually with loss of ankle jerks.

Osteoporosis

Loss of bone mass begins in the late twenties and thirties. One woman in three and one man in eight develops osteoporosis. Factors include the following:

- Age
- Early menopause
- Family history of osteoporosis
- Low BMI (under 19) or previous anorexia nervosa
- Drugs (e.g. steroids)
- Rheumatoid arthritis
- Hyperthyroidism
- Smoking
- Heavy drinking.

Symptoms include pain, deformity and fractures (often vertebral, with kyphosis).

Investigations

While a plain X-ray may show osteoporosis and a typical vertebral fracture, the gold standard test for bone density is dual energy X-ray absorptiometry (DEXA).

The World Health Organization has developed a fracture risk assessment tool (**FRAX**) to help identify an individual's risk of fracture.

Management

Bisphosphonates are the mainstay of treatment (see NICE guidelines).

Osteomalacia

Osteomalacia ('bone softening') is loss of bone mass from poor mineralisation. The cause is either vitamin D deficiency or a defect in vitamin D metabolism.
- Lack of sunlight: over half the UK adult population have low levels of vitamin D, and 16% have severe deficiency during winter and spring (worse in Scotland). The elderly and those with pigmented skin are at high risk, especially if they keep covered up.
- Malabsorption (e.g. coeliac disease).
- Renal or liver disease.
- Treatment with anticonvulsants, rifampicin or anti-retroviral drugs.

Symptoms can be vague and insidious, but look for these pointers:
- The patient may feel unwell.
- Weak quads and gluteus muscles, with a waddling gait and difficulty getting up from a chair.
- It's said that Porosis hurts Part of the time, and Malacia hurts Most of the time.

Investigations

Tests should aim to diagnose the condition, and establish the underlying cause.

X-rays may show demineralisation. If available, vitamin D assay is diagnostic. Levels under 50 nmol/L (125 µg/L) suggest supplements are needed.

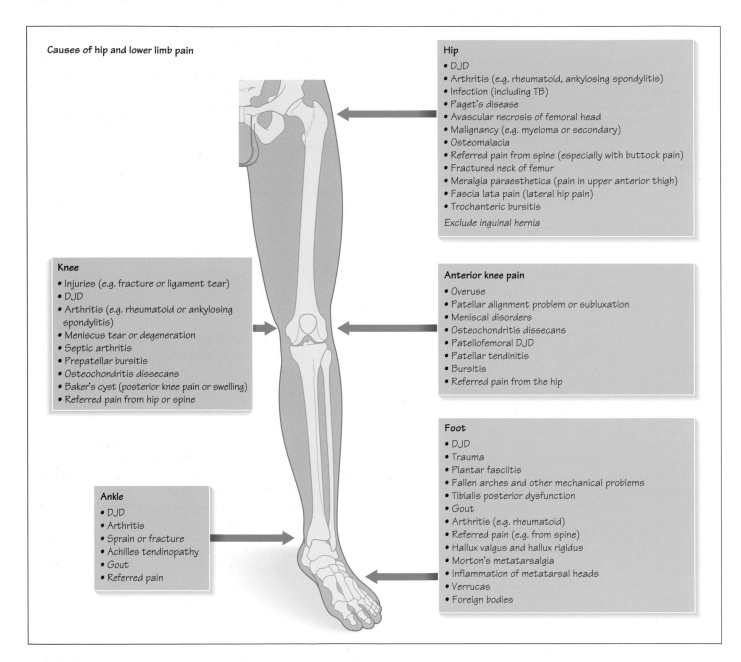

Causes of hip and lower limb pain

Hip
- DJD
- Arthritis (e.g. rheumatoid, ankylosing spondylitis)
- Infection (including TB)
- Paget's disease
- Avascular necrosis of femoral head
- Malignancy (e.g. myeloma or secondary)
- Osteomalacia
- Referred pain from spine (especially with buttock pain)
- Fractured neck of femur
- Meralgia paraesthetica (pain in upper anterior thigh)
- Fascia lata pain (lateral hip pain)
- Trochanteric bursitis

Exclude inguinal hernia

Knee
- Injuries (e.g. fracture or ligament tear)
- DJD
- Arthritis (e.g. rheumatoid or ankylosing spondylitis)
- Meniscus tear or degeneration
- Septic arthritis
- Prepatellar bursitis
- Osteochondritis dissecans
- Baker's cyst (posterior knee pain or swelling)
- Referred pain from hip or spine

Anterior knee pain
- Overuse
- Patellar alignment problem or subluxation
- Meniscal disorders
- Osteochondritis dissecans
- Patellofemoral DJD
- Patellar tendinitis
- Bursitis
- Referred pain from the hip

Foot
- DJD
- Trauma
- Plantar fasciitis
- Fallen arches and other mechanical problems
- Tibialis posterior dysfunction
- Gout
- Arthritis (e.g. rheumatoid)
- Referred pain (e.g. from spine)
- Hallux valgus and hallux rigidus
- Morton's metatarsalgia
- Inflammation of metatarsal heads
- Verrucas
- Foreign bodies

Ankle
- DJD
- Arthritis
- Sprain or fracture
- Achilles tendinopathy
- Gout
- Referred pain

The hip

Take a careful history, including general health and lifestyle:
- 'Where is the pain?' Pain from the hip is usually felt in the groin, less often in the lateral or anterior thigh. It can also be referred to the knee. If your patient has buttock pain, the source is probably the lumbo-sacral spine.
- What makes it better or worse? Significant morning stiffness suggests inflammation. Degenerative joint disease (DJD) is usually worse on activity.
- Ask about trauma and other joint symptoms.
- Understand the impact of hip symptoms on your patient's daily life, whether it is on work or on activities like cutting toenails.

▶ Night pain can occur in DJD – and in malignancy. Secondary bone tumours are more common than primary.

Examination
- There may be a limp.
- Leg shortening suggests advanced DJD, but also occurs in fracture. Patients can sometimes walk on an impacted femoral neck fracture, but the leg is often externally rotated and shorter.
- Check range of movements (ROM), comparing with the other leg. Full ROM is unlikely in advanced hip disease.
- Exclude inguinal hernia too.

Investigations

- FBC, ESR, CRP, rheumatoid factor for inflammatory arthritis.
- X-ray hips or whole pelvis if you suspect Paget's disease.

Management

If you can't make a diagnosis, your patient is well and without a limp, and the hip moves well, you could prescribe NSAIDs and review in 2 weeks.

Mild DJD is very common. Weight loss, physiotherapy (or gentle exercise like swimming) and analgesics often help.

Severe symptomatic DJD merits surgery. Pain and loss and function are the usual reasons for hip replacement. Surgeons often use a scoring system (e.g. Oxford Hip Score) to assess symptoms pre-operatively and postoperatively.

The knee

Knee symptoms are very common in general practice and there are many possible causes. Acute pain is often sports related. Chronic pain is more likely to be DJD.

History

- Is there pain? If so, use SOCRATES. The exact site matters: medial joint line pain suggests a meniscal problem. Pain behind the knee may be a popliteal cyst.
- **Stiffness** points to an inflammatory cause (rheumatoid or psoriatic arthritis, ankylosing spondylitis).
- **Swelling** can be synovitis, effusion or a bursa.
- 'Does the knee give way?' **Instability** suggests ligament injury.
- **Locking** means inability to straighten knee fully. It may mean a trapped fragment of torn meniscus, or a loose body.
- Enquire about trauma ('What exactly happened?'), symptoms in other joints, general health, occupation, leisure and medication. Septic arthritis often causes ▶ systemic symptoms and is more common in ▶ immunosuppression, including steroid therapy.

Examination

- How does the patient walk?
- Is there quads wasting? This usually suggests a knee problem, but it can be neuropathic.
- Is the knee in varus or valgus?
- What about swelling or ▶ redness?
- Check for joint line tenderness (suggesting meniscal injury).
- Is there an effusion or synovitis?
- Check ROM. Are movements painful?
- Test the stability of the knee. Perform tests for ligament integrity.
- Remember to examine the hip too.

Investigations

Blood tests are rarely needed for chronic knee pain. X-rays show osteoarthritis in up to 70% of those with knee pain, but are unnecessary for confirming a clinical diagnosis of DJD.

Refer if there are red flags:
▶ Significant trauma – there may be an intra-articular fracture.
▶ Possible sepsis. If the knee is swollen and hot, septic arthritis needs to be excluded by aspirating under aseptic conditions.
▶ Knee instability especially if acute (but timing of any repair depends on the patient's activities).

Management

- Meniscal injuries are usually treated conservatively at first.
- Refer patients with effusion, unless you can confidently and aseptically aspirate it.
- Mild to moderate DJD symptoms improve with weight loss, regular exercise and analgesia. Modify lifestyle. Warn your patient against squatting with the knee bent to more than 90 degrees. Glucosamine and/or chondroitin supplements may help some.
- Severe symptomatic DJD merits surgery, as for the hip, and there are similar scoring systems.
- Anterior knee pain is often chronic, poorly localised and hard to diagnose (see Figure 48). Management should focus on quads exercises, especially the medial quadriceps component.

> TIP
>
> Most knee problems other than fracture benefit from quads exercises.

Ankle and foot pain

The ankle

Sprains (inversion or eversion) are the most common cause of ankle pain and swelling, but bear in mind fractures, DJD, gout and sepsis.

Achilles tendinopathy is common in athletes but anyone can develop it. The main symptom is pain and stiffness just above the heel, and there may be swelling. Ultrasound helps in diagnosis but some need MRI. Ice and stretching can relieve symptoms.

The foot

- DJD is common.
- Morton's metatarsalgia (due to interdigital neuroma) usually causes increasing attacks of neuralgic pain or pins and needles in the third and fourth toes when walking. Orthoses help. Otherwise, refer to orthopaedics for steroid injection or excision.
- Acute inflammation of metatarsal heads tends to affect women. It causes burning or throbbing pain, often linked with wearing a favourite pair of high heels. Changing footwear and/or adding cushioned insoles relieves the problem.
- Plantar fasciitis causes pain anywhere along the plantar fascia, but there's often a tender spot just anterior to the heel. Rest, a change of footwear, heel pads, arch supports, NSAIDs, gentle stretching exercises and steroid injection can all help.

History

Ask about trauma, general health and symptoms in other joints.

Examination

- Look for valgus (or varus) ankle, state of circulation (ischaemic pain), bunion or other deformity (DJD), verrucas. Glance at the shoes – the style may give away the problem.
- Feel for exquisite tenderness (gout), tender anterolateral ankle (typical sprain), tender metatarso-phalangeal joints (inflammation or DJD), tender plantar fascia or heel (plantar fasciitis).
- Which movements worsen pain? Is the big toe immobile (hallux rigidus)? Watching your patient walk can help diagnosis.

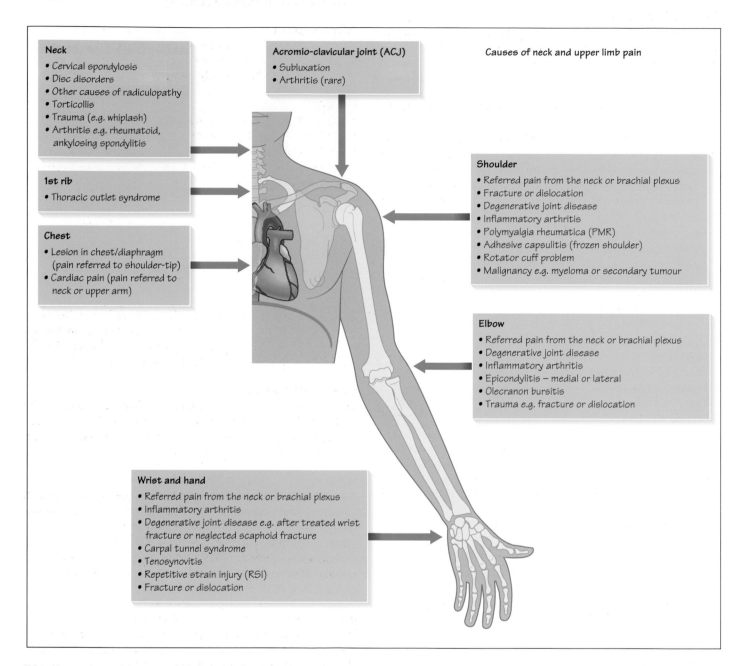

Causes of neck and upper limb pain

Neck
- Cervical spondylosis
- Disc disorders
- Other causes of radiculopathy
- Torticollis
- Trauma (e.g. whiplash)
- Arthritis e.g. rheumatoid, ankylosing spondylitis

1st rib
- Thoracic outlet syndrome

Chest
- Lesion in chest/diaphragm (pain referred to shoulder-tip)
- Cardiac pain (pain referred to neck or upper arm)

Acromio-clavicular joint (ACJ)
- Subluxation
- Arthritis (rare)

Shoulder
- Referred pain from the neck or brachial plexus
- Fracture or dislocation
- Degenerative joint disease
- Inflammatory arthritis
- Polymyalgia rheumatica (PMR)
- Adhesive capsulitis (frozen shoulder)
- Rotator cuff problem
- Malignancy e.g. myeloma or secondary tumour

Elbow
- Referred pain from the neck or brachial plexus
- Degenerative joint disease
- Inflammatory arthritis
- Epicondylitis – medial or lateral
- Olecranon bursitis
- Trauma e.g. fracture or dislocation

Wrist and hand
- Referred pain from the neck or brachial plexus
- Inflammatory arthritis
- Degenerative joint disease e.g. after treated wrist fracture or neglected scaphoid fracture
- Carpal tunnel syndrome
- Tenosynovitis
- Repetitive strain injury (RSI)
- Fracture or dislocation

Neck pain

One of the most common symptoms in general practice, this is often degenerative (cervical spondylosis), but there are other causes.

History

► 'Have you had an accident lately?' Trauma is significant.
- Ask about mode of onset, relieving and aggravating factors (SOCRATES).
- Ask about lifestyle (e.g. carrying infants, heavy work, sports).

Examination

- Look for stiff tender trapezius muscle on one side in torticollis.
- Check active movements – they may be normal or reduced in cervical spondylosis.
- Look for ► long tract signs – refer if you find any.

Except after trauma, X-rays are usually unhelpful. By the age of 50, at least 50% of people have neck X-ray changes, and they correlate poorly with symptoms.

Management

- Try simple analgesia. Muscle relaxants relieve spasm, but can be habit forming.
- Lifestyle advice (e.g. sleeping with one pillow, a lighter handbag or case, adjusting height of monitor, hourly breaks from the PC). Laptops stress the neck unless used with an external keyboard.
- Physiotherapy, especially for persistent pain.

Patients often ask about manipulation, particularly by complementary practitioners. This can be hazardous.

Shoulder pain

After back and neck pain, shoulder disorders are the most common musculoskeletal problem in general practice. Most improve within 3 months, but some become chronic.

History

• Ask about pain. Pain from the shoulder joint itself is usually felt in the lateral upper arm.
• Is there loss of movement, disturbed sleep or difficulty with daily activities? It's not always possible to relieve them all, so establish which symptom troubles your patient most. Is the patient right or left-handed? Always ask with any upper limb symptoms.
• Find out about other joint problems, a history of trauma or dislocation, and occupational and leisure activities.
• Enquire after general health, as heart disease and diabetes are linked with adhesive capsulitis.
• Ask about red flag symptoms:
▶ Acute onset of severe weakness (probable rotator cuff tear)
▶ History of cancer
▶ Fever or weight loss.

Examination

• Is there deformity, asymmetry or bony protrusion?
• Wasting above the scapular spine suggests neck problem.
• Compare active and passive movements. Both are usually reduced (and painful) in adhesive capsulitis ('frozen shoulder'), especially external rotation. Passive movements are near-normal in rotator cuff disorders.
▶ Unexplained deformity or lump (could be infection, malignancy or dislocation)
▶ Any signs of infection, such as warmth or fever
▶ Wasting, or muscle or sensory deficit (could be cervical radiculopathy)
▶ Inability to support the abducted arm suggests a significant rotator cuff tear, which may need surgery.

> **TIP**
>
> If the patient can touch his or her ear, the opposite shoulder and the back of the head, it's not a shoulder problem.

Investigations

Consider FBC, fasting glucose, ESR, CRP. X-rays rarely help, but consider chest X-ray if you suspect lung cancer.

Management

Are there red flags? Refer.

Do you suspect a rotator cuff problem (other than tendon rupture)? Try analgesics and/or NSAIDs. Consider subacromial steroid injection especially if you find a painful arc of movement.

Is it adhesive capsulitis? Analgesics and/or NSAIDs help. Reassure the patient: it will be painful and very stiff for 6 months, followed by loss of pain. Movement gradually recovers over 18–24 months. Steroid injection gives symptom relief only. Physiotherapy isn't curative either but can help maintain mobility. Physio-

therapy and exercise are more helpful later, to improve shoulder mobility.

Some patients have mixed pathology.

Elbow pain

The most common causes are tennis elbow (lateral epicondylitis) and golfer's elbow (medial epicondylitis), but pain can also come from the neck, especially with bilateral symptoms.

History

• Ask about pain, weakness, impact on daily life.
• Are there also neck symptoms?
• What are your patient's job and leisure pursuits? (Note that one needn't play tennis to have tennis elbow. The same goes for golfer's elbow – and for athlete's foot.)

Examination

• Look for olecranon bursa and any signs of infection.
• Check for epicondylar tenderness.
• Check neck movements. Do extremes of neck movement worsen elbow symptoms? If so, it's referred pain.

Management

Steroid injections help tennis and golfer's elbow, but are best kept for patients with well-localised tenderness. Olecranon bursitis usually improves with NSAIDs, but sometimes infection needs treating. If you don't know what it is, seek advice.

Hand and wrist

There are many possible causes, among them degenerative joint disease of the hand, affecting 20% of people over 55 years of age. Carpal tunnel syndrome (CTS) is also common, especially in pregnancy, diabetes and hypothyroidism.

History

• Ask about numbness or tingling. CTS often causes numbness in the lateral fingers on waking, and makes it hard to perform fine tasks.
• Is the patient pregnant?
• Enquire about new and old injuries, general health, current and previous occupation and leisure, family history of diabetes or thyroid disease.

Examination

▶ Wasting occurs in brachial plexus problems (less often in CTS).

Can your patient make a fist? If not, it may be arthritis of interphalangeal and/or metacarpo-phalangeal joints. It can also be tenosynovitis, in which case you may feel crepitus in the palm.

Is there synovitis (could be inflammatory arthritis) or bony prominences at the joints (degenerative joint disease)?

Look for tophi on knuckles (gout) and nail-pitting (psoriasis).
▶ After a fall onto the hand, always check for scaphoid tenderness by pressing into the anatomical snuffbox.

Management

Depending on the cause, it can help to adjust the work environment (repetitive strain injury [RSI]), check inflammatory markers (synovitis or tenosynovitis), X-ray the wrist or hand (new or old injury), take blood for glucose or thyroid function (CTS).

If you don't know what's wrong, someone else will, so ask or refer.

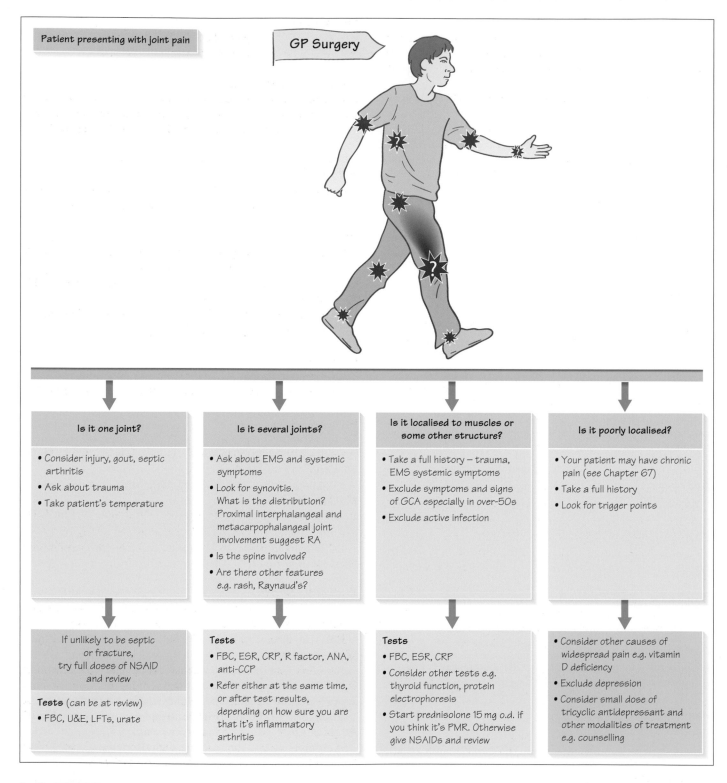

Patient presenting with joint pain

GP Surgery

Is it one joint?

- Consider injury, gout, septic arthritis
- Ask about trauma
- Take patient's temperature

If unlikely to be septic or fracture, try full doses of NSAID and review

Tests (can be at review)
- FBC, U&E, LFTs, urate

Is it several joints?

- Ask about EMS and systemic symptoms
- Look for synovitis. What is the distribution? Proximal interphalangeal and metacarpophalangeal joint involvement suggest RA
- Is the spine involved?
- Are there other features e.g. rash, Raynaud's?

Tests
- FBC, ESR, CRP, R factor, ANA, anti-CCP
- Refer either at the same time, or after test results, depending on how sure you are that it's inflammatory arthritis

---

Is it localised to muscles or some other structure?

- Take a full history – trauma, EMS systemic symptoms
- Exclude symptoms and signs of GCA especially in over-50s
- Exclude active infection

Tests
- FBC, ESR, CRP
- Consider other tests e.g. thyroid function, protein electrophoresis
- Start prednisolone 15 mg o.d. if you think it's PMR. Otherwise give NSAIDs and review

---

Is it poorly localised?

- Your patient may have chronic pain (see Chapter 67)
- Take a full history
- Look for trigger points

- Consider other causes of widespread pain e.g. vitamin D deficiency
- Exclude depression
- Consider small dose of tricyclic antidepressant and other modalities of treatment e.g. counselling

---

Inflammatory arthritis

Inflammation is the underlying pathology in many types of arthritis – rheumatoid arthritis (RA), ankylosing spondylitis, psoriatic arthritis and lupus. RA is the most common. Some 690,000 people in the UK have RA, so every GP has several patients.

However, in primary care most patients with joint pain don't have inflammatory arthritis. **The challenge is to spot those who do and refer them promptly, as early treatment with disease-modifying anti-rheumatic drugs (DMARDs) has lasting benefits.**

The hallmarks of inflammatory arthritis are:

General Practice at a Glance, First Edition. Paul Booton, Carol Cooper, Graham Easton, and Margaret Harper.
106 © 2013 Paul Booton, Carol Cooper, Graham Easton, and Margaret Harper. Published 2013 by Blackwell Publishing Ltd.

▶ Several joints involved, often in typical distribution of RA
▶ Marked early morning stiffness (EMS), usually >1 hour
▶ Systemic symptoms – feeling unwell, tired or losing weight.

History

• Establish whether there is pain, stiffness, loss of movement and/or swelling, in which joints, and the time-course. Inflammatory arthritis often begins suddenly, although the onset can be insidious.
• Family history is important for RA, psoriatic arthritis and ankylosing spondylitis.
• Ask about Raynaud's phenomenon or photo-sensitivity: 'Do your fingers go cold and blue?' and 'Do you get a rash from the sun?' These suggest lupus.

Examination

• Look for synovitis (tender swollen joints).
• Is there a rash? Check knees, elbows and scalp for psoriasis. A butterfly rash on the face points to lupus.
• Back involvement in ankylosing spondylitis and psoriatic arthritis.

Investigations

• FBC may be normal.
• ESR is often raised but not always. CRP is usually raised.
• Rheumatoid factor can be raised without RA. Anti-cyclic citrullinated peptide (anti-CCP) is more specific for RA.
• Anti-nuclear antibody is often positive with lupus.
• HLA-B27 won't help diagnose ankylosing spondylitis, and won't change the outcome if your patient has it.
• X-rays are often pointless. They can show erosions, but your aim is to refer before then.

Management

Refer to an early arthritis clinic if available. If you're sure it's inflammatory arthritis, refer without waiting for results.

Meanwhile, start a NSAID. With its long half-life, naproxen is more useful for EMS than diclofenac or ibuprofen. If your patient has upper gastrointestinal symptoms, add a PPI.

Reassure your patient. It's scary to have arthritis develop rapidly, and patients may fear a future confined to a wheelchair.

Gout

An inflammatory arthritis caused by urate crystals in the joint, gout is excruciating painful but attacks are self-limiting. Typically, the big toe becomes shiny, swollen, red and hot – but any joint can be a focus for gout.

Always look for possible risk factors:
• Increased uric acid production – high purine intake, psoriasis, leukaemia, cytotoxic treatment – and alcohol.
• Decreased uric acid excretion – renal impairment, low dose aspirin, diuretics, hypothyroidism – and alcohol.
• Attacks can be triggered by starvation, dehydration or stress.

Investigations

Uric acid levels are often normal during an attack, but raised between attacks. U&E may reveal risk factors.

The gold standard diagnostic test for gout is aspirating the joint and finding urate crystals on microscopy, but it's rarely done.
▶ Before treating, think: 'Could this be septic arthritis?'

Septic arthritis is more common in children, the elderly and the immunocompromised. Fever can be high.
If in any doubt, refer promptly.

Management

For an acute attack, prescribe NSAIDs or colchicine. If you can't use either, consider 30 mg prednisolone o.d. for 5 days.

Long-term management

If your patient has hyperuricaemia, prescribe allopurinol to lower urate, titrate to achieve your target level and cover initial treatment with an NSAID. Treat underlying factors (e.g. alcohol).

Polymyalgia rheumatica and giant-cell arteritis

Polymyalgia rheumatica (PMR) is the most common inflammatory rheumatic disease, but diagnosis can be a challenge.

History

• The patient, usually aged 50 or more, has aching in both shoulders or thighs, along with EMS of an hour or more.
• Try to exclude active infection somewhere. Ask 'How did this all start?' and look for signs of infection.
• ▶ If your patient has headache, visual disturbance, jaw pain or scalp tenderness, it could be GCA.

Examination

Look for tender upper arm muscles and check movements.
▶ Is there tenderness over the temporal arteries or the scalp?

Investigations

ESR is often over 40.
CRP is almost always raised. ▶ If very high, it could be GCA.
Consider other tests (e.g. TFTs).

Management

If you suspect GCA, refer immediately. Otherwise, start NSAIDs while waiting for results. If tests also point to PMR, then start 15 mg/day prednisolone. A clinical response within days clinches the diagnosis.

Osteoarthritis

Also called degenerative joint disease (DJD), this very common condition is often described as wear-and-tear of cartilage.

DJD can affect almost any joint but is most likely to develop in joints subject to heavy loads.

It becomes more common with increasing years and is the most frequent reason for replacement arthroplasty (e.g. hip or knee replacement). Women are more often affected and there can be a family history. In some people, symptoms and signs of DJD progress rapidly over a period of a year or less.

Symptoms include pain, swelling and deformity. **If your patient is systemically unwell, it is probably not osteoarthritis.**

Management

The mainstay of treatment is to keep active and use pain relief as necessary. Simple analgesics are often enough.

Evidence shows that appropriate exercise relieves pain rather than making it worse. Weight loss is often a good idea too.

Sore throat

History

As for URTI. You must also ask about the onset and severity of the soreness on swallowing, what makes it better or worse, other associated symptoms such as hoarseness and fever and exclude **red flag** symptoms:

▶ **Trismus** – inability to open the mouth (think of a peritonsillar abscess/quinsy)
▶ **Hoarseness** persisting for >3 weeks
▶ **Unexplained persistent sore or painful throat**
▶ **Dysphagia** – difficulty swallowing, with drooling of saliva (consider epiglottitis)

Examination

As for URTI. Is the patient systemically unwell? Look out for the presence of skin rashes (consider streptococcal infection), presence of exudates (pus) on the tonsils/pharynx, drooling and inability to speak. Infectious mononucleosis (glandular fever) is a common cause of sore throats in adolescents
Check for **red flag** signs:

▶ **Respiratory distress** – with added inspiratory sounds suggests **stridor** (think of epiglottitis)
▶ **Epiglottitis** – is a medical emergency – transfer the patient calmly to urgent care – do not use a tongue depressor to examine such a patient's throat as you can precipitate laryngeal spasm and obstruction
▶ **Peritonsillar abscess**

Red flags present → **Refer urgently to ENT**

No red flags →

Apply Centor criteria

These criteria were developed to predict bacterial infection (Group A Beta-Haemolytic Streptococcus [GABHS]) in people with acute sore throat. The four Centor criteria are:

1. Presence of tonsillar exudate
2. Presence of tender anterior cervical lymphadenopathy or lymphadenitis
3. History of fever
4. Absence of cough

Consider throat swab or rapid antigen testing

(Centor RM, Witherspoon JM, Dalton HP, Brody CE & Link K (1981). The diagnosis of strep throat in adults in the emergency room. Medical Decision Making 1 (3): 239–246

0 or 1 Centor criteria →

Antibiotics unlikely to be helpful

80% chance that patient does not have GABHS, and antibiotics unlikely to be needed

3 or 4 Centor criteria

Consider prescribing antibiotics

May have GABHS (40–60% chance) and may benefit from antibiotic treatment

Antibiotic prescribing in URTI and sore throat

NICE guidelines suggest three options when considering antibiotic prescribing in patients with sore throats and respiratory tract infections:

1. **Give antibiotics immediately** if the patient has signs of severe illness, or fits a high risk category:
   - Child <2 yrs with bilateral acute otitis media or
   - Child with otorrhoea and otitis media
   - Patient with acute sore throat/acute pharyngitis/acute tonsillitis & centor score >3

   For patients with mild to moderate illness, NICE recommends guidance on symptomatic relief, and gives you a choice of:

2. **Delayed antibiotic prescription** (advising the patient to wait for few more days to re-assess symptoms before starting antibiotics) or
3. **No antibiotic prescription** and instead educate the patient about the natural course of the disease, and follow up if symptoms persist

(Adapted from NICE Clinical Guideline 69. London: NICE, 2008. http://www.nice.org.uk/CG69)

Average total illness length of common URTIs

- Acute otitis media: 4 days
- Acute sore throat/acute pharyngitis/acute tonsillitis: 1 week
- Common cold: 1.5 weeks
- Acute rhinosinusitis: 2.5 weeks
- Acute cough/acute bronchitis: 3 weeks

(Adapted from NICE Clinical Guideline 69. London: NICE, 2008. http://www.nice.org.uk/CG69)

(a) Acute tonsillitis: reddened tonsillar tissue with surface discharge

(Reproduced with kind permission from Rila Publications Ltd, London)

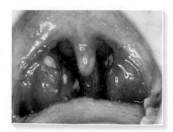

(b) Quinsy (peritonsillar abscess), arrow marks the spot: swollen left tonsil/oropharynx and very oedematous uvula pushed to the opposite side

(Reproduced with kind permission from Rila Publications Ltd, London)

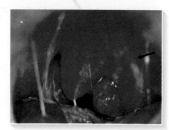

Upper respiratory tract infection

Upper respiratory tract infection (URTI) is one of the most common reasons for people to see their GP. It is a massive public health problem and leads to more loss of time from work than any other condition. On average an adult may suffer from two to three such infections a year. It is the most common illness affecting children. Most URTIs are mild and resolve completely without specific treatment. Inappropriate antibiotic prescribing adds to the problem of antibiotic resistance. There are clinical decision-making tools to help GPs decide whether or not to request additional tests or provide antibiotics when the illness may appear to be more complex.

Definition

A URTI is an inflammatory and usually infectious condition of the upper respiratory tract: the throat, nose, nasal sinuses, tonsils, pharynx or larynx.

Pathology

URTIs are caused by infection of the upper respiratory tract by any one of a number of viruses such as rhinovirus, coronavirus, parainfluenza, adenovirus, enterovirus or respiratory syncytial virus. The largest reservoir of viruses is in young children; transmission occurs through either inhalation of airborne respiratory droplets or by direct contact with infectious secretions by hand contact with people infected with the virus.

History

A patient may present with any of the following symptoms:
- Headache and sinus pains (over the face)
- Burning of eyes
- Nasal obstruction or discharge
- Loss of smell and taste
- Sore throat
- Hoarseness of voice
- Cough.

Cough tends to occur in 30% of cases, usually on the fourth or fifth day, when nasal symptoms have subsided. There may be a mild increase in temperature.

URTIs usually lasts up to 7 days but 25% of cases last up to 14 days. If symptoms exceed 2 weeks you must reconsider your diagnosis, and invite the patient back for a clinic review. Expect the illness to be prolonged in patients who are smokers or who have a history of respiratory co-morbidities such as asthma or chronic obstructive pulmonary disease (COPD). Possible complications to look out for include otitis media, croup, bronchiolitis (especially in infants) and sinusitis or pneumonia in older children and adults.

Examination

A thorough examination of the patient should begin with assessment of the vital signs:
- Temperature
- Respiratory and heart rates
- Blood pressure and oxygen saturation (pulse oximetry).

Then examine:
- Ears, nose, throat and pharynx
- Palpate lymph nodes along the cervical chains (anterior and posterior)
- Auscultate the lungs
- Throat swabs are no longer taken routinely as they rarely alter clinical management.

Management

For **uncomplicated URTIs**, treatment is aimed at symptomatic relief and adequate hydration. Paracetamol is a first choice medication to relieve pain and fever. Other alternatives are ibuprofen (in children and adults) and aspirin (in adults). Non-pharmacological cough mixtures (e.g. honey and lemon, or simple linctus) may be advised for symptom relief but there is little empirical evidence of benefit.

Many patients use **over-the-counter (OTC) medicines**, such as nasal decongestants containing norephedrine, oxymetazoline or pseudoephedrine. These may offer short-term relief from nasal congestion for up to a week, but often cause rebound congestion after they are stopped. Antihistamines may be used to improve runny nose and sneezing, although overall effect is insignificant and drowsiness is a common side effect. Echinacea, steam inhalation, vitamin C and zinc (intranasal gel or lozenges) have been tested for symptomatic relief in common cold. Evidence for their efficacy beyond placebo effect is limited.

For uncomplicated URTI, explain to the patient that:
- URTIs such as the common cold or sore throat are **self-limiting illnesses.**
- **Antibiotics will not influence the course of the disease** significantly or reduce complications.
- Antibiotics can cause problems like diarrhoea and antibiotic resistance.
- Offering a **delayed prescription** only to use if needed after 24–48 hours has been shown to cut antibiotic use and keep patients satisfied, without affecting outcomes.

For sinusitis, an antibacterial is usually only used for persistent symptoms and purulent discharge lasting at least 7 days, or if symptoms are severe.

The GP as risk manager

Although most URTIs are self-limiting, GPs must be alert for the unusual serious case or complication such as pneumonia. URTI is a good example of how GPs have to spot the rare high risk case amongst the low risk patients. GPs often take a focused history to exclude any red flag features, and then target their examination and investigations accordingly. To reduce clinical errors GPs must carefully record their findings and management plans in the notes. Finally, GPs often tell patients that they would like to see them again if **symptoms are not improving**, if there is concern about **deterioration** (it is important to be specific about what to look out for) or if **symptoms persist** beyond the expected duration (see Figure 51). This is an example of what Roger Neighbour, a GP expert on the consultation, termed **safety netting.**

(a) Normal ear drum

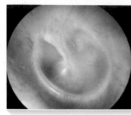

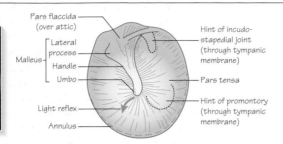

Pars flaccida (over attic)

Hint of incudo-stapedial joint (through tympanic membrane)

Lateral process

Malleus — Handle

Umbo

Pars tensa

Light reflex

Hint of promontory (through tympanic membrane)

Annulus

(b) Otitis media: a featureless red and bulging tympanic membrane

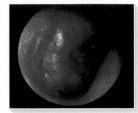

(Reproduced with kind permission from Rila Publications Ltd, London)

Table 52.1 Common causes of ear ache due to external ear conditions are outlined in the table below

Otitis externa (OE)	• Inflamed pinna, external auditory canal & outer surface of ear drum • Caused by infections (e.g. bacterial or fungal), allergy to irritants (hair products, ear plugs, hearing aids etc.) or inflammatory conditions • Common cause of earache in adults, especially swimmers • Generally good response to treatment with good clinical prognosis		
		Clinical features	**Management**
Acute OE	Localised infected furuncle	Fever, tender to examine canal, acute pain relief as it pops	• Pain control • Local heat application • Topical antibiotic drops
	Diffuse otitis externa	• Fever, LNs, swollen pinna, itching, pain with jaw movement • Canal and external ear are swollen and inflamed with scaly shedding of the skin • Clear discharge	• Pain control • Water protection • Antibacterial or steroid ear drops for 7 days • Ear canal is packed with wick/ribbon gauze soaked with steroids or an astringent (usually secondary care)
Chronic OE (months/ years)	Diffuse otitis externa	External canal skin is dry and thickened, narrowing the canal with evidence of pus	• Identify the underlying cause. (explore noncompliance with topical antibiotics, continued trauma, swimming, underlying skin disease, hearing aids, ear plugs or anatomical problems • Aural hygiene • Topical acetic acid 2% + steroid drops may be considered 7/7 • Referral to ENT may be needed

Table 52.2 Common causes of ear ache due to inner ear conditions

Acute otitis media (AOM)	• Inflammation of the middle ear, associated with URTIs. Bacterial or viral cause • Peak incidence: 0.5–1.5 years • Pathogens cross from pharynx to middle ear due to angle between eustachian tube and pharynx		• Most cases resolve spontaneously • Perforation of TM is common	
	Clinical features		**Management**	
	• Ear ache • Irritability • High fever (risk of convulsion) • Red +/– bulging ear drum • Vomiting & loss of appetite	• Common complication arising from AOM is a perforation of tympanic membrane (TM) or otitis media with effusion	• Pain & fever control • Avoidance of overdressing • 2% lidocaine ear drops • Antibiotics not recommended except in susceptible patients: – *Children <2 years	• *Bilateral AOM • *Systemically ill • *Evidence of severe infection • Sign of pus due to ruptured TM • Amoxicillin is first line Rx. • See delayed script (URTI)
Perforated tympanic membrane	Typically an irritable baby/child who stops crying suddenly and soon after discharge/pus appears from the outer ear		• First line antibiotics (amoxicillin) • Water prevention • Review in 3 weeks for healing	
Otitis media with effusion (glue ear)	• Inflammation and accumulation of fluid in the middle ear in the absence of any symptoms of acute inflammation • Commonest cause of acquired hearing loss in children • Risk factors include: male children, history of recurrent URTIs, children whose parents smoke, who attend day cares and winter season • 50% resolve in 3 months and 95% in 1 year (Lancet 1989)			
	Clinical features		**Management**	
	• Often no symptoms or signs of ear pain • Ear ache and hearing loss may/may not be present • Behavioral problems should alert the GP to assess a child for OM with effusion • Examination of the TM may reveal any of the following: increased opacity, a loss or disturbance to light reflex, • in drawing or retraction of TM, evidence of fluid level or air bubbles behind the TM		• Educate parents on diagnosis • Reduce risk of passive smoking • If, history <1 month; advise parents to bring child for re-examination at 1 month • If >1 month; refer for formal hearing assessment and consult ENT specialist if hearing loss is significant • Children 4 years + can benefit from 'watchful waiting' where the child is re-examined after 3 months with repeat hearing test. It is not recommended for children at risk; with disabilities, Down syndrome, cleft palate • Surgical options include insertion of grommets and /or adenoidectomy. Risks of GA and other surgical complications must be considered before opting for surgery **	

General Practice at a Glance, First Edition. Paul Booton, Carol Cooper, Graham Easton, and Margaret Harper.

Ear ache (otalgia)

Ear ache often triggers a visit to the GP; for children it is the most common cause for an out-of-hours call. The common causes seen in general practice are otitis media (middle ear infection) and otitis externa (infection of the outer ear canal). Otitis media with effusion ('glue ear') can cause niggly, short-lived ear pain. Remember that, particularly in adults, ear ache can come from outside the ear – referred from, for example, tonsils, dental abscess or trigeminal neuralgia.

History

- Assess the usual features of **pain**, including how severe it is, when it came on and if anything makes it better or worse.
- Ask about **discharge**: this may be thick and scanty in otitis externa or copious and mucoid through perforation from acute middle ear infections.
- **Deafness** can accompany both otitis media and externa, and pain on swallowing might suggest referred pain from the pharynx or tonsils.
- Ask whether the patient uses cotton buds – 'cleaning' the ear canal can traumatise the canal and introduce infection triggering otitis externa. A history of recent swimming or diving could indicate otitis externa, and pain during a flight points towards barotrauma.

Examination

See Table 52.1.

Management

Ear ache can be excruciating so adequate analgesia is the focus for treatment. Management then depends on the cause (see Table 52.1).

Otitis media is usually a self-limiting condition, so most patients do not need antibiotics. GPs sometimes offer a delayed prescription (only start antibiotics if needed after 24–48 hours). The evidence suggests that the following may benefit from antibiotics:

- Child under 3 months (or under 2 years of age with bilateral acute otitis media)
- Systemically very unwell, including high temperature (above 38.5°C) or vomiting
- Those at risk of complications (e.g. heart disease or immunocompromised)
- Acute otitis media (AOM) symptoms already lasted 4 days or more

Otitis externa often responds well to local antibiotic and/or steroid drops in the ear canal. Advise the patient to avoid getting water in the ear and not to use cotton buds. In most patients no underlying cause is found and the problem resolves quickly. **Refer** to a specialist when there are queries over diagnosis, if symptoms are not settling, or if there are red flag features. Sometimes, meatal swelling must be reduced by inserting a medicated ribbon gauze into the canal.

Ear discharge (otorrhoea)

The common conditions causing discharge in primary care are chronic otitis externa (from the outer ear) and AOM with perforation of the tympanic membrane. Most cases seen in primary care settle with simple treatment, but beware occasional serious causes such as cholesteatoma (a destructive growth of keratinising squamous epithelium in the middle ear) or cerebrospinal fluid (CSF) discharge (e.g. after head injury). Ask about the duration of discharge, the possibility of foreign bodies (including grommets), head injury and the presence of co-morbidities (especially immunosuppression and diabetes mellitus).

Begin examination by **feeling** behind the ear (for mastoid or lymph node tenderness), inspect the pinna (for colour, temperature and test for pain by pulling it up and backwards) and inside the canal for evidence of inflammation, foreign bodies or growths. Examine the discharge focusing on its colour (bloody: trauma or cancer; clear: may be CSF leak; pus: infection; mucoid: middle ear discharge from the mucus glands) and odour. Finally, try to see the tympanic membrane: if there is a perforation, is it central (generally 'safe') or marginal (at the edge – generally 'unsafe' and may imply cholesteatoma for example).

Often no investigations are needed – most cases settle with empirical treatment. Swab of ear discharge may help to guide treatment in refractory cases (for management options for different conditions see Table 52.2).

Hearing loss

Hearing loss can cause educational problems in children and worry their parents, and in adults considerable disability and even stigmatisation. Always take a careful history from the patient including how the deafness is affecting them, and listen to parental concerns about a child's deafness. History and examination should help sort out the most common types of hearing loss. Whispered voice testing is a useful screen, and tuning fork tests such as Weber's and Rinne's tests can sort out sensorineural from conductive deafness. Refer for audiometric testing to quantify deafness, determine the type of hearing loss and inform decisions about the need for hearing aids.

Common causes seen in general practice:

- **Ear wax:** easy to spot with an otoscope and simple to treat with olive oil drops to soften wax and then either ear syringing or microsuction.
- **Presbycusis (age-related hearing loss)** is usually bilateral and progressive, multi-factorial and related to environmental exposure to noise. Hearing speech is often affected first as high frequency hearing is lost. Management includes reassurance, education and amplification by hearing aids or cochlear implants.
- **Glue ear (otitis media with effusion) or eustachian tube dysfunction** is particularly common in children, and can present with behavioural problems. Because of fluid behind the ear drum, the tympanic membranes may be dull, indrawn or concave with loss of light reflex. If hearing loss lasts more than a month then refer for ENT assessment – treatment is either grommet insertion, adenoidectomy or both.

▶ Unilateral deafness, especially with tinnitus, vertigo or neurological symptoms or signs – consider acoustic neuroma
▶ Sudden onset deafness (e.g. vascular, infection, neurological)
▶ Cholesteatoma
▶ Mastoiditis
▶ Unilateral unexplained pain in the head and neck area for more than 4 weeks, associated with otalgia (ear ache) but a normal otoscopy.

Table 53.1 Symptoms, signs and management of 'the red eye'

Condition	Related conditions	Pain/ discomfort	Vision	Unilateral or bilateral	Discharge	Pattern of redness	Pupil affected?	Management
Bacterial conjunctivitis	Blocked nasolacrimal duct	Nil-mild discomfort	Unaffected	Unilateral (commonly) or bilateral	Mucopurulent	Diffuse 'pink eye'	No	Simple cleansing +/– topical antibiotics
Viral conjunctivitis	Some acute viral illnesses e.g. measles, coryza	Nil-mild discomfort	Unaffected +/– mild photophobia	Bilateral	Eyes may water	Diffuse 'pink eye'	No	No treatment
Allergic conjunctivitis	Hayfever Atopy	Itch	Unaffected	Bilateral	Eyes may water	Diffuse 'pink eye'	No	Includes oral or topical antihistamines
Traumatic conjunctivitis/ foreign body/ chemical irritant		Irritation/ grittiness	May be blurred if cornea affected +/– photophobia	Unilateral or bilateral (depending on cause)	Eyes may water	Diffuse 'pink eye'	Only if severe injury	Irrigation (for chemical irritation)
Subconjunctival haemorrhage	High blood pressure Anticoagulant therapy	Nil	Unaffected	Unilateral	No	Well defined bright red patch that fades	No	Reassurance
Keratitis	Dry eyes	Irritation/ grittiness	May be blurred if cornea affected +/– photophobia	Unilateral	No	Ciliary flush (circumcorneal injection)	May be constricted and unreactive	Topical steroids
Anterior uveitis (also known as iritis)	Connective tissue and systemic inflammatory disorders	Irritation, orbital pain and headache	Often blurred and photophobia	Typically unilateral	Eye(s) may water	Ciliary flush (circumcorneal injection)	If there are synechiae (adhesions of iris to lens or conjunctiva)	Topical steroids
Acute glaucoma		Severe 'boring' orbital pain, headache, nausea and vomiting	Often blurred, haloes around lights and photophobia	Unilateral	No	Ciliary flush (circumcorneal injection)	Dilated (may be oval) and unreactive	Ophthalmic emergency
Episcleritis		Usually mild	Unaffected	Unilateral or bilateral	No	Localised or diffuse	No	No treatment or topical steroids
Scleritis	Connective tissue disorders	Moderate to severe 'boring' pain	May be blurred if cornea affected	Unilateral or bilateral	No	Typically diffuse	Only if associated keratitis	Topical steroids
Blepharitis	Seborrhoeic dermatitis	Lids may be sore or may itch	Unaffected	Bilateral	May have a light 'sticky' discharge	Lids may be red, crusted and/or scaling	No	Lid hygiene advice +/– topical or oral antibiotics
Meibomian cyst/ chalazion		No/minimal discomfort	Unaffected	Unilateral	No	May be local or extensive lid erythema	No	Excise if lesion does not resolve spontaneuosly
Stye/hordeolum		Mild discomfort			Not usually but may be purulent discharge	May be local or extensive lid erythema		No treatment or drainage +/– topical or oral antibiotics

Causes of a 'red eye'

Chalazion

Conjunctivitis 'pink eye' (typically the whole of the visible sclera is involved)

Ciliary flush seen in anterior uveitis, keratitis & glaucoma

Stye

Tarsal/allergic conjunctivitis

Dilated oval pupil seen in acute glaucoma

Subconjunctival haemorrhage

Episcleritis

Blepharitis

General Practice at a Glance, First Edition. Paul Booton, Carol Cooper, Graham Easton, and Margaret Harper.

'Red eye' is one of the most common reasons for consulting a GP. Patients often present acutely and may be apprehensive, fearing visual loss. Fortunately, many of the causes are mild and self-limiting, such as bacterial conjunctivitis. However, delay in diagnosis can have a profound impact on vision in more serious cases. Acute glaucoma, for instance, can lead to blindness if untreated.

Figure 53 summarises the features and management of some of the more common and important causes of red eye.

History

Try to avoid making a 'spot diagnosis' simply because the patient is presenting with a physical sign. You will make a more precise diagnosis by taking a quick but structured history. The eye is essentially an **extension of the brain** and the history is as critical here as it is in neurology. Listen to your patients. They bring their own expert perspective to the consultation.
• Can the patient tell you the diagnosis? The child may be prone to recurrent **bacterial conjunctivitis**. The adult may have the **seasonal conjunctivitis** of **hay fever**. Contact lenses may be causing irritation. There could be recurrent **herpes simplex keratitis**.
►A **foreign body** can cause a **corneal abrasion**.
►Chemical exposure can lead to **conjunctivitis or keratitis**.
• Are there systemic features? In shingles (herpes zoster) there may be a high temperature and ipsilateral forehead rash and neuralgia. Or there may be a history of a connective tissue disease such as rheumatoid arthritis in a patient presenting with uveitis.
• Is there discomfort (as in the itch of hay fever) or pain?
►Pain can be serious, for instance the 'boring' orbital pain of acute angle glaucoma (angle closure glaucoma, AAG).
• Are the eyelids crusty or flaky? These are typical features of blepharitis which particularly affects patients with a history of seborrhoeic dermatitis or rosacea.
• Are the eyes unusually sensitive to light? Photophobia is a feature of many eye and CNS conditions, including acute anterior uveitis (iritis) and of course meningitis.
• Do symptoms affect one or both eyes? Bacterial conjunctivitis often affects one eye whereas viral usually affects both.
• Has there been any discharge or are the eyes sticky on waking? A mucopurulent discharge suggests bacterial conjunctivitis.
• Is vision affected?
►Loss of acuity is often linked with the more serious causes, although patients with watery eyes sometimes also say they do not see well.
• Is the presentation acute, chronic or recurrent? This is relevant for subconjunctival haemorrhage (acute but can recur), anterior uveitis (can be chronic) and allergic conjunctivitis caused by hay fever (usually recurrent every year).
• How much of the eye is affected? With subconjunctival haemorrhage, only part of the globe is involved. In uveitis there is circumcorneal injection, while acute conjunctivitis affects the whole eye.

Examination

Depending on the history, you may need to include:
• Check the **visual acuity** (VA) of each eye
• Use an **ophthalmoscope** to examine each eye 'front to back'
• Check **pupillary reflexes**
• Test **visual fields** by confrontation if you suspect a field defect.

When documenting VA, record the smallest standard word processor font size for near vision and use a Snellen chart for distance vision.

Using the ophthalmosope, first check the red reflex, then rotate the lens wheel to focus down on lids, surrounding skin, conjunctiva, cornea, sclera and iris then compare the pupils and perform fundoscopy. Remember the acronym PERLA: 'Pupils Equal and Reactive to Light and Accommodation'.

If there is a history of foreign body in the eye or you suspect a corneal abrasion or ulcer (e.g. herpes simplex dendritic ulcer), fluorescein dye will highlight the defect in blue light.

Eye pressure measurement with a tonometer and in-depth examination with a slit lamp microscope are of great value in certain situations, but seldom possible in general practice.

Investigations

An **eye swab** (for bacterial culture and sensitivity) is the only investigation commonly undertaken in general practice.

Management

In many situations, simple reassurance is all that is necessary (e.g. subconjunctival haemorrhage, mild bacterial and viral conjunctivitis).

Antibiotics (drops and ointment) are often prescribed for conjunctivitis. Arguably, they are over-prescribed but they have a place for some cases of bacterial conjunctivitis, blepharitis (eyelid inflammation and infection) and superficial abrasions.

Ophthalmologists often prescribe topical steroids to reduce inflammation in many types of keratitis, anterior uveitis and scleritis. These must be avoided if an infective cause has not been ruled out. Herpes simplex keratitis, for instance, will get worse.

Some cases of 'red eye' are caused by eyelid disorders such as meibomian cyst (chalazion), stye (hordeolum) and blepharitis (see Figure 53). Ectropion typically affects the lower lid and is caused by muscle weakness in old age. The eye appears red as the inside of lower lid (tarsal conjunctiva) is exposed. Entropion is caused by inversion of the lid causing the eyelashes to rub on the conjunctiva and cornea, and it can result in an irritant conjunctivitis or keratitis.

Some 'red eye' red flags

►**Reduced visual acuity** in any patient presenting with 'red eye'.
►**Orbital cellulitis.** The lids and surrounding skin may be inflamed too, and the eye may bulge (proptosis).
►A history of **penetrating foreign body** (e.g. metal fragment from grinding).
►**Subconjunctival haemorrhage** when associated with a head injury and no posterior margin to the haemorrhage is visible.
►**Dendritic ulcer** caused by **herpes simplex keratitis**. This will flare if topical steroids are applied.
►**Ophthalmic zoster.** Always consider shingles if there are features like a peri-orbital or frontal rash, which may not look typically vesicular at first.
►**Acute 'boring' headache**, often with nausea and vomiting, blurred vision and fixed oval pupil. These are typical of AAG.

THINK it through!

Visual symptoms can be due to anything that influences:

1. The passage of light from the front to the back of the eye (conjunctiva to retina): such as a cataract or posterior vitreous detachment
2. The relay of information from the retina to visual cortex in the occipital lobe: such as a brain tumour or stroke
3. The subsequent processing and subjective interpretation of this data: such as migraine, hallucinogenic drugs, the delirium of a high fever or alcohol withdrawal (delirium tremens)

(a) Visual pathway from eye to occipital cortex

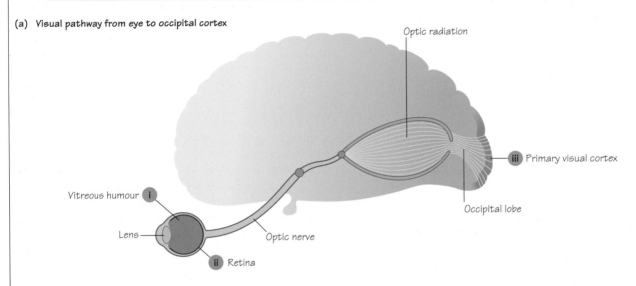

Optic radiation

iii Primary visual cortex

Occipital lobe

Optic nerve

Vitreous humour i

Lens

ii Retina

(b) Floaters seen as most clearly visible against a light background

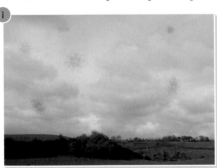

(c) Central scotoma seen in age-related macular degeneration (ARMD)

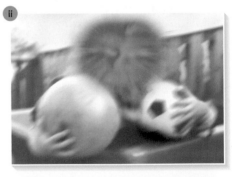

(d) Distorted Amsler gridlines in ARMD

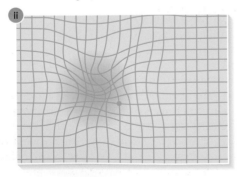

(e) Scintillating scotoma seen in the visual aura that precedes the headache of classical migraine

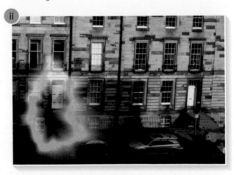

Patients often present with visual symptoms, and are understandably concerned that they may be going blind. There are many local and systemic causes, and some are very serious. You need to assess your patient carefully, reassure where possible and refer promptly if the condition may be serious.

History

As with any neurological condition, it is critically important to take a comprehensive history:
• Can the patient describe their symptoms?
• Was the onset acute or gradual? Are symptoms permanent, transient or recurrent?
• Is one or are both visual fields affected?
• Is the image blurred, dim, distorted, double?
• Do the symptoms and signs resonate with any of the conditions described below?
►Diplopia is a relatively common and important symptom. It can be a manifestation of an underlying neurological (e.g. multiple sclerosis) or neuromuscular (e.g. myasthenia gravis) disorder.

Examination

Examine your patient as in Chapter 53. You must also assess the visual fields using a finger or hat pin (confrontation).

A full neurological or cardiovascular examination may be needed – or both, for instance if you suspect a stroke may be causing the visual symptoms.

Summary of conditions presenting with visual symptoms in primary care

We all see **floaters**, especially on looking at a bright, even background such as a blue sky. Although some are embryonic deposits, they increase with age as degenerative changes involve the vitreous and retina.

Patients frequently present with a typical history of **classical migraine** with a visual aura (usually their first attack). Some patients have an aura with little or no headache. Migraine without visual symptoms is much more common, and some 75% of patients have this common form of recurrent headache. Many visual symptoms are associated with **migraine**. A **scintillating scotoma** (fortification spectra) is the classic visual aura of migraine. Typically, it begins as a spot near to the centre of the field of vision. It then evolves into a shimmering and enlarging zigzag peripheral arc (usually bilateral) before resolving.

Patients presenting with **cataract** are usually older and may have been referred by an optician. Cataracts are more common in diabetes. Cataract surgery is now one of the most common operations in the elderly.

Primary/chronic open angle glaucoma (POAG) has an insidious onset and can present late with tunnel vision.
► Loss of peripheral vision may present with a tendency to trip over, miss the kerb or steps or bump into things.
Visual loss is caused by irreversible damage to the optic disc and retina. Raised pressure without visual loss is called ocular hypertension.

Posterior vitreous detachment affects some 75% of over-65-year-olds. As the jelly-like vitreous ages, it liquefies centrally and this pulls the vitreous cortex from the retina. Patients may describe floaters and ►flashes (photopsia from stimulation of retinal receptors by the pull of the vitreous cortex).

Patients with **retinal tears** and **detachments** often report ►a marked increase in the number of floaters (dots if there is haemorrhage) or ►flashes seen. If there is full detachment, the patient may have a ►curtain or shadow coming across the field of vision. If the macula is involved, visual loss is profound.

The circulation to the retina can be compromised (e.g. from a **carotid artery embolus**). Ischaemia is **transient** in **amaurosis fugax** which has an annual incidence of 1 in 10,000. The patient may give a history of a brief (seconds or minutes) painless unilateral loss of vision, typically a shade or curtain coming across the eye. Sudden (over seconds) **permanent** visual loss in one eye is a feature of **central** and **branch retinal artery occlusion (CRAO** and **BRAO**, respectively). Acuity is typically reduced to counting fingers.

A **stroke (cerebrovascular accident [CVA])** involving the optic radiation may be associated with the abrupt onset of typically binocular visual loss (which is **temporary in a transient ischaemic attack [TIA]**). As in retinal detachment, the patient may describe a curtain coming across part of the visual field, but both eyes are usually affected, not one. The pattern of field loss is determined by the site of the vascular insult. The patient may have other systemic features.

Focus on age-related macular degeneration

One consequence of the growing elderly population is the relentless rise in **age-related macular degeneration (ARMD)**. Some 30% of over-75-year-olds are affected and ARMD is the most common cause of blindness in the UK. There is an association with smoking.

There are two forms:
1 'Dry' (90% of cases) ARMD is slowly progressive and caused by atrophy of retinal cells.
2 'Wet' (10% of cases) ARMD is caused by neovascularisation and may cause sudden blindness. It can be diagnosed by fluorescein angiography.

History

Because the macula is involved, a **central scotoma** can develop. Patients may complain that it is difficult to focus on objects and to read. Straight lines and objects appear distorted.
► Sudden central visual loss can occur resulting from haemorrhage from new vessels in the exudative 'wet' form.

Examination

If you show your patient an Amsler grid (printed on a piece of paper) he or she may see distorted lines in the centre of the grid. With an ophthalmoscope you may see:
• Drusen – yellow deposits – around the macula
• Pale patches at the macula
• Patchy hyperpigmentation
• Dot and flame haemorrhages.

Management

These patients need referral to the eye clinic for assessment.

There is no specific treatment for the dry form, but giving up smoking may halt progression of the disease. Vitamin and mineral supplements may also slow progression in some people.

For the wet form, there are now options. The anti-vascular endothelial growth factors (anti-VEGFs) such as ranibizumab (Lucentis®) and bevacizumab (Avastin®) show most promise. Anti-VEGF is injected into the vitreous humour monthly.

Skin problems in general practice

At least 15% of all GP consultations concern the skin but as many as 80% of people with skin problems do not seek medical advice. Although they are so common, confident diagnosis of skin conditions remains a challenge even to experienced GPs. While this is a visual specialty, don't make a 'spot' diagnosis. Take a careful focused history and never under-estimate the psychological impact of a skin condition which may not correlate with severity.

The history should include the following:
- When and where it started?
- Has the rash spread? If so where?
- Features of the rash (e.g. itch, pain, blistering, weeping).
- Systemic symptoms associated with the rash.
- Past and family history (e.g. atopy or chronic diseases).
- Drug history including topical, oral and OTC preparations, alcohol and smoking.
- Psychosocial history, occupation, hobbies, recent travel and sun exposure.

When examining patients, expose and inspect all areas of skin and carefully describe any skin changes seen. Using correct terminology and accurate descriptions helps establish a diagnosis and communication with colleagues.

Eczema

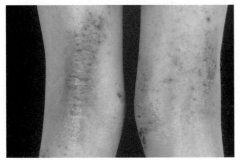

(a) Eczema

The terms eczema and dermatitis (inflammation of the skin) are often used interchangeably. **Atopic eczema** is common as part of the atopic syndrome of eczema, hay fever and asthma. It affects about 1 in 6 children and 1 in 20 adults and usually develops around 3–12 months of age. The distribution changes with age and moves from the face, neck, scalp and extensor surfaces in infants to flexures, particularly the popliteal and antecubital fossae, in older children and adults. Ninety per cent of children 'grow out' of their eczema by puberty. **Contact dermatitis** may be caused by **allergy** (e.g. latex gloves or nickel in jewellery, watches and buttons) or **irritant** from chronic contact with substances that remove natural skin oils such as washing up liquid. Eczema, like many skin diseases, can have a significant effect on quality of life, can lead to low self-esteem and limit day-to-day activities – exploring the patient's ideas and concerns is essential.

History and examination

Ask about site – is it the typical atopic distribution or a local distribution such as around the neck from nickel sensitivity or perfume (bergamot oils)? Ask about the treatments they have tried, frequency of application, occupation, exacerbating triggers (including stress) and family history. On examination look for vesicles (these are often not seen but the patient may tell you about them), dry skin and poorly defined areas of a pink scaly rash. There may also be evidence of weeping or oozing and crusting. Look for areas of excoriation from itching which can lead to lichenification (thickened leathery skin) and check for any infected areas.

Management

There are three important aspects to the management of eczema:
1 **Avoid triggers:** avoid soaps and biological washing powders, wear loose cotton clothing and avoid getting too hot or cold. Other triggers include food allergies, house dust mites, stress, pollens, pets, mould, habitual scratching and changes in the weather. Avoiding these may not be practicable.
2 **Emollients** are the mainstay of treatment. They prevent the skin from becoming dry, reduce itch and reduce the number of flare ups of inflamed patches of eczema. They must be applied regularly (at least twice daily) as part of a daily routine to prevent dry skin, even when eczema is well controlled. Emollients come as lotions, creams, ointments or bath and shower additives. The more greasy it is the more effective, but the less well tolerated.
3 **Topical steroids** are used in short courses for flare ups of eczema. Use the lowest strength necessary for the shortest course possible to treat the area. One finger tip is enough to treat an area of skin the size of the palm of the hand. Emollients should be continued.

Other medications

Eczema can become infected requiring topical or oral antibiotics. Antihistamines decrease the itch and are particularly useful at night. For severe and refractory eczema topical tacrolimus or pimecrolimus creams are steroid sparing, as are oral immune moderators such as ciclosporin and azathioprine, which require secondary care advice.

Psoriasis

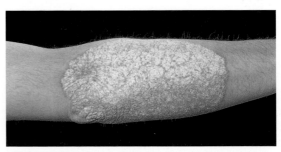

(b) Psoriasis

Psoriasis is an autoimmune skin condition characterised by scaly plaques resulting from epidermal hyperproliferation. There is a 2% prevalence, equal sex ratios, a higher incidence in Caucasians, and onset can occur at any age.

Environmental triggers include stress, skin trauma (Koebner's phenomenon), smoking, alcohol, throat infections and some medications. Psoriasis often improves with sun exposure. There is no relationship to diet.

Psoriasis can have a significant impact on patients' psychosocial well-being, so ask patients about the impact on their life, including work and relationships.

Chronic plaque psoriasis is the most common type (90%). Well demarcated plaques with white scale typically occur over extensor surfaces, trunk and scalp, although can occur anywhere. It tends to be symmetrical and plaque size varies. Guttate psoriasis often affects young people, 30% following streptococcal throat infection. Widespread small (<1 cm) plaques usually resolve spontaneously, typically in 2–3 months. Pustular psoriasis is less common and affects palms and soles. Erythrodermic psoriasis with increasing numbers of unstable, poorly demarcated plaques is a medical emergency.

Look for nail changes – pits, onchylosis and thickening. Some 1–2% of people with psoriasis have joint symptoms, including arthritis mutilans. An increased risk of CVD is associated with psoriasis.

Management

Focus on controlling symptoms and managing flare ups. Most patients are managed with topical treatments which are time-consuming and sometimes messy to apply so compliance is often poor. Patients may prefer to use no treatment if they have mild symptoms.

Emollients soften scales, reduce irritation and may reduce proliferation. They may be all that is required in mild disease. Adding a keratolytic (e.g. salicylic acid) to reduce scale allows other medications to work. Vitamin D analogues (e.g. calcipotriol) are well tolerated and non-staining, but may take up to 12 weeks to work. Crude coal tar cream is effective but messy and smelly: refined creams are more acceptable but less effective. Dithranol and the newer tazarotene are effective, but may be irritant and the former stains clothes. Steroids may be useful in the short term but can cause rebound on cessation and provoke erythroderma. For the scalp try a tar-based shampoo first, which can be combined with salicylic acid, potent steroids or calcipotriol scalp application. Provide patients with written information about how to apply the topical treatments, when to come for review and give details of local support groups.

Skin cancers
Malignant melanoma

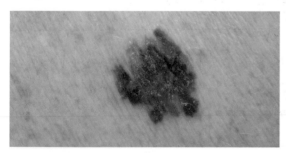

(c) Malignant melanoma

One-third of all melanomas develop from pre-existing naevi so take a careful history of changes in the lesion. Moles tend to increase in number and size following sun exposure, during puberty and pregnancy. When taking a history consider risk factors: fair skin, history of sun burn, multiple moles (especially atypical moles) and family or personal history of malignant melanoma. Assess moles using the ABCDE rule: Asymmetry, Border (is it irregular), Colour (are there multiple colours), Diameter (>6 mm), Evolution/Elevation (has it changed and is it raised). Because early diagnosis and treatment has an important influence on prognosis, rapid referral of suspicious lesions to a dermatologist is vital.

Prevention: use sun protection factor (SPF) 30+ sun cream, avoid sun exposure and stay in the shade in the middle of the day.

Basal cell carcinoma

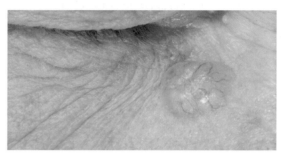

(d) Basal cell carcinoma

Basal cell carcinomas (BCCs) are the most common form of skin cancer occurring in sun exposed areas, often on the face. They are slow growing with a rolled pearly white edge, telangiectasia and an ulcerated centre. They do not metastasise and treatment is by local excision.

Squamous cell carcinoma

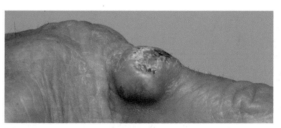

(e) Squamous cell carcinoma

A malignant skin tumour arising from sun damaged skin. They are faster growing than BCCs and produce keratin so can have a horny surface and later ulcerate. Treatment is by surgical excision. Solar (actinic) keratosis is a pre-malignant form of this lesion.

Seborrhoeic keratoses

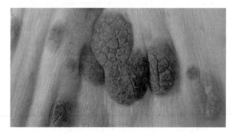

(f) Seborrhoeic keratoses

Common, benign, warty-like lesions that appear 'stuck on' to the skin. They increase in number and pigmentation with age. They are benign and included here because they are so common and may be confused with pigmented lesions. No treatment is necessary but they can be removed by curettage and cautery or freezing if required.

Acne

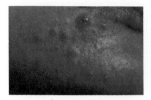

a. Acne.

Spotty skin will affect most teenagers at some point, and usually improves into their twenties. Spots occur on the face, neck, chest or back and can have a significant effect on quality of life irrespective of severity. Acne is caused by increased sebum secretion, blockage of pilosebaceous ducts, colonisation with *Propionibacterium acnes* and release of inflammatory mediators. In teenagers increased androgen is the main trigger.

Ask women about their use of the combined oral contraceptive pill. Some worsen acne, others may be used to treat it. Enquire about OTC medications and consider steroid use (topical, systemic and anabolic all exacerbate). Look for open comedomes (blackheads – dilated pores with keratin plug), closed comedomes (whiteheads), inflammatory papules, pustules, nodules, cystic areas and scarring.

Mild acne can be treated topically with benzoyl peroxide, with or without topical antibiotics, or retinoids. It takes 6–8 weeks before benefit is seen. Moderate acne involves papules and pustules and often requires oral antibiotics (first line treatment tetracycline) which should be continued for 2–3 months usually with topical treatments. Severe acne is nodular cystic. Anti-androgens (e.g. Dianette®) can be considered in females who haven't responded to treatment.

Indications for referral to secondary care include patients with severe nodular cystic acne, scarring or acne not responding to 6 months of oral treatment. Appropriate patients will be considered for oral retinoid (isotretinoin) treatment, which is teratogenic and needs regular blood monitoring.

Acne rosacea

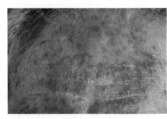

b. Acne rosacea.

This is a chronic condition affecting the forehead, cheeks and nose, characterised by redness, papules, pustules and telangiectasia. Patients may complain of blushing easily, and will often identify triggers for flares of their symptoms such as stress, alcohol, spicy foods, extremes of temperature, and it usually gets worse in direct sunlight. Ask about eye symptoms as it can cause rosacea keratitis. It mostly affects fair-skinned and middle-aged people, more commonly in women but more severe in men. Treatments aim for control, not cure, and include topical metronidazole, oral tetracyclines and camouflage creams to hide redness. Avoid triggers (e.g. alcohol) and irritants (e.g. soaps).

Seborrhoeic dermatitis

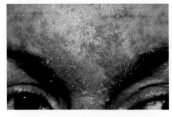

c. Seborrhoeic dermatitis.

This commonly presents in general practice as a sudden rash over the face and chest, which produces red areas of skin with greasy looking white or yellow scales. It is also the most common cause of dandruff and commonly affects the nasolabial folds, forehead, scalp, also beard area in men, and chest. It may affect the eyelashes (blepharitis) and ears (otitis externa). It commonly occurs in babies and throughout adult life. The aim of treatment is to control, not cure. The cause is not fully understood, but it responds to anti-fungal preparations (which kill commensal yeast cells) supplemented by short courses of steroid creams. Remember, it is also one of the most common skin manifestations of HIV.

Pityriasis versicolor

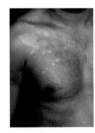

d. Pityriasis versicolor.

This produces a patchy rash over the shoulders and trunk. 'Pityriasis' is a fine scale, and 'versicolor' means colour changing. It is a common rash, mostly affecting young people, and is caused by the overgrowth of commensal yeast cells. It often appears pale on darker skins and darker on pale skins. It can be mildly itchy but often goes unnoticed. Anti-fungal shampoos (e.g. selenium) as a body wash often work well, oral anti-fungals are reserved for rashes that don't respond or are very widespread. Warn patients that pale patches of skin may take several months to return to their normal colour even though treatment has been successful.

Pityriasis rosea

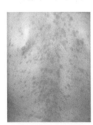

e. Pityriasis rosea.

A scaly and pink rash which goes away after about 8 weeks. The cause is unknown, and it tends to affect young adults and children. The initial rash is as a small pink scaly oval usually on the trunk (the Herald patch), and may be preceded by feeling mildly unwell. After a few days the rash changes to form the 'Christmas tree rash' on the trunk, formed of lined up elongated oval shapes like the branches of a Christmas tree. This rash evolves over a few weeks, then fades with no permanent skin changes. No treatment necessary, only reassurance that it is self-limiting.

General Practice at a Glance, First Edition. Paul Booton, Carol Cooper, Graham Easton, and Margaret Harper.

Fungal infections

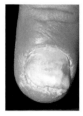

f. Fungal infections.

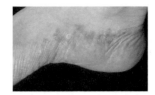

g. Tinea corporis.

Fungal infections are usually scaly, itchy, red, asymmetrical and often annular with a well-defined active spreading outer edge and pale centre. They can usually be diagnosed visually, but skin scrapings or hair or nail microscopy can be used to confirm the diagnosis. This is important in nail infections as treatment takes months. They are traditionally given Latin names after their site of occurrence. Tinea pedis (athlete's foot) causes white flaking skin and fissuring between the toes. Tinea corporis (ringworm) causes circular eyethematous lesions more or less anywhere on the body but typically trunk, groin, hands and scalp (tinea capitis). Tinea unguium causes discolored and thickened (onycholysis) nails. Most fungal skin infections can be treated with topical anti-fungals. Nail lacquers (e.g. 5% amorolfine) can be used for nail infections; however, oral terbinafine is more effective (but treatment takes months and it can cause derangement of liver function).

Warts

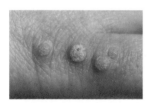

h. Warts.

Warts are very commonly seen in general practice, particularly in children. The lesions can be raised or flat and commonly present on the hands or soles of the feet in the form of verrucas. They are contagious and easily spread. They are caused by the human papilloma virus (HPV), are benign and normally resolve within 1–2 years and therefore do not require treatment. However, patients often find them distressing and treatments include salicylic acid preparations (wart paints) or cryotherapy although the evidence base is poor.

Molluscum contagiosum

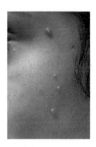

i. Molluscum contagiosum.

The rapid appearance of white or pink papules with a central punctum, usually in children, is typical of molluscum. They are viral and spread by direct contact and scratching. The lesions typically spontaneously resolve within 2–3 months but occasionally longer and usually reassurance is all that is required.

Cold sores

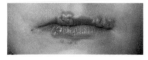

j. Cold sores.

Most patients recognise cold sores although they can occur intra-orally as mouth ulcers. Herpes simplex virus (HSV) infection causes a vesicular rash. The blisters de-roof, ulcerate and then finally crust over.

Primary infection often occurs in childhood and produces a more severe reaction; recurrences are a result of re-activation. Common triggers for re-activation are stress, fever, sunlight, respiratory infections, menstruation or local trauma. Treatment involves avoiding possible triggers and topical or oral aciclovir if required.

Shingles

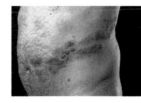

k. Shingles.

This is caused by re-activation of the varicella zoster virus which lies dormant in the dorsal root ganglion following primary infection with varicella virus (chickenpox). It is more common in people over the age of 50 years and often presents with a prodome of pain, burning or tingling. A vesicular erythematous rash then appears which is unilateral and confined to one or two neighbouring dermatomes. The rash can take 2–4 weeks to crust over. The ophthalmic branch of the trigeminal nerve and thoracic dermatomes are most commonly affected. If lesions develop on the tip of the nose (Hutchinson's sign) or there are any eye symptoms, an urgent ophthalmology opinion is indicated.

Treatment with oral aciclovir (started within 48 hours of the rash) can reduce the incidence of post-herpetic neuralgia, a common complication especially in the elderly.

Impetigo

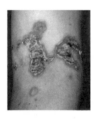

l. Impetigo.

This is a common childhood infection that is highly infectious and presents as a vesiculo-pustular rash that forms honey-coloured crusts. It is caused by *Staphylococcus aureus*, *Streptococcus pyogenes* or a combination of both. Treatment involves removal of the crusts followed by topical antibiotics, such as mupirocin (Bactroban®).

Scabies

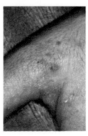

m. Scabies.

This is a skin infestation by the human scabies mite, *Sarcoptes scabiei*. It typically causes very itchy skin and an inflammatory papular rash, although some people are asymptomatic. It is a common problem in general practice and the prevalence is rising. The itching tends to be worse at night. Ask about other household members. The mites burrow under the skin, causing track marks often seen in the finger web spaces and wrists, and nipples and groin are also affected. All household members must be treated with a lotion (permethrin) applied to the whole body and left overnight, and repeated in 1 week. Itching may persist for some weeks despite successful treatment.

See also Chapter 55 Eczema, psoriasis and skin tumours.

High-risk groups for depression

- Social issues (relationship difficulties, financial or housing problems, unemployment, bereavement)
- Chronic physical illnesses or terminal illnesses (heart disease, chronic lung disease, malignancy)
- Hormonal changes (pregnancy, postnatal, menopause)
- Previous episode of depression or other psychiatric disorders (anxiety disorder, drug or alcohol misuse, eating disorders, dementia)
- Drugs (beta-blockers, calcium channel blockers, anticonvulsants, oral contraceptives)
- Family history

Key features in depression history

- Pervasive low mood
- Loss of interest and enjoyment (anhedonia)

Additional features

- Disturbed sleep (insomnia, hypersomnia or early morning wakening)
- Change in appetite or weight
- Reduced energy, fatigue
- Poor concentration, indecisiveness
- Sense of worthlessness or guilt
- Feeling of hopelessness
- Psychomotor agitation/retardation
- Ideas or acts of self-harm or suicide

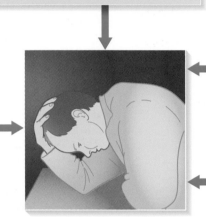

High-risk groups for suicide

- Male
- Advancing age
- Divorced > widowed > never married > married
- Social isolation
- Unemployment
- Certain professions (e.g. vets, pharmacists, farmers, doctors)
- Alcohol and substance misuse
- Psychiatric disorder (depression, schizophrenia, personality disorder especially with history of deliberate self-harm)
- Admission/recent discharge from psychiatric hospital
- Previous suicide attempt(s)
- Institutionalised (e.g. prison, army)
- Serious medical illness (e.g. cancer)

Treatment

NB: Physical exercise has been shown to improve mood and reduce anxiety (aim for 30 minutes, five times a week)

Mild depression

- Active monitoring (follow-up at regular intervals without formal intervention)
- Low intensity psychosocial intervention (e.g. guided self-help, computer-based or group cognitive behavioural therapy [CBT])
- Do not use antidepressant medication routinely

Moderate depression

- Low intensity psychosocial interventions plus
- Antidepressant medication
- Consider high intensity psychosocial intervention if symptoms persist despite above measures (e.g. individual CBT, psychotherapy)

Severe depression

- High intensity psychosocial intervention plus
- Antidepressant medication
- Consider referral to secondary care
- Urgent referral if high risk of suicide, psychotic symptoms, severe agitation or self-neglect
- Electroconvulsive therapy (ECT) may be considered in severe, unresponsive depression

Bereavement: The Five Stages of Grief

Elisabeth Kubler-Ross introduced a model describing five 'Stages of Grief'. It is important to remember that everyone responds differently to loss and that people may progress through the stages in a different order, or skip stages entirely. Up to a third of bereaved people go on to develop a depressive illness. While you should reassure patients that certain emotions are to be expected after bereavement, it is important to recognise depressive illnesses in bereaved people

1. **Denial** – feel shocked, 'numb' and refuse to believe what has happened
2. **Anger** – directed towards medical professionals, family/friends, or the person who has died
3. **Bargaining** – may occur during an illness or after a death; irrationally attempt to 'make deals' in order to change what has happened
4. **Depression** – all of the typical features may be experienced as part of the bereavement process
5. **Acceptance** – begin to think about other things and goals for the future

General Practice at a Glance, First Edition. Paul Booton, Carol Cooper, Graham Easton, and Margaret Harper.

Depression in primary care

Depression affects around 2.3 million people in the UK at any one time and is the third most common reason for people going to see their GP. The diagnosis is not always straightforward: patients may be concerned about the stigma of mental illness (particularly in certain cultures) or they may **somatise** (experience their depression as a physical symptom such as generalised body pain). It is therefore extremely important that GPs are alert to the possibility of depression, particularly in high risk groups (see Figure 57).

History

As with other mental health problems, a good history is key to diagnosis and may also be therapeutic for the patient. Start with open questions and allow the patient time to explain how they are feeling in their own words. They may feel able to tell you everything straight away, or it may take a few consultations to establish rapport. They may cry and there may be long periods of silence. Allow the patient to direct the history, but ensure that you have covered the key points:

- Clarify what the patient means by 'depressed'.
- Any obvious events that may have triggered these feelings?
- How long have they been feeling this way?
- Do they no longer enjoy things that they used to get pleasure from?
- Has sleep and/or appetite changed?
- Is concentration or memory affected?
- Do they feel fatigued, lethargic or 'slowed down'?
- Any physical symptoms, such as sexual dysfunction, headaches, pain or digestive problems?
- Is the way that they feel impacting on their functioning at work or home?
- Who is at home with them? Are they aware?
- Ask specifically about self-harm or suicidal ideation.
- Any similar episodes before and how were they treated?
- Any other psychiatric illnesses or chronic physical illnesses?
- Clarify current medication, alcohol and illicit drug use.
- Any history of mental illness in the family?

Examination

While taking your history, you should be carrying out a **mental state examination:**

- **Appearance** may be normal, or there may be evidence of self-neglect, weight loss or gain or a smell of alcohol. The patient may be tearful, avoid eye contact or appear distant, anxious or fidgety.
- **Speech** may be monotonic, slow or hesitant and the patient may appear distracted or lose track of the conversation.
- **Mood** may be both subjectively and objectively low, or there may be a disparity between the feelings they are describing and their affect.
- In very severe depression there may be **psychotic** features (such as auditory hallucinations), with loss of **insight**.

Investigations

Certain physical illnesses can cause symptoms like depression (such as hypothyroidism and anaemia). Try to avoid unnecessary investigations but it may be appropriate to do some baseline tests such as full blood count and thyroid function tests to exclude these conditions.

Management

Treatment can be based on psychosocial interventions and/or drug treatment, depending on severity and patient choice (see Figure 57). It is important that you agree a shared management plan with the patient in order to improve concordance and outcome.

Non-drug treatments

- **Information and self-help:** leaflets, websites, books, exercise, diet
- **Counselling or psychotherapy:** reflective listening
- **Cognitive behavioural therapy (CBT):** group, individual or self-directed via books or computer programmes.

Drug treatments

The most commonly used group of antidepressants are **selective serotonin reuptake inhibitors (SSRIs; e.g. citalopram, fluoxetine, paroxetine)**. These are used first line because they are better tolerated and safer in overdose than other classes of antidepressants. SSRIs can take 2 weeks or more to start having an effect, and can worsen anxiety, agitation and suicidal ideation in the early weeks, so regular review is important. Medication should be continued for 6 months following remission and withdrawn gradually to avoid withdrawal effects which may be severe in some cases.

Other antidepressants include **venlafaxine, mirtazepine**, tricyclic antidepressants (e.g. **lofepramine, amitriptyline**). Be aware that some patients may take the popular herbal remedy St John's Wort; it is on sale to the public but can have important interactions with conventional medications.

Assessing suicide risk

Assessing suicide risk is crucial when seeing someone with depression. Although it may feel uncomfortable, there is no evidence that asking someone about suicidal intentions makes them any more likely to commit suicide. Ensure that you prepare the patient by signposting clearly what you are about to ask and why, and explain that these are routine questions. Use a gradual approach, starting with questions such as: 'Do you ever feel like harming yourself? And, depending on the patient's answers, working up to a more direct question such as 'Do you ever feel that you would be better off dead?'

Ask the patient to describe their **suicidal thoughts**, and assess their level of intent. Ask if they have made **active plans** (such as hoarding tablets, writing a note) and look for evidence of hopelessness, guilt or high impulsivity. Has there been an accumulation of **psychosocial stressors** (work/money/relationship) that have triggered their current feelings? Check if something is **stopping them from acting** (such as the impact on their family) and ask about **previous suicide attempts or self-harming behaviours**, other **mental health issues** or **abuse of alcohol and/or illicit drugs**. Certain groups are at increased **risk of suicide** (see Figure 57), which must also be considered part of your risk assessment. It may also be appropriate to briefly check for thoughts of harm toward others.

If you feel that they are low risk, offer regular contact, psychosocial intervention or drug treatment as indicated and signpost to suicide prevention charities. If you have concerns about patient safety, refer urgently to mental health specialists who will attempt to support the patient in the community but admit them to hospital if necessary.

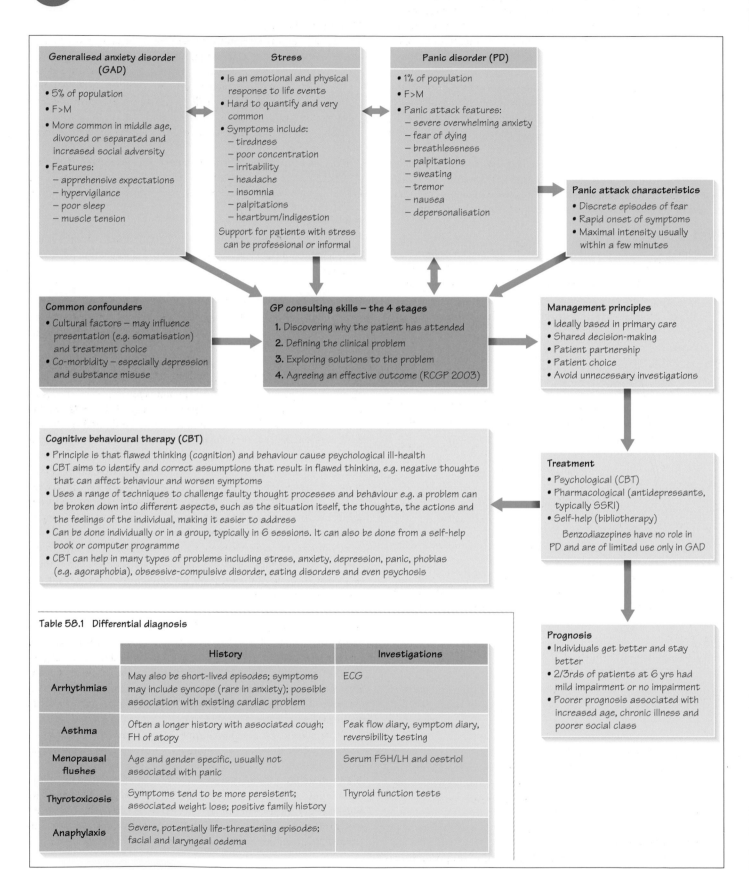

Generalised anxiety disorder (GAD)

- 5% of population
- F>M
- More common in middle age, divorced or separated and increased social adversity
- Features:
  – apprehensive expectations
  – hypervigilance
  – poor sleep
  – muscle tension

Stress

- Is an emotional and physical response to life events
- Hard to quantify and very common
- Symptoms include:
  – tiredness
  – poor concentration
  – irritability
  – headache
  – insomnia
  – palpitations
  – heartburn/indigestion

Support for patients with stress can be professional or informal

Panic disorder (PD)

- 1% of population
- F>M
- Panic attack features:
  – severe overwhelming anxiety
  – fear of dying
  – breathlessness
  – palpitations
  – sweating
  – tremor
  – nausea
  – depersonalisation

Panic attack characteristics

- Discrete episodes of fear
- Rapid onset of symptoms
- Maximal intensity usually within a few minutes

Common confounders

- Cultural factors – may influence presentation (e.g. somatisation) and treatment choice
- Co-morbidity – especially depression and substance misuse

GP consulting skills – the 4 stages

1. Discovering why the patient has attended
2. Defining the clinical problem
3. Exploring solutions to the problem
4. Agreeing an effective outcome (RCGP 2003)

Management principles

- Ideally based in primary care
- Shared decision-making
- Patient partnership
- Patient choice
- Avoid unnecessary investigations

Cognitive behavioural therapy (CBT)

- Principle is that flawed thinking (cognition) and behaviour cause psychological ill-health
- CBT aims to identify and correct assumptions that result in flawed thinking, e.g. negative thoughts that can affect behaviour and worsen symptoms
- Uses a range of techniques to challenge faulty thought processes and behaviour e.g. a problem can be broken down into different aspects, such as the situation itself, the thoughts, the actions and the feelings of the individual, making it easier to address
- Can be done individually or in a group, typically in 6 sessions. It can also be done from a self-help book or computer programme
- CBT can help in many types of problems including stress, anxiety, depression, panic, phobias (e.g. agoraphobia), obsessive-compulsive disorder, eating disorders and even psychosis

Treatment

- Psychological (CBT)
- Pharmacological (antidepressants, typically SSRI)
- Self-help (bibliotherapy)

  Benzodiazepines have no role in PD and are of limited use only in GAD

Prognosis

- Individuals get better and stay better
- 2/3rds of patients at 6 yrs had mild impairment or no impairment
- Poorer prognosis associated with increased age, chronic illness and poorer social class

Table 58.1 Differential diagnosis

	History	Investigations
Arrhythmias	May also be short-lived episodes; symptoms may include syncope (rare in anxiety); possible association with existing cardiac problem	ECG
Asthma	Often a longer history with associated cough; FH of atopy	Peak flow diary, symptom diary, reversibility testing
Menopausal flushes	Age and gender specific, usually not associated with panic	Serum FSH/LH and oestriol
Thyrotoxicosis	Symptoms tend to be more persistent; associated weight loss; positive family history	Thyroid function tests
Anaphylaxis	Severe, potentially life-threatening episodes; facial and laryngeal oedema	

General Practice at a Glance, First Edition. Paul Booton, Carol Cooper, Graham Easton, and Margaret Harper.

122 © 2013 Paul Booton, Carol Cooper, Graham Easton, and Margaret Harper. Published 2013 by Blackwell Publishing Ltd.

Anxiety disorders cover a wide spectrum of illness including presentations of acute overwhelming anxiety (e.g. panic attacks) or more generalised persistent anxiety (e.g. generalised anxiety disorder). Panic attacks may be related to specific situations or stimuli (e.g. phobias) or may have no obvious precipitant (e.g. panic disorder).

Panic disorder (PD; see also Chapter 38) is where the patient experiences regular panic attacks without any obvious precipitant, in the absence of any other psychiatric illness. Generalised anxiety disorder (GAD) refers to patients who have persistent anxiety symptoms (>6 months) without panic attacks, agoraphobia or other marked phobic symptoms.

These are all common in primary care. The impact of anxiety disorders is significant for both the affected individual and society in terms of distress, loss of work and productivity and use of NHS resources. There is a genetic predisposition for both GAD and PD.

History

The challenge in taking a history is to disentangle 'the chaos of the first presentation' into a clinical syndrome that allows a management plan to be developed (NICE). There are no validated screening tools that reliably identify anxiety disorder so you need high level consulting skills to make an accurate diagnosis. Patients with anxiety disorders often fear they are suffering from a physical illness and it may take many consultations to arrive at a proper diagnosis. Panic attacks are usually relatively easy to diagnose although more generalised anxiety may be harder to identify (see Figure 58).

As with all psychological problems, the **therapeutic alliance** between patient and clinician is critical. Start with open questions to establish the nature of the problem.
• Take time to establish their concerns and expectations. 'What was the worst thing you thought was happening?' and 'What were you hoping I might do for you?'
• Are there obvious precipitating causes (e.g. going outside)? This suggests a phobic disorder.
• Establish a personal history, including any self-medication.
• Have they attended A&E? If so, what investigations were done?
• Is there a family history of anxiety disorders?
• Presentations can vary and diagnosis can be made more difficult by cultural factors (some patients are more likely to somatise) and co-morbidity (particularly anxiety with depression and substance misuse). Take time to elicit a thorough social history including drug and alcohol consumption.
• Be sure you understand the impact of the patient's symptoms on their social functioning.

Examination

As you talk to the patient, assess their mental state (see Chapter 57).

Differential diagnosis

Common conditions that might be mistaken for panic attacks include those shown in Table 58.1. Some patients are suffering from stress rather than anxiety or panic disorder. Stress can also be a trigger or a result of mental illness.

Investigations

You may need to exclude physical illness with appropriate investigations. If needed, these tests are best performed from primary care, not A&E. Avoid unnecessary or untargeted investigations as they can reinforce the patient's belief that there is physical illness.

Management

There are clear advantages to services being based in primary care as they are more acceptable to patients and associated with lower non-attendance rates. But there may be instances when a particular intervention is not available locally or the patient turns it down.

Where significant co-morbidities exist, identify the biggest problem and treat that first.

When anxiety and depression co-exist, always treat depression first (see Chapter 57).

It is especially important to uphold the principles of shared decision-making, patient partnership and patient choice as these improve concordance and outcomes.

Treatment

In addition to continued and sensitive patient support, treatment options (in order of long-term effectiveness) include the following.

Psychological help (CBT)

Cognitive behavioural therapy (CBT) is the treatment of choice. This is ideally delivered by a trained therapist, in weekly sessions of 1–2 hours over a 4-month period.

Pharmacological therapy (SSRI antidepressants)

Benzodiazepines have **no** role in the management of panic disorder, and are of limited short term use only (2–4 weeks) in the treatment of GAD. Drug treatment should be limited to the use of antidepressants with a licence for anxiety disorder, usually a selective serotonin reuptake inhibitor (SSRI). The choice of drug depends on a number of variables including possible interactions, previous response to therapy and likelihood of self-harm. Discuss possible side effects and withdrawal symptoms but reassure your patient that the drugs are not addictive. For drugs with equal effectiveness, consider cost too. Titrate the dose to the response.

Monitor your patient's response, and be ready to change treatments if necessary. Most SSRIs take 4–6 weeks to work. If there is no benefit after 12 weeks, consider another antidepressant from a different group.

Self-help (bibliotherapy, self-help groups)

Give your patient (and if appropriate the family too) literature about anxiety disorder and panic attacks. This should be jargon-free and based on CBT principles. There is some evidence for the use of computerised CBT as a self-help tool and some patients prefer it. Remember that exercise benefits mental health, so discuss this too.

There should be a stepped approach to care, with referral to secondary care should two or more interventions not prove helpful.

Prognosis

Individuals do get better and remain better. Two-thirds of patients with anxiety disorder followed up at 6 years reported either mild impairment or no impairment at all. Poorer prognosis was associated with increased age, chronic illness and lower social class.

Table 59.1 Effects of alcohol and drug use

Effect of excess alcohol	Effects of drug use
• **Brain:** – Short-term – elation, slurred speech, malco-ordination, agression – Long-term – tiredness, neglect and reduced motivation, dependence, depression and anxiety, CVA, Wernicke's encephalopathy and Korsakoff's Syndrome – Withdrawal – anxiety, fits, delirium tremens • **Face:** – Jaundice, facial injury, rhinophyma, premature ageing – Throat – mouth and larynx cancer • **Chest:** Spider naevi, breast cancer, reduced immunity – colds, pneumonia • **Heart:** Hypertension, cardiomyopathy, heart failure • **Upper abdomen:** Dyspepsia, gastritis, ulcer disease, oesophageal cancer, varices, pancreatitis, diabetes • **Central abdomen:** Central weight gain, ascites, malnutrition, caput medusa • **Hands:** Tremor, Dupuytren's contracture • **Pelvis:** Erectile dysfunction, infertility, low birth weight babies, fetal alcohol syndrome • **Legs/bones:** Myopathy Haematological dysfunction, thrombocytopenia, anaemia • **Feet:** Peripheral neuropathy	• **Brain:** – Inappropriate behaviour – impulsive, drowsy, aggressive – Neglect and reduced motivation – Chaotic behaviour – Psychiatric illness – overdose (accidental or deliberate); depression/anxiety; schizophrenia • **Face:** – Short term – pupil constriction/dilation (opiate/ stimulants) – Longer term – nasal discharge, septal perforation (stimulants esp cocaine) • **Chest:** – Short term – (stimulants, opiate withdrawal): tachycardia and tachypnoea – Short term – (opiates, depressants): respiratory depression – Long term – (drug smoking): lung damage • **Arms:** Track marks (IV use – potential HIV, Hep B and C) • **Abdomen:** Weight loss and malnutrition, (withdrawal and overdose): diarrhoea, vomiting, abdominal pain • **Liver:** Fatty liver, cirrhosis, hepatitis, hepatomegaly, cancer • **Hands:** – Short term – (stimulants, withdrawal opiates and benzodiazepines): tremor/twitches • **Pelvis:** Sexually transmitted disease, high risk sexual practices

Figure 59.1(a) Alcohol units

Drink
25 ml single spirit shot (40%) = 1 unit
125 ml glass wine (12.5%) = 1.5 units
568 ml pint of beer (4%) = 2 units
750 ml bottle of wine (12.5%) = 9 units
750 ml bottle of spirits (12.5%) = 30 units

Government advises alcohol consumption should not regularly exceed:

♂ **Men**
3–4 units daily

♀ **Women**
2–3 units daily

(source: Office for National Statistics)

► Child at risk – is the patient with the alcohol or drug problem responsible for any children?
► Does the patient ever drive while under the influence of alcohol or drugs (see DVLA guidance)?
► Delirium tremens: major withdrawal symptoms after dependent drinker stops drinking.
► Wernicke's encephalopathy (nystagmus, ophthalmoplegia, ataxia) and Korsakoff's syndrome (confabulation) – both secondary to thiamine deficiency in excessive alcohol use.
► Decompensated liver disease: signs of acute liver disease (encephalopathy, ascites, jaundice). often triggered after binge drinking.
► Infection from injecting drugs with a dirty needle or unsterile diluent.

(b) Fast Alcohol Screening Test (FAST)

Scoring – a total of 3+ indicates hazardous or harmful drinking					
Question	0	1	2	3	4
1. How often do you have 8(men) / 6(women) or more drinks on one occasion?	Never	Less than monthly	Monthly	Weekly	Daily or almost daily
Only answer the following questions if your answer to the question above is monthly or less ...					
2. How often in the last year have you not been able to remember what happened when drinking the night before?	Never	Less than monthly	Monthly	Weekly	Daily or almost daily
3. How often in the last year have you failed to do what was expected of you because of drinking?	Never	Less than monthly	Monthly	Weekly	Daily or almost daily
4. Has a relative/friend/ doctor/health worker been concerned about your drinking or advised you to cut down?	No		Yes, but not in the last year		Yes, during the last year

(Adapted from Hodgson R. et al. The FAST alcohol screening test. Alcohol & Alcoholism 2002;37 (1); and Institute of Health & Society, Screening Tools for Alcohol Related Risk 2006, Newcastle University)

General Practice at a Glance, First Edition. Paul Booton, Carol Cooper, Graham Easton, and Margaret Harper.

124 © 2013 Paul Booton, Carol Cooper, Graham Easton, and Margaret Harper. Published 2013 by Blackwell Publishing Ltd.

GPs have an important role in recognising, assessing and supporting people with problem alcohol or illicit drug misuse. Patients can behave in challenging ways; it is important to adopt a patient-centred and non-judgemental approach.

Alcohol

Alcohol misuse is becoming a major public health problem. Twenty-six per cent of the UK population drink more than government limits, either by regular over-consumption or by binge drinking (large amounts of alcohol in a short space of time). Some patients become dependent on alcohol; physical and psychological addiction can then disrupt their life. It can also be dangerous when these patients stop drinking suddenly.

History

Remember risk factors for alcohol misuse:
• Previous personal or family history of alcohol misuse
• Unemployment or alcohol at work (e.g. publican)
• Social/personal/financial/legal problems
• Lack of social support or drug use.

Patients are often coy about their alcohol consumption, so it's important to be non-judgemental and sensitive. It may help to explain that asking about alcohol is routine for all patients. Screening tools (e.g. questionnaires such as FAST, see Figure 59b) can help spot problem drinkers.

Examination

Alcohol misuse can cause a huge range of signs and symptoms (see Table 59.1 for potential presentations and complications of alcohol misuse and what to look out for on examination).

Investigations

• **FBC:** MCV ↑, platelets ↓
• **LFTs:** gamma-glutamyl transpepsidase (GGT) ↑, aspartate aminotransferase (AST) ↑, bilirubin ↑
• **Lipids:** total cholesterol ↑ (1–2 units a day → ↑ high density lipoprotein [HDL] cholesterol)
• **Ultrasound:** fatty liver → hepatitis → cirrhosis.

Management

Prevention is better than cure – identifying alcohol problems early is important.

Non-dependent drinkers, brief advice can help 1 in 8 people reduce their drinking (e.g. discussing with patients the risk of their current consumption, the benefits of cutting down and negotiating a realistic plan together).

Dependent drinkers are at risk of withdrawal symptoms if they stop drinking suddenly so they may need medical management of assisted withdrawal (e.g. using a reducing dose of chlordiazepoxide over 7–14 days). **Mild or moderately dependent** drinkers can often be managed by GPs in the community. For **more severe dependence**, specialist input is required – usually from community support workers or drug and alcohol centres. The patient will need dietary supplementation with vitamins (especially thiamine) and they may need admission for intravenous thiamine replacement if they have signs of Wernicke's encephalopathy or Korsakoff's syndrome. Multi-disciplinary support is key to prevent relapse (psychosocial interventions, Alcoholics Anonymous, family and carer support). Consider medications such as acamprosate (helps to maintain abstinence) or disulfiram (causes unpleasant reactions to even small amounts of alcohol).

Drugs

The definition of drug misuse varies according to personal perspective, cultural and political beliefs, and local legislation. In the UK about 10% of adults (16–59 years), 22% of young adults (16–24 years) and 15% of young people (11–15 years) report illicit drug use in the last year. Cannabis is the most likely drug to be used across all age groups, but of those presenting for help and treatment, opioids are the main drug of abuse. Drug use for recreational purposes is particularly common today and may be relevant to many of your patients.

History

The risk factors for drug misuse are similar to those for alcohol misuse (see above). If you think your patient may be using drugs, consider:
• **Basic details:** identification, address (or homeless).
• **Social set up:** co-habiters, family (partner/children at risk), employment, finances, criminal background.
• **Medical background:** infectious diseases, psychiatric illness, overdose history.
• **Drug use:** details of current and past use, awareness of/exposure to risks (e.g. sexually or intravenously transmitted disease).
• **Other signs that may alert you to substance misuse:** atypical use of services frequently late or non-attendance; heavy out-of-hours attendance; work and/or school trouble, sickness, poor performance, truancy, family disruption or criminal involvement, self-neglect, frequent or atypical physical symptoms.

Examination

Patients often present with physical symptoms that mimic other diseases (for potential presentations of drug use and misuse see Table 59.1).

Investigations

• Consider urine toxicology to confirm drug misuse.
• FBC, LFTs, hepatitis B, C and HIV (counselling and consent first).

Management

Negotiating contracts or agreements with the patient and boundary setting can help you overcome some of the challenges of caring for drug users. Your aim is to reduce drug-related morbidity and mortality – you can encourage health checks, promote general care (contraception, cervical screening) and reduce infectious disease related to habits:
• Education-safer use of drugs (e.g. needle exchange), sex education, self-help groups (e.g. Narcotics Anonymous).
• Prevention: hepatitis B immunisation if currently unaffected.
• Treatment options (often lead by specialist GPs):
   ○ abstinence –help the patient stop taking drugs altogether
   ○ manage dependence (e.g. methadone for opiate dependence or detoxification).
• Maintenance: as with alcohol, multi-disciplinary support is key to prevent relapse.

(a) Anorexia nervosa and bulimia nervosa

Aetiology of anorexia nervosa (AN): Includes
- Sociocultural factors-idealisation of thinness
- Peer pressure
- Academic or job pressures
- Genetic
- Family influences – high expectations
- Personality – perfectionist, obsessive
- In children think of child abuse

Diagnosis of anorexia nervosa – female : male ratio 10:1
– There are 4 main criteria for diagnosis:
- **BMI <17** (not so useful for children and adolescents)
- **Intentional weight loss by** dieting, self-induced vomiting, taking laxatives, slimming pills or diuretics. In Type 1 diabetics-reducing insulin. Excessive exercise
- **Distorted body image** – see themselves as being fat even when they are thin
- **Widespread endocrine disorder** of the pituitary-hypothalamic axis leading to amenorrhea in women (note if they take OC will have bleeds), loss of libido in men and poor growth or delayed puberty in children

Physical signs
- Thin and emaciated BMI<17.5
- Dry skin, lanugo hair (fine hair over the upper body and face)
- Feel the cold
- Signs of repeated vomiting – dental decay
- Anaemia
- CVS – orthostatic hypotension, bradycardia, arrhythmias (secondary to electrolyte imbalance)
- Osteoporosis
- Poor growth in children –or static wt. during a growth spurt – delayed puberty

The patient is at high risk
- BMI <13.5 (Note BMI and blood tests alone are not adequate markers of risk)
- Excess exercise plus low weight
- Rapidly fluctuating weight
- Medical complications – electrolyte imbalance – cardiac arrhythmias
- Depression, risk of suicide
- Associated substance abuse or self-harm

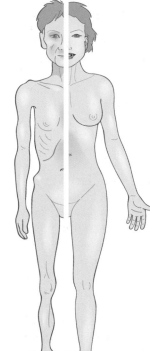

Aetiology of bulimia nervosa: Includes
- Sociocultural factors
- Parental or childhood obesity
- Criticism of weight
- Family – dieting in the family/mental health problems, parents obese
- Adverse life events
- History of anorexia
- History of sexual abuse

Diagnosis of bulimia nervosa: Includes
- Abnormal fear of getting fat
- Preoccupied with food
- Binging with loss of self-control
- Prevention of weight gain by self-induced vomiting
- Use of slimming pills, laxative abuse, thyroid preparations
- Diabetics – reduction of insulin

Physical signs
- Maybe none with normal weight
- Complications of repeated vomiting – dental decay, sore throat. Gastro-oesophageal reflux
- Haematemasis
- Abdominal pain
- Arrhythmias secondary to electrolyte disturbance from vomiting
- Osteoporosis
- Depression, signs of self-harm

The patient is at high risk
- Electrolyte disturbances
- Especially If there is low potassium due to vomiting leading to cardiac arrhythmias
- Risk of suicide

Examination and investigations
- Exclude other causes of weight loss – thyroid disease, inflammatory bowel disease, malignancy, diabetes (all rare). Do a physical examination
- Weigh regularly. Measure height and weight and calculate BMI, for children plot growth
- Take BP lying and standing
- Take the temperature and pulse
- Assess hydration
- Squat test – assesses muscle strength – Pt should be able to stand from squatting without holding on or using arms. Useful indicator of severity of AN

Tests – Fbc, ESR, U&E, TFT, LFT, blood glucose, urinanalysis, CPK. ECG especially if evidence of cardiac problems like bradycardia or electrolyte abnormalities

(b) SCOFF questionnaire

1. Have you ever felt so uncomfortably full that you have had to make yourself **Sick**?
2. Do you worry that you have ever lost **Control** over what you eat?
3. Have you recently lost or gained more than **One** stone in a three month period?
4. Do you believe yourself to be **Fat** when others think you are thin?
5. Would you say that **Food** dominates your life?

Score one point for each question. A score of two or more suggest anorexia or bulimia

(c) Obesity

Complications
- Orthopaedic problems
- Sleep apnoea – daytime tiredness
- Type 1 diabetes
- Dyslipidaemia
- Hypertension
- Increased incidence of ischaemic heart disease and strokes, certain cancers
- Worsening of asthma
- Psychological – low self-esteem, depression

Aetiology – multifactorial involving:
- The patient – less physical activity – car to school, sedentary activities – TV and computer time
- Family habits – type of diet, eating in front of TV, sedentary hobbies, obese parents. Bottle feeding/early weaning
- Nutrition – large food portions, high calorie snacks, TV suppers, ready meals
- Environment – lack of playing fields/safe play areas
- Advertising and food industry
- Genetic – not fully understood – leptin and ghrelin implicated
- Social and psychological problems leading to compensatory comfort eating
- Medical problems – rare e.g. Cushings, hypothyroidism, medication

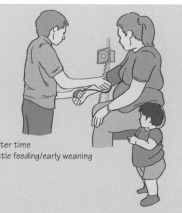

General Practice at a Glance, First Edition. Paul Booton, Carol Cooper, Graham Easton, and Margaret Harper.

Eating disorders are chronic conditions that usually start in adolescence and have profound effects on the patient's physical and mental health, employment, education, social and family life. Anorexia nervosa has the highest mortality of any psychiatric disorder, death being due to suicide or complications of starvation. In both anorexia and bulimia there is a pathological fear of becoming fat coupled with an obsession about body size and shape.

A practice with 10,000 patients will have two patients with anorexia nervosa and about 18 with bulimia. Younger children are now presenting with eating disorders and these can be the cause of poor weight gain or delayed puberty. Men can also develop eating disorders, often under-diagnosed. An early diagnosis improves outcome.

Because patients tend to deny their illness it can be difficult to spot in general practice unless you are alerted by worried parents, friends or the school. Patients may present with non-specific symptoms like lethargy, headaches and abdominal symptoms. Suspect the possibility of an eating disorder if a patient comes to see you with:

• A BMI <17.5 with no other cause. In children and adolescents do not rely on BMI – look at growth pattern. BMI >15% of expected BMI is more useful in children.
• Constipation, abdominal pain, signs of starvation or vomiting.
• Amenorrhoea for more than 3 months (bulimics may have amenorrhoea with a normal weight).
• Request for a diet when their weight is patently normal.
• Poorly controlled type 1 diabetes – may be using reduction of their insulin dose to lose weight.
• Children with poor weight gain or delayed puberty.

The SCOFF questionnaire is useful as a screening tool. NICE recommends that GPs should be responsible for the initial diagnosis, participate in shared care and recognise any emergency.

History

Taking a history in patients with anorexia or bulimia is not easy. **They may have faced criticism about their condition so your first task is to gain the patient's confidence and trust, to be supportive and non-judgemental.**

It can be difficult to ask direct questions. Ask:
• How the patient sees their weight and ideal weight.
• Diet and exercise.
• Vomiting or bingeing, laxative abuse, diet pills.
• Any physical symptoms like constipation, abdominal pain, menstrual or dental problems?
• Family history including family dynamics, any mental illness or stress in the family.
• Is there employment or educational pressures?
• Has the patient ever self-harmed or abused drugs or alcohol? This is common in bulimia.
• Enquire about depression, suicidal ideation and mood disturbances.

Management

Anorexia nervosa

• Refer to a specialist eating disorder clinic unless the condition is mild and responding to supportive measures.
• Support the patient and the family. Explain that the length of treatment varies but may be for years.
• Look after the physical health. Monitor diabetics carefully.
➤ Recognise medical emergencies and refer serious complications.

• Screen for osteoporosis.
• Look for risk factors and substance misuse.
• Medication has not been shown to be of any benefit.
• With children and adolescents family therapy has been shown to be effective.
• Short-term therapy is of little value but longer term therapy has been shown to be of value.

Bulimia nervosa

• Provide support and information (leaflets and books on self-help). A food diary may helpful. Refer for counselling or CBT-BN (specially adapted cognitive behaviour therapy for bulimia).
• Drug treatment – usually SSRIs.
• **Be alert to substance and alcohol misuse, depression and the possibility of suicide.**
• Look after physical problems.
• Refer to secondary care if there is failure to respond treatment. Refer immediately if the bulimia is severe.

Obesity

Obesity is a major health problem. In adults it is defined as a BMI >30 and in children a BMI >98th centile plus your clinical judgement. Obesity carries the risk of chronic medical problems. The psychological impact can be huge, with social isolation and poor self-esteem.

Childhood obesity

One in 10 children are obese by school age. The child may present because:
• Parents' own request or via the school nurse or health visitor.
• Because the child has been teased at school.
• Opportunistic screening.

Many parents do not appreciate their child is obese or the associated health risks. The consultation needs tact and support from the GP. Take a full history, including the weight of family members. Explore their eating habits. Ask about exercise, TV and computer time. Assess the motivation for change. Plot the height and weight. Test the urine. If indicated carry out a physical examination to exclude rare organic causes of obesity. Look for risk factors like asthma and psychological distress. Involve the child and family in a management plan with **realistic** goals. A food diary may help. Consider referral to a dietitian.

Prevention: During antenatal care, target high risk families (e.g. obesity in the mother or father) and continue education for obesity throughout the Child Health Programme. Promote facilities for exercise, safe play areas, education in nurseries and schools.

Adult obesity

Patients may self-refer or be picked up because of an associated medical problem. Enquire why they want to lose weight, and assess their motivation. Take a history asking about their lifestyle, diet, employment and if they smoke. Identify any underlying cause that may cause weight gain like medication, underlying disease (e.g. hypothyroidism). Are there any psychological, social problems or depression that may lead to comfort eating?

Calculate the BMI, measure the BP, lipid profile and blood sugar.

Management is not easy and includes weight management clinics, education about diet, supportive psychotherapy and CBT. Drugs only have a limited value. In severe obesity refer for possible bariatric surgery.

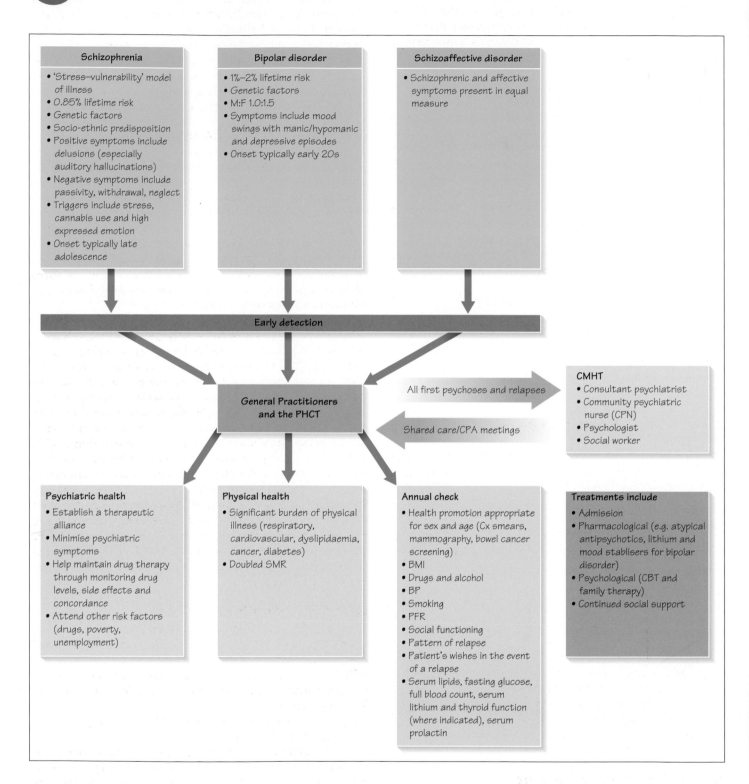

Schizophrenia

- 'Stress–vulnerability' model of illness
- 0.85% lifetime risk
- Genetic factors
- Socio-ethnic predisposition
- Positive symptoms include delusions (especially auditory hallucinations)
- Negative symptoms include passivity, withdrawal, neglect
- Triggers include stress, cannabis use and high expressed emotion
- Onset typically late adolescence

Bipolar disorder

- 1%–2% lifetime risk
- Genetic factors
- M:F 1.0:1.5
- Symptoms include mood swings with manic/hypomanic and depressive episodes
- Onset typically early 20s

Schizoaffective disorder

- Schizophrenic and affective symptoms present in equal measure

Early detection

General Practitioners and the PHCT

All first psychoses and relapses

Shared care/CPA meetings

CMHT

- Consultant psychiatrist
- Community psychiatric nurse (CPN)
- Psychologist
- Social worker

Psychiatric health

- Establish a therapeutic alliance
- Minimise psychiatric symptoms
- Help maintain drug therapy through monitoring drug levels, side effects and concordance
- Attend other risk factors (drugs, poverty, unemployment)

Physical health

- Significant burden of physical illness (respiratory, cardiovascular, dyslipidaemia, cancer, diabetes)
- Doubled SMR

Annual check

- Health promotion appropriate for sex and age (Cx smears, mammography, bowel cancer screening)
- BMI
- Drugs and alcohol
- BP
- Smoking
- PFR
- Social functioning
- Pattern of relapse
- Patient's wishes in the event of a relapse
- Serum lipids, fasting glucose, full blood count, serum lithium and thyroid function (where indicated), serum prolactin

Treatments include

- Admission
- Pharmacological (e.g. atypical antipsychotics, lithium and mood stablisers for bipolar disorder)
- Psychological (CBT and family therapy)
- Continued social support

General Practice at a Glance, First Edition. Paul Booton, Carol Cooper, Graham Easton, and Margaret Harper.

With a prevalence of 5 per 1000, the psychoses pose significant challenges to patients, their families, the NHS and Social Services. Following the closure of large old-fashioned asylums in the 1980s and 1990s, national policy dictates that consultant psychiatrists and their community mental health teams (CMHTs) take the lead in the management of psychosis in the community ('care in the community').

However, it would be wrong to assume that primary care has a minor role. Patients with psychosis are significant users of general practice. Given the close contact GPs enjoy with their patients (they see 70–75% of their list at least once a year), first presentations are often made in primary care. Some 25% of patients with schizophrenia only see their GP and have no contact with CMHTs. Patients with psychosis also have a significantly increased risk of physical illness with double standardised mortality ratios (SMR).

Actively engaging with patients and CMHTs, GPs can ensure those with schizophrenia, bipolar disorder and schizo-affective disorder receive timely and effective support, keeping them as well as possible and out of hospital. Apart from the stress of an acute admission, schizophrenia alone is estimated to cost 5% of the NHS inpatient budget.

Key aims for primary care include the following:
1 Early detection of first episode and relapses
2 Early referral for treatment
3 Continued engagement over time
4 Reducing psychiatric symptoms
5 Improving and monitoring physical health
6 Relapse prevention.

Early detection of first episode and relapses

The psychoses are 'stress–vulnerability' models of illness, with genetic factors and social stressors both having a role in aetiology. There are ethnic variations, with higher prevalence in the African-Caribbean and black African communities as well as in the refugee population generally.

Typically presenting in late adolescence, those who develop schizophrenia often have a prodromal period during which their families and friends notice:
▶ Uncharacteristic behaviour
▶ Social withdrawal
▶ Lack of interest and motivation.
When families express these concerns, GPs must consider the possibility of an early psychotic illness.

The duration of undiagnosed psychosis is an important concept. Early detection and treatment leads to a much better longer term prognosis. The first 2 years following a psychotic event are critical. If the patient can be kept well on therapy, they are much less likely to have a relapsing pattern of illness. Patients with chronic illness often have a typical pattern of relapse (e.g. increasing persecutory delusions) which GPs are well placed to notice.

Early referral for treatment

It is the GP's role to facilitate prompt referral to secondary care services for initiating therapy. The patient may be happy to be referred, or the GP may need to take part in a formal mental health assessment ending in a compulsory admission. Most mental health trusts have assertive outreach and crisis resolution teams that will see and assess patients in their own homes.

Continued engagement over time

Unfortunately, relapses are common with both schizophrenia (80%) and bipolar disorder (90%). Repeated relapses are invariably associated with further decline in social functioning, compounding problems. A good therapeutic alliance with the patient helps keep patients engaged and well. Many patients find primary care follow-up more acceptable and less stigmatising. Working closely with CMHTs and the care programme approach (CPA) also allows GPs to share information, and can target care more effectively.

Reducing psychiatric symptoms

While it may be impossible to eliminate all symptoms of psychosis, careful follow-up of drug tolerability and side effects can significantly improve concordance. Atypical antipsychotics are a vast improvement on older drugs, with fewer extra-pyramidal side effects (especially tardive dyskinesia). Bipolar patients on lithium and other mood stabilisers need regular serum monitoring to ensure the drug remains in the therapeutic range. Cognitive behavioural therapy (CBT, see Chapter 58) can help those patients with persistent delusions. Families caring for patients can also be helped to lower 'expressed emotion'. Remember that 10% of all patients with schizophrenia commit suicide.

Improving and monitoring physical health

All chronic psychoses are associated with long-term physical problems. Up to 90% of patients with relapsing schizophrenia smoke. They may also have problems from drug and alcohol use (dual diagnosis). With unemployment and associated poverty, lifestyle choices may be limited, making healthy eating and exercise harder. Rates for respiratory disease, cardiovascular disease and cancer are all higher. The newer atypical anti-psychotic drugs, while helping to control psychiatric symptoms, predispose patients to both diabetes and dyslipidaemia. Lithium therapy predisposes to hypothyroidism. Studies show that, despite being frequent consulters and having greater medical needs, these patients do not get the same level of health promotion input of other patients. It is to be hoped that this clinical despondency has been challenged by the Quality and Outcomes Framework (QOF 2004) targets for mental health requiring structured physical examination and assessment of risk (see Figure 61).

Relapse prevention

Given the distress and social decline linked with relapses, it's vital to do everything to reduce this risk. Several factors are associated with better outcomes:
• Early detection of first episodes and early treatment
• Maintenance of anti-psychotic medication for at least 2 years following a first psychosis
• Psychological interventions (CBT and family therapy)
• Continued social support.

Social support, including supportive accommodation, is extremely important as patients with chronic relapsing illness often function very poorly. GPs are well placed to look out for the signs of neglect. Home visits offer a good insight into social functioning. Working closely with CMHTs, GPs can help identify and treat other risk factors, such as stress and substance misuse. Unemployment is very high in this population so helping patients re-engage with their lives, through restarting work or study, is also constructive.

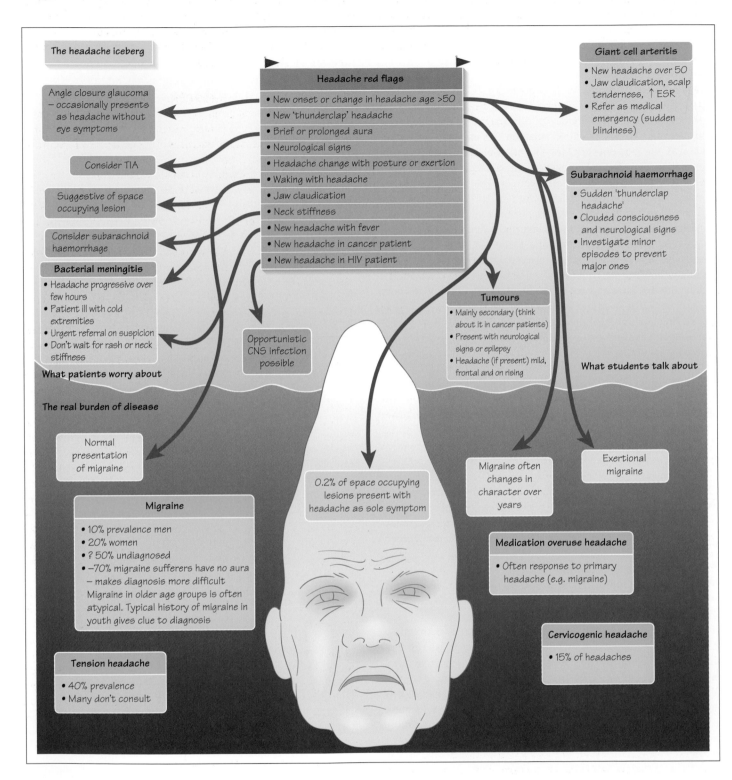

The headache iceberg

Headache red flags
- New onset or change in headache age >50
- New 'thunderclap' headache
- Brief or prolonged aura
- Neurological signs
- Headache change with posture or exertion
- Waking with headache
- Jaw claudication
- Neck stiffness
- New headache with fever
- New headache in cancer patient
- New headache in HIV patient

Giant cell arteritis
- New headache over 50
- Jaw claudication, scalp tenderness, ↑ ESR
- Refer as medical emergency (sudden blindness)

Angle closure glaucoma – occasionally presents as headache without eye symptoms

Consider TIA

Suggestive of space occupying lesion

Consider subarachnoid haemorrhage

Bacterial meningitis
- Headache progressive over few hours
- Patient ill with cold extremities
- Urgent referral on suspicion
- Don't wait for rash or neck stiffness

Opportunistic CNS infection possible

Subarachnoid haemorrhage
- Sudden 'thunderclap headache'
- Clouded consciousness and neurological signs
- Investigate minor episodes to prevent major ones

Tumours
- Mainly secondary (think about it in cancer patients)
- Present with neurological signs or epilepsy
- Headache (if present) mild, frontal and on rising

What students talk about

What patients worry about

The real burden of disease

Normal presentation of migraine

0.2% of space occupying lesions present with headache as sole symptom

Migraine often changes in character over years

Exertional migraine

Migraine
- 10% prevalence men
- 20% women
- ? 50% undiagnosed
- ~70% migraine sufferers have no aura – makes diagnosis more difficult
Migraine in older age groups is often atypical. Typical history of migraine in youth gives clue to diagnosis

Medication overuse headache
- Often response to primary headache (e.g. migraine)

Cervicogenic headache
- 15% of headaches

Tension headache
- 40% prevalence
- Many don't consult

General Practice at a Glance, First Edition. Paul Booton, Carol Cooper, Graham Easton, and Margaret Harper.

Headache is an enormously common presenting symptom in general practice. Headaches are a cause of great anxiety to patients, so exploring their concerns over the meaning of the headache is crucial. Meningitis or tumours are frequent concerns. Diagnosis is by history, with examination and investigations having a relatively minor role. A careful history is therefore critical and a headache diary (with medication use) is very helpful.

Migraine

To many patients migraine means any severe headache. So explore their symptoms and don't accept the diagnosis at face value. Equally, much mild headache is migraine: it is important to appreciate that migraine is a type, not a severity, of headache. Migraine is extremely common in practice, often undiagnosed or wrongly diagnosed, sometimes for many years. Understanding migraine and its treatment is essential for GPs.

There are a number of more or less distinct varieties of migraine.

Migraine with aura (previously classic migraine). Around 30% of patients get an aura, usually fortification spectra or a scotoma, less often paraesthesiae or rarely hemiplegia, the headache starts shortly after. The pain is unilateral, often felt as a pulsing headache behind the eye, but the pain may be temporal or occipital and may be across the whole head. Migraines may last 3 days or more; the duration is diagnostically helpful. Nausea, vomiting and photophobia (and sometimes phonophobia) are common. Patients avoid normal physical activity – typically lying down in a darkened room. Migraine commonly occurs on waking, often after a period of stress. Excess sleep, the 'Sunday morning headache' (often mistaken for a hangover) is common. This classic pattern may be lost in older age groups who may present with atypical headaches apparently for the first time. A careful exploration will often reveal typical migraine in their youth which is the clue to their present symptoms.

Migraine without aura (previously common migraine) can have all the above features except aura. It can also be a more vaguely described headache and as such more difficult to diagnose.

Exercise migraine is relatively uncommon presenting either as a generalised headache during or after exercise or more dramatically as an explosive headache coming (typically) at the climax of sexual intercourse. It is frightening and may require investigation for subarachnoid haemorrhage which it can closely resemble.

Treatment

Treatment for migraine involves lifestyle, preventative and acute aspects. A 'regular' lifestyle, regular bed and getting up times help Sunday morning headaches. Tiredness is a common precipitant, as is hypoglycaemia which may be a correctible factor in exercise migraine. Alcohol excess is a precipitant although often not temporally related, unlike the various food triggers for migraine (e.g. coffee, red wine, cheese, chocolate) where there is a clear relationship between trigger and symptoms (patients usually recognise this without medical prompting). Oestrogen-based contraceptives often worsen migraine. In acute treatment of migraine, simple analgesics (aspirin, or other NSAID in a hefty dose) taken in combination with an anti-emetic (domperidone – to counter gastric stasis, even if there are no gastric symptoms) is effective, especially if taken early. **Beware excessive analgesic use** (see chronic daily headache below). A short sleep often aborts an attack if the patient is able to do so. For patients with more severe symptoms Triptans administered either orally or parenterally (e.g. via nasal spray or injection), may abort acute attacks. If headaches are severe or frequent enough prophylaxis is useful but only effective in around 50% of patients. Beta-blockers or tricyclic antidepressants are most commonly used.

Other types of headache

Cluster headache is rare and probably overdiagnosed. It is most common in middle-aged males presenting with brief (15 minutes to a few hours) episodes of excruciating unilateral pain recurring over 2–3 weeks before remitting sponataneously.

Anxiety/tension headache is unsurprisingly common in primary care and with it the risk of over-diagnosis. Stress needs to be present, although may be unrecognised by the patient (such as the unsupported carer or high pressure business environment). The headache is classically described as a tight band round the head, although diagnostically more usefully is a (often diffuse) headache coming on through the day (and absent, or less severe on days when the pressure is relieved). While simple analgesics offer relief, removal of the cause or coping better with the stressor (perhaps through counselling) is a better solution.

Depression on occasion presents with headache, and headaches (and other aches and pains) are a frequent accompaniment of psychological malaise. Classically, the headache is described as a pressure on top of the head 'the weight of the world bearing down on you'. In the author's experience it is uncommon, but always check for depression.

Medication overuse headache is an important and under-recognised cause of sometimes debilitatingly severe headaches. Because analgesics are frequently taken for headaches it is easy to confuse the original cause with the effects of the treatment. The headache evolves over a few weeks with both symptoms and analgesic use becoming more frequent until headaches are more or less continuous and medication may be being taken pre-emptively. Patients taking painkillers more than 15 days a month (or 10 days for opiates) are at risk. Persuading patients to stop taking medication gives an immediate worsening of headache, but then improvement over the next 12 weeks.

Headaches arising from other structures. Headaches commonly present from radiation of **upper neck pain**, usually in older people from cervical spondylosis. Pain will typically be exacerbated by strain on the neck (e.g. from lifting). Tenderness in the neck may be present (as it may with tension type headaches). An X-ray of the cervical spine is unhelpful as there is little correlation between spondylitic changes and symptoms. Headaches are often wrongly blamed on **sinuses**, but only acute sinus disease causes pain. Refractive errors are commonly blamed but unusual in practice; a quick trip to the optician sorts this out one way or the other. Dental problems and temporo-mandibular dysfunction cause facial pain and sometimes headache.

Serious causes of headache

Patients and doctors worry about these **commonly**: they arise **rarely** (see Figure 62).

1. **'How do you feel when you first wake up in the morning?'**
   - Physical tiredness tends to be best after rest and worst after exertion
   - Psychological causes often bad all the time
   - Depressive illness symptoms often worse in the mornings

2. **'Do you have any sleep problems?'**
   - Early waking (depression) or difficulty getting off to sleep (anxiety), but any disturbed pattern of sleep may represent psychological morbidity
   - Sleep apnoea syndrome is becoming more common through increasing levels of obesity. Ask a partner for details of snoring or stopping breathing during sleep
   - Physical illness frequently disturbs sleep through interference with circadian rhythms (e.g. asthma and commonly in serious illnesses e.g. malignancy)
   - Elderly patients need less sleep, but may report this as a problem. Lifestyle pattern with sleeping in the day (consider in the elderly and unemployed) often result in insomnia and daytime sleepiness. (see Chapter 64)

3. **'What do you mean by tired/how does the tiredness affect you?'** – shortness of breath? physical weakness? mental exhaustion?

4. **'For how long have you felt tired?'** – was there a precipitating illness (e.g. influenza), event (e.g. a funeral), or change in social circumstances (e.g. birth of a child)? – Patients may fail to make the connection between life events and their symptoms
   - **'Have you had anything like this before?'** – explore previous symptoms and energy levels. **'Is this a new problem?'** – don't accept 'it's just my age' as a reason
   - **'What medication do you take?'** – many drugs produce tiredness (e.g. beta-blockers) or related symptoms (e.g. muscle fatigue from statins). OTC medications and alternative remedies all have side effects which the patient (or unwary doctor) may not expect. Alcohol in moderate doses can affect sleep adversely (which is important as many patients use it to help them sleep). Enquire for illicit drug use
   - **'Any other symptoms?'** – this is a situation where a full systems review may be useful. Unexplained weight change, precipitants of anaemia (such as heavy periods) and sleep disturbance and mood are particularly relevant. Always consider diabetes, though the classic symptoms of thirst and polyuria are often absent in type 2 disease. Remember 'silent cancers' – caecum and ovary particularly in older age groups
   - **'What else is going on in your life?'** – lifestyle factors: long working hours, a new child in the family, caring for an elderly relative can be physically and mentally exhausting and affect sleep. Patients may not have made the link or have unrealistic expectations about their ability to cope with life's stresses.
   - **'What do you think this is about?'** – the patients ideas about their illness may be revealing and may be entirely unexpected from the doctor's viewpoint, their concerns over what the symptoms represent can worsen the symptoms themselves (e.g. anxieties about cancer). With somatising patients the refusal to countenance any psychological explanation for their symptoms is itself revealing

Box. 63.2 Conditions where tiredness may be the main symptom

- Anaemia
- Hypothyroidism, and thyrotoxicosis (in the elderly the symptoms of both may be subtle)
- Obesity
- Numerous medications
- Depression & anxiety
- Chronic fatigue syndrome
- Sleep apnoea
- Chronic diseases, e.g. cancer, renal, liver and cardiac disease, autoimmune diseases (e.g. rheumatoid disease)
- Diabetes
- Infectious mononucleosis
- Haematological malignancies
- This list is not exhaustive!

Assessing anaemia
- Start with an FBC: – Is there anaemia? – If so what is the MCV and MCH?

MCV	MCH	Appearance	Likely diagnosis	Follow up
Low	Low	Hypochromic, microcytic	• Fe deficiency	Ferritin (low – reflects depleted Fe stores), Low Fe, High TIBC
High	High	Megaloblasts in peripheral blood (when severe)	• Folate, B12 deficiency • Chronic liver disease & hypothyroidism cause macrocytosis without anaemia • Recent blood loss: increased reticulocytes give high MCV (but should be identified on blood film)	B12 and folate (red cell folate more reliable), LFTs and TFTs for macrocytosis without anaemia
Anaemia with normal or confusing indices?				
Normal	Normal	Normal	• Anaemia of chronic diseases/renal disease	Ferritin (normal or raised), Low Fe, low TIBC
Variable	Variable	Variable	• Haemoglobinopathy	Hb electrophoresis will reveal most haemoglobino-pathies, but further investigation may be required

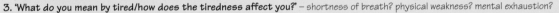

Tiredness is a common symptom in primary care, with causes ranging from psychological to social and physical (25%). It is a symptom common to many diseases where the overall pattern of symptoms makes the diagnosis relatively straightforward. Nevertheless patients may not realise the link between their illness and their tiredness and will be helped by a careful explanation.

History

The history is crucial: see Figure 63.

Examination

Look for pallor (an unreliable indicator of anaemia), obesity, hypothyroidism and thyrotoxicosis (and don't forget rare endocrine conditions like Cushing's and Addison's). Weight loss may be indicative of malignancy or thyrotoxicosis (although is most commonly psychosocial). Measure the patient's weight and calculate the BMI. Examination should be directed by the findings in the history.

Investigations to be considered in primary care: FBC (and vitamin B12, folate, serum iron and ferritin if warranted); U&E and LFT for renal and liver disease; TFT for thyroid problems; fasting glucose for diabetes; Monospot or Paul–Bunnell tests for infectious mononucleosis; vitamin D levels commonly reveal deficiency and may present with non-specific aches and pains or weakness. ESR/CRP are non-specific tests of inflammation and may be helpful in differentiating physical from psychological disease.

Chronic fatigue syndrome (CFS)

A relatively new syndrome of as yet unclear and contended aetiology. CFS can affect all sexes, races, socio-economic groups and ages, including children, but young and middle-aged women are most commonly affected. The symptoms are of protracted tiredness, particularly after exertion and often delayed for 24 hours. Onset may be acute after an illness (e.g. flu) or a stressful event, or may come on slowly. Symptoms are similar to those found in depression: sleep disturbance, muscle aches, palpitations, dizziness, cognitive problems (e.g. poor concentration), headaches, flu like symptoms. There is no diagnostic test available. NICE guidance (August 2007) describes a constellation of symptoms that should be present before making the diagnosis. The syndrome ranges in severity from mild to those who are wheelchair bound. The management recommended by NICE is a combination of physical therapy (graded exercise) and psychological (cognitive behaviour therapy) for both of which there is an evidence base. Symptomatic pharmacological treatment of pain (simple analgesics) and sleep disturbance (e.g. low dose tricyclics) may be helpful. Antidepressants and other psychopharmacological agents are often given, but evidence for their effectiveness is poor.

Obstructive sleep apnoea syndrome

A syndrome only identified 40 years ago characterised by irregular breathing at night caused by physical obstruction of the airway and excessive sleepiness during the day. It is most commonly seen in males of middle age (55–59 years) and somewhat less in women (60–64 years). Obesity, smoking and excess alcohol consumption are all risks.

Suspect the diagnosis with a story of excessive sleepiness, impaired daytime concentration and a sense of being unrefreshed by sleep. A history from a partner is very helpful and may reveal restlessness, snoring, choking in sleep and episodes of apnoea. Drugs may cause or exacerbate. Both sedatives and stimulants (including caffeine and alcohol) are associated with OSA as are beta-blockers and SSRIs.

Examination findings are non-specific. Obesity is common, but 50% of OSA patients are not clinically obese. Neck circumference is a much stronger predictor: a neck circumference of <37 cm has a very low risk, >48 cm a very high one. However, most men fall between these extremes and COPD patients with OSA do not have large necks.

Suspicion of the condition requires specialist assessment – polysomnography (a sleep EEG) is used to identify apnoeic and hypopnoeic episodes. Warn your patient of the risks of driving: the patient should declare their diagnosis symptoms to the DVLA. Any sleepiness while driving is (obviously) dangerous and falling asleep while driving a criminal offence.

Management includes sleep hygiene measures (e.g. reducing alcohol and sedatives, raising the bed head), stimulant drugs, ENT surgery to remove physical obstructions and continuous positive airways pressure (CPAP) ventilation.

Managing anaemia

Overwhelmingly, the most common anaemia seen in general practice is due to iron deficiency, with folate and B12 deficiencies some way behind. The improved longevity of chronic disease patients means GPs see more anaemia of chronic disease. Other anaemias are uncommon and generally require specialist help.

Iron is poorly absorbed by humans, stores are low and are quickly diminished. Menstruating women are most commonly affected because of menstrual iron loss with inadequate dietary replacement. You need neither overt menorrhagia nor an obviously poor diet for this to occur. Inadequate diet alone is an extremely common cause: faddy eaters, fast food eaters, the poor and the elderly are most at risk. A dietary history will help confirm this, but particularly in older age groups other causes should be excluded. The classic presentation of caecal carcinoma, of unexplained iron deficiency anaemia due to small but persistent gastrointestinal blood loss, is not uncommon, but is also true of any chronic, low grade bleeding. Oral iron replacement may be unpleasant – constipation and black stools (greenish black, unlike the brownish black of melaena) are common. Remember, many OTC remedies do not contain sufficient iron for adequate replacement.

Folic acid deficiency is normally dietary in origin except for pregnant women who have increased requirements. Beware the patient who when treated with folic acid quickly uses up stores of other haematinics, provoking other deficiencies e.g. subacute combined spinal degeneration (B12 deficiency).

While B12 deficiency may be nutritional, it is most commonly autoimmune due to destruction of gastric parietal cells and occasionally due to failure of absorption in the terminal ileum. A Schilling test is usually not necessary and simple replacement via regular intramuscular injections all that is required.

Haemoglobinopathies are common in ethnically diverse communities.

Anaemias of chronic diseases are usually secondary to chronic infection (e.g. TB), inflammation (especially the connective tissue diseases) and neoplasia. The anaemia of chronic renal failure is similar, but more directly linked to failure of renal erythropoietin production.

Sleep advice for patients

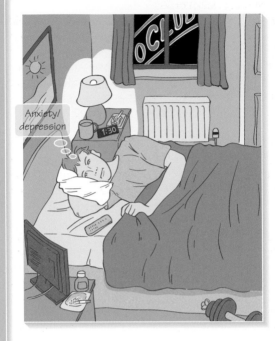

- **Limit stimulants and alcohol**
  - do not take caffeine or cigarettes (nicotine) six hours before bedtime. Cutting out caffeine completely may help. Some people use alcohol to relax but it may cause awakenings later

- **Do not have a large meal** just before bedtime; a light snack may be helpful

- **No strenuous exercise within four hours of bedtime** to avoid arousal, but exercise earlier in the day is helpful

- **Do not sleep or nap during the day** – even if tired, to establish a routine of wakefulness during the day and sleepiness at night

- **Avoid going to bed until drowsy** in the late evening to avoid the frustration of lying awake

- **If not asleep after 20 minutes** – then get up and go into another room to do something else, such as reading or watching TV, rather than brooding in bed. Go back to bed when sleepy. Repeat this as often as necessary until asleep

- **Sleep hygiene and stimulus control** are both offered as behavioural approaches to treat primary insomnia and have considerable overlap in their approaches

- **The bedroom** should be a quiet, relaxing place to sleep
  - it should not be too hot, cold, noisy or not comfortable
  - earplugs and eye shades may be useful
  - the bedroom should be dark; switch the light off once you get into bed and fit good curtains to stop early morning sunlight
  - do not use the bedroom for work, eating or television, to avoid stimulation before bedtime
  - consider moving alarm clock out of sight to prevent 'clock watching'
  - use an alarm to always get up at the same time each day of the week, however short the time asleep. Resist the temptation to 'lie-in' even after a poor night's sleep. Do not use weekends to 'catch up' on sleep, as this may upset the natural body rhythm that you have got used to in the week

- **Mood and atmosphere** – try to relax and 'wind down' with a routine before going to bed e.g. a stroll followed by a bath, some reading, and a warm drink (without caffeine) may be relaxing in the late evening

- **Get up at the same time every day** – any sleep deficit will increase the pressure for sleep the subsequent night, thereby helping establish more routine sleep

Box 64.1 Causes of insomnia

Primary Insomnia
a diagnosis of exclusion
- Without a co-morbid condition
- Accounting for around 30% of chronic insomnia cases

Secondary Insomnia
- Accounting for around 70% of chronic insomnia cases
  e.g. anxiety, depression, nocturia, arthritis, pain, sleep apnoea, dyspnoea, chronic illness, drugs and alcohol

- **Psychosocial stressors**
  - situational stress: occupational, relationships, financial, academic, medical
  - environmental stressors: noise
  - bereavement
- **Psychiatric disorders**
  - mood disorders: depression, bipolar disorder, dysthymia
  - anxiety disorders: generalised anxiety disorder, panic disorder, post-traumatic stress disorder
  - psychotic disorders: paranoia, schizophrenia, delusional disorder
- **Medical illness**
  - cardiovascular: angina, congestive heart failure
  - respiratory: chronic obstructive pulmonary disease, asthma
  - neurological: Alzheimer's disease, Parkinson's disease, head injury
  - endocrine: hyperthyroidism
  - rheumatological: fibromyalgia, chronic fatigue syndrome, osteoarthritis
  - gastrointestinal: gastroesophageal reflux disease, irritable bowel syndrome
  - parasomnias (sleep disorders): restless legs syndrome, sleep apnoea, circadian rhythm disorders
- **Drug and substance use**
  - excessive use of alcohol
  - after stopping heavy drinking sleep may be disturbed for several weeks
  - tobacco
  - recreational drugs
- **Medications**
  - antihypertensives: beta-blockers
  - lipid lowering: statins
  - antidepressants: selective serotonin reuptake inhibitors, venlafaxine, bupropion, duloxetine, monoamine oxidase
  - hormones: oral contraceptive pills, cortisone, thyroid supplement
  - sympathomimetics: albuterol, salmeterol, theophylline, pseudoephedrine

Box 64.2 Hypnotic drugs

Benzodiazepines
- Shorter acting – loprazolam, lorazepam, lormetazepam and temazepam
- Longer acting – diazepam, nitrazepam, and flurazepam not recommended because they may cause next day residual effect

Z-Drugs
- Zolpidem, Zopiclone, Zaleplon

General Practice at a Glance, First Edition. Paul Booton, Carol Cooper, Graham Easton, and Margaret Harper.

134 © 2013 Paul Booton, Carol Cooper, Graham Easton, and Margaret Harper. Published 2013 by Blackwell Publishing Ltd.

Insomnia can be very distressing and affects 10–30% of the population. It is more common in women and increases with age. Most adults require 7–9 hours sleep a night, although some people say they function on as little as 4 or as much as 10 hours. Key roles for the GP are to establish any underlying reasons for the insomnia such as depression, anxiety, medication side effects, lifestyle choices, sleep apnoea or chronic disease (see Box 64.1), and advise on sleep hygiene (see Figure 64).

Insomnia is either **primary** (no other contributing cause) or **secondary** (caused or affected by an underlying condition).

History

The following questions should help you to define the nature of the sleep problem:

• **Describe your sleeping difficulty.** Identify secondary causes of insomnia: look specifically for symptoms of anxiety and depression.

• **Describe your bedtime routine. What time do you go to bed? How long does it take getting to sleep? How long do you stay asleep?** If the time spent in bed is more than a few hours longer than the time spent sleeping the cause may be primary insomnia. Restricting the time in bed can improve sleep quality. Computer screen exposure may also delay sleep.

• **Any associated symptoms with awakenings?** Look for signs of a secondary cause (e.g. sleep apnoea). Physical problems may account for around 40% of cases of insomnia.

• **What time do you wake up?** Early morning awakening may be a symptom of depression.

• **When did problems start?** Have you had any other problems or difficulties during this time? Do symptoms correlate with other events (e.g. relationship breakdown or bereavement)? This may indicate anxiety, low mood or depression.

• **What is your usual or desired sleep duration?** Some patients may feel that they do not get enough sleep but are still able to function well during the day: this is not insomnia.

• **Do you sleep during the day?** This may reduce sleep pressure at night. Consider obstructive sleep apnoea which accounts for 9% of patients reporting poor sleep; symptoms include heavy snoring, pauses in breathing and gasping.

• **Do you drink tea/coffee/cola/alcohol or take tobacco/drugs?** Caffeine as well as prescription and non-prescription drugs may interfere with sleep (e.g. beta-blockers, selective serotonin re-uptake inhibitors, diuretics and sympathomimetic drugs).

Examination

Physical examination is useful in identifying secondary causes of insomnia; for example, high BMI (≥30) and neck circumference of ≥40 cm increase the risk of obstructive sleep apnoea.

Investigations

• Directed at secondary causes of insomnia (e.g. thyroid function tests to check for hyperthyroidism).
• EEG recordings made in a sleep laboratory may be useful if continuing concerns about the nature and extent of the insomnia.
• Sleep studies (polysomnography) are useful for assessing obstructive sleep apnoea as well as some types of parasomnias (encompass a range of neurological conditions including periodic limb movements, restless legs, sleep talking, sleep walking, sleep terrors, bruxism (or teeth grinding)).

Management

Treatment of secondary insomnia (where a cause is identified) is directed at the underlying condition, but advice about non-pharmacological techniques for primary insomnia is often also beneficial.

Non-pharmacological treatments

• Sleep hygiene advice and stimulus control therapy (see Figure 64).
• Cognitive behavioural therapy (CBT): the aim is to change the incorrect beliefs and attitudes regarding sleep which may worsen insomnia.
• Relaxation therapy: as well as massage and a warm bath.
• Sleep restriction: restricting the time spent in bed to the actual time spent sleeping, so rather than lying in bed for 8 hours but only sleeping for 6, patients are advised to only spend 6 hours in bed. In practice this usually means going to bed later.
• Exercise, but not in the few hours before bedtime, may be beneficial in some patients.

Pharmacological treatments

Hypnotics: the use of hypnotic drugs, such as benzodiazepines and z-drugs, to treat insomnia has been problematic. They can be associated with tolerance and addiction; abuse and black market selling; missed diagnoses of depression and anxiety; withdrawal effects and rebound insomnia; adverse effects, such as falls; and overdose. Despite these problems, hypnotic drugs are still used for insomnia. In the short term, they decrease sleep latency (time taken to go to sleep) and increase total sleep time. However, psychological and behavioural approaches offer the same or better short-term improvements compared with hypnotic drugs, but have ongoing benefits which also improve with time.

Hypnotic drugs should only be given after careful assessment, education and appropriate non-drug measures have proved insufficient. Patients should be told of risks of dependence and advised to take them only for very short periods (e.g. for no more than three consecutive nights). Patients should be warned that they need to be very cautious about driving the day after taking any hypnotic. To minimise residual next-day sedative effects, a short-acting drug, given in the lowest effective dose, is preferable to a longer acting drug (see Box 64.2).

Many long-term users of benzodiazepine hypnotics are able to reduce or stop their use of these medications, with benefit to their health and without detriment to their sleep, if given simple advice and support during dose tapering.

Melatonin is secreted by the pineal gland in darkness, signalling sleep onset. It may be used in the short term to treat circadian rhythm sleep disorders, jet lag and shift work.

Sedating antidepressants such as amitriptyline, doxepin and trazodone may be useful in patients who have insomnia and depression. They can cause daytime sedation, have anticholinergic side effects and toxicity in overdose.

Antihistamines: sedating antihistamines, such as promethazine, may have a minimal effect in inducing sleep. In some patients they may cause increased agitation.

(a) **Epipen** showing instructions on side

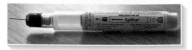

(c) **Medic Alert bracelet** (with permission from Medic Alert UK)

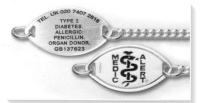

(b) Nasal polyposis

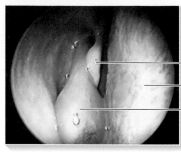

- Middle turbinate
- Septum
- Nasal polyp arising from the middle meatus

(d) Skin prick allergy testing

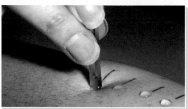

Box 65.1   Advice to patients with rhinitis – allergen exposure reduction tips

Dust mites	Animal dander from pets	Fungal spores/moulds
Use wood or hard wood floors, not carpets	Keep pets outdoors as much as possible	Keep windows closed to reduce entry to house
Use blinds not curtains	Wash your pets every 2 weeks	Use dehumidifier to reduce moisture in air
Vacuum cleaner with HEPA filter	Install HEPA filter at home	Install HEPA filter
Use synthetic pillows and duvets	If your pet is indoors; keep it in the same room without any carpets	Check around water pipes, radiators, boilers and A/C units. Use fungicidal sprays
Dust surfaces using damp cloth	Castrate male cats/dogs	Use hard vinyl/wooden floors

Box 65.2   Warning – drug induced rebound nasal congestion

Many nasal decongestants can be bought over the counter all over the world. Be careful with prolonged use of nasal decongestants (more than 5-7 days), as they contain substances which induce rebound congestion (e.g. pseudoephedrine, xylometazoline etc), and can make symptoms worse

Box 65.3   Differential diagnosis of anaphylaxis

- **Life-threatening:**
  - septic shock: look for petichial/purpuric rash
  - severe asthma: especially in children
- **Non-life threatening:**
  - vasovagal (fainting spell)
  - breath holding episode in a child
  - idiopathic urticarial or angio-oedema

Box 65.5   Long term management of patient with history of anaphylaxis

- Refer the patient to an allergy specialist
- Prescribe and educate patient on self-use of the EpiPen (0.3 ml of 1:1000 for adults) & (0.3 ml of 1:2000 for children aged >12 years)
- Encourage Medic Alert bracelet endorsed by a doctor

Box 65.4

How might anaphylaxis present?	How to manage acute anaphylaxis	
▶ Minutes to hours after exposure to allergen	Call for help. Start resuscitation (remember ABCDE)	IMMEDIATELY
▶ Itchiness with blotchy rash all over body	Provide high flow oxygen (>10 L/min)	
▶ Swelling of the face, eyes, lips, tongue, throat and upper airways	Lie patient flat – raise legs if possible	
▶ Sensation of impending doom	Administer adrenaline intramuscularly to anterolateral aspect of thigh	
▶ Feeling of sickness and abdominal cramps	**Adult:** Adrenaline 0.5 ml of 1:1000 **Pediatrics:** >12 years: 0.5 ml of 1:1000 >6–12 years: 0.3 ml of 1:1000 <6 years: 0.15 ml of 1:1000	
▶ Reddening of face, speeding of heart rate, drop in blood pressure that can cause fainting or collapse – due to arterial dilatation	After help has arrived begin: • Fluid replacement • Chlorphenamine • Hydrocortisone • Monitor O_2 saturation, blood pressure and ECG • Transfer patient to hospital	AFTER
▶ Difficulty breathing, wheezing sounds due to airway obstruction & swelling of the throat		

General Practice at a Glance, First Edition. Paul Booton, Carol Cooper, Graham Easton, and Margaret Harper.

GPs see many allergy-related disorders, including asthma, rhinitis, conjunctivitis, eczema (particularly in young children), occupational asthma and food intolerance. Rarely, a GP may be faced with a patient with life threatening asthma or anaphylaxis and should know how to recognise and manage this.

Type 1 immunoglobulin E (IgE) mediated response accounts for the majority of these.

Hay fever (seasonal allergic rhinitis)

History

Symptoms are caused by sensitivity to various pollens, and thus worst in spring and early summer. Patients typically complain of a runny, itchy or blocked nose, sneezing and watery and itchy red eyes. It is common, self-limiting and recurs yearly at the same season. It tends to run in families and hay fever patients who also have **eczema** and **asthma** are said to be **atopic**.

Examination

In addition to a general ENT examination, look out for evidence of **allergic shiner** – dark shadows around eyes – and **nasal polyps** which indicate that the nasal mucosa is inflamed (seen best when the nasal cavities are inspected with a nasal speculum).

Diagnosis

Hay fever diagnosis is usually clinical but skin prick tests or serum IgE levels may be indicated.

Management

Patients often require symptomatic relief and advice on how to minimise exposure to allergens (see Box 65.1). Oral antihistamines manage both nasal and ocular symptoms effectively. Newer generation antihistamines (e.g. cetirizine or loratadine) are less sedating. They are effective within hours, but not suitable when pregnant or breast-feeding. If antihistamines are insufficient, intranasal corticosteroid sprays or drops, or antihistamine or mast cell stabilising eye drops may be added.

Perennial rhinitis

Perennial rhinitis is caused by hypersensitivity to indoor allergens such as dust mites, fungus spores, pets/animal danders and wood dust, latex and chemicals which may be found in the workplace. Perennial rhinitis symptoms are divided into early and late phase and can happen at any season of the year.

History and examination

Patients describe sneezing, runny or blocked nose, itchiness and irritation of the eyes, nose and throat, and sometimes facial pains and headache immediately after exposure to an allergen. After a few hours typically the nasal mucus and congestion increase, and the patient complains of fatigue, sleepiness and feels unwell. With time, these patients may report total loss of sense of smell and taste.

Examine as for hay fever. Check for nasal polyps.

Diagnosis

Skin prick allergy tests and a blood sample for IgE antibodies may be needed to confirm the diagnosis.

Management

Treat as for hay fever patients but where a single causative allergen has been identified, desensitising **immunotherapy** may be offered. It takes several years to be effective, and is contraindicated in patients with severe asthma or immune suppression.

Food allergies and intolerance

Food allergies are caused by an IgE mediated response. They commonly occur in the first year of life, or when any new food is introduced. Reactions may be mild (e.g. a red rash around the mouth, nausea, vomiting, abdominal discomfort or eczema), but severe life-threatening reactions like angioedema (swelling of lips, tongue and oropharynx ▶) and anaphylaxis can occur rapidly after ingestion. Foods associated with such reactions include milk, eggs, fish and seafood, peanuts and wheat. People may be allergic to more than one single food protein and the reaction usually comes on rapidly.

Food intolerance is not allergic, although immune mechanisms may play a role. It may have metabolic, toxic, psychological or pharmacological causes.

- **Lactose intolerance** is a **metabolic** food intolerance, where patients develop abdominal pain and diarrhoea after ingesting milk due to lactase deficiency which may be genetic (common in Chinese) or temporary following gut infection.
- **Food poisoning** is an example of **toxic** food intolerance, where food contaminated by viruses, bacteria, parasites or toxins causes nausea, vomiting or diarrhoea.
- **Psychological** reactions are known as 'food aversions' where people express an emotional response to a particular food.
- **Pharmacological** reactions from food additives and chemicals (e.g. foods containing monosodium glutamate) may cause headaches, flushing and abdominal pains.

Diagnosis is made after taking a careful history from the patient, including dietary habits. Physical examination should assess for growth (in children) as well signs of atopy. Patients are asked to keep a diet diary and may need skin patch testing or blood tests for IgE antibodies. Patients may benefit from seeing a dietitian who can help with both diagnosis and management of food allergies.

Anaphylaxis

Anaphylaxis is a sudden severe systemic allergic reaction, affecting multiple organs. The number of people who develop severe systemic reactions is estimated at 1–3 per 10,000 in the UK, and is increasing.

It is most often provoked by stinging insects (bees or wasps), foods (such as peanuts, shellfish, eggs and milk) and drugs (such as antibiotics, opioids, NSAIDs, intravenous contrast medium and anaesthetics).

Patients will often have a history of previous sensitivity to an allergen, or have a recent exposure to a drug or vaccination. Box 65.3 lists the differential diagnosis to consider and Box 65.4 outlines the clinical manifestations and immediate management of any patient in whom anaphylaxis is suspected. Box 65.5 lists what a patient can do to manage a future life-threatening attack.

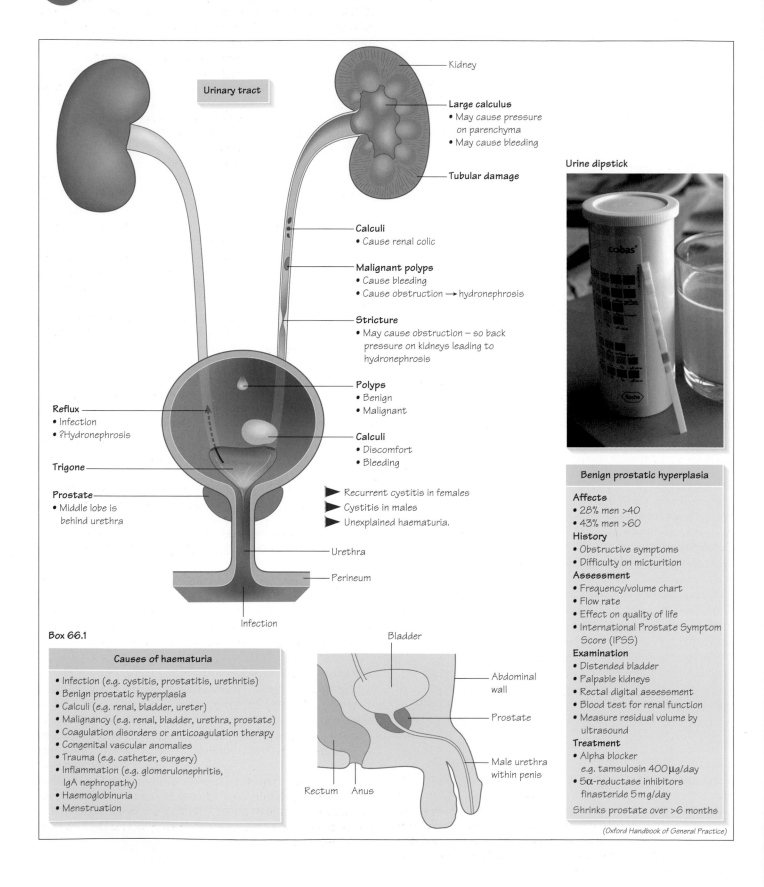

Urinary tract

Kidney

Large calculus
• May cause pressure on parenchyma
• May cause bleeding

Tubular damage

Calculi
• Cause renal colic

Malignant polyps
• Cause bleeding
• Cause obstruction → hydronephrosis

Stricture
• May cause obstruction – so back pressure on kidneys leading to hydronephrosis

Polyps
• Benign
• Malignant

Calculi
• Discomfort
• Bleeding

► Recurrent cystitis in females
► Cystitis in males
► Unexplained haematuria.

Reflux
• Infection
• ?Hydronephrosis

Trigone

Prostate
• Middle lobe is behind urethra

Urethra

Perineum

Infection

Urine dipstick

Benign prostatic hyperplasia

Affects
• 28% men >40
• 43% men >60

History
• Obstructive symptoms
• Difficulty on micturition

Assessment
• Frequency/volume chart
• Flow rate
• Effect on quality of life
• International Prostate Symptom Score (IPSS)

Examination
• Distended bladder
• Palpable kidneys
• Rectal digital assessment
• Blood test for renal function
• Measure residual volume by ultrasound

Treatment
• Alpha blocker e.g. tamsulosin 400 μg/day
• 5α-reductase inhibitors finasteride 5 mg/day

Shrinks prostate over >6 months

Box 66.1

Causes of haematuria

• Infection (e.g. cystitis, prostatitis, urethritis)
• Benign prostatic hyperplasia
• Calculi (e.g. renal, bladder, ureter)
• Malignancy (e.g. renal, bladder, urethra, prostate)
• Coagulation disorders or anticoagulation therapy
• Congenital vascular anomalies
• Trauma (e.g. catheter, surgery)
• Inflammation (e.g. glomerulonephritis, IgA nephropathy)
• Haemoglobinuria
• Menstruation

Bladder

Abdominal wall

Prostate

Male urethra within penis

Rectum   Anus

(Oxford Handbook of General Practice)

Urinary symptoms are very common in general practice. Women are affected more often than men.

Haematuria

Whether the patient notices blood in their urine (macroscopic), or it is picked up on dipstick or microscopy testing (microscopic), haematuria usually needs prompt and full investigation to exclude serious causes (see Box 66.1). In primary care it is helpful to exclude transient causes first such as UTI, menstruation in women or exercise-induced haematuria. Further investigations will be guided by any associated history, but patients may be asymptomatic.

Infection
History

Patients typically give a short history of frequency and burning pain on passing urine and often suprapubic discomfort. It occurs commonly in females because of the shortness of urethra. Recurrent infection must be investigated. In otherwise healthy women presenting with symptoms of both dysuria and urinary frequency, the probability of UTI is >90%. Infection is unusual in men and if confirmed should **always** be investigated. With advancing age the prostate gland will enlarge and may well cause urgency and frequency. This may be accompanied by infection because the obstruction leads to incomplete emptying.

Investigations

The diagnosis is primarily based on symptoms and signs. Presence of white cells (leucocytes) with or without nitrites on urine dipstick suggests infection. In a mid stream urine sample (MSU), large numbers (>100,000 organisms/ml) of organisms are strong evidence of infection but (except in pregnancy) bacteriuria alone is rarely an indication for antibiotic treatment.

Treatment
Lower urinary tract infection

A brief course of antibiotics (e.g. trimethoprim 200 mg b.d. for 3 days) is usually successful. Where the infections are frequent and **an underlying cause has been excluded** many authorities recommend an extended course. Although the common infecting organism is *Escherichia coli*, probably transferred from the perineum, remember that other more pathogenic organisms may be responsible. In debilitated patients or those with instrumentation (e.g. an in situ catheter), *Pseudomonas* is a frequent cause and TB should always be remembered especially in the immunocompromised.

Upper urinary tract infection (e.g. pyelonephritis)

Infection of the kidney may occur, usually by the ascending route. Patients are unwell, with high fever and tenderness in the loin. Dysuria may not be present. Treatment with broad spectrum antibiotics should be started as soon as possible in order to minimise damage to the kidneys.

Renal colic

Renal colic caused by kidney stones affects about 10–20% of men and 3–5% of women. Typically, the pain is severe, colicky, may radiate from loin to groin and may be accompanied by haematuria or infection. **Management** is adequate pain control, usually with i.m. or p.r. NSAIDs. Surgical removal may be necessary. After the acute problem has settled investigate for risk factors to prevent further episodes.

Prostate

With age the prostate grows larger (benign prostatic hyperplasia [BPH]), affecting the quality of life of about one-third of men over 50 years, the numbers increasing markedly with years (see Figure 66). As the median lobe enlarges it pushes on the urethra. Symptoms include increased frequency of micturition, urgency, hesitancy, stopping and starting during urination (intermittency), incomplete bladder emptying, nocturia and a weak urinary stream. The International Prostate Symptom Score (IPSS) is a quick screening tool that assesses these symptoms, and effect on patient's quality of life (see Further reading). Eventually, obstruction of the urethra may cause acute retention of urine.

Prostate cancer is the fourth commonest cancer in the UK. It should be suspected in older men (3/4 are over 65 at diagnosis) with lower urinary tract symptoms or UTI. A rectal examination may reveal a prostatic nodule. PSA is unreliable as a screening test, but useful as part of the assessment of possible cases. The condition is however problematic as it exists very commonly in a more or less benign form (most elderly men will have foci of carcinoma of prostate) which is difficult to differentiate from the much smaller numbers of aggressive, metastatic forms requiring vigorous treatment.

Patients frequently request PSA testing from their GP. This should be approached cautiously as the test has many limitations (see Further reading).

Urinary incontinence

Urinary incontinence is common, especially in women, with 1 in 5 affected over the age of 40 years. Symptoms can range from occasional dribbling to regular flooding of urine, and can cause distress and hygiene problems. The history often points towards one of the three main types and keeping a bladder diary for a few days can be helpful:
- **Stress incontinence** is the most common type. Triggered by coughing, laughing, sneezing or exertion. More common in women who have had several pregnancies, the obese and the elderly.
- **Urge incontinence** (or overactive bladder) is an urgent desire to pass urine, often leaking before reaching the toilet. Cause is often unknown.
- **Mixed incontinence** is a combination of stress and urge incontinence.
- **Overflow incontinence**: for example, prostatic enlargement may lead to outflow obstruction with overflow. Constipation can distort the bladder neck and interfere with micturition.

Investigation in primary care usually includes urine dipstick testing for infection, glucose or haematuria, and examination of rectum and/or vagina to assess strength of pelvic floor or state of prostate. Possibly ultrasound scan to assess residual urine in bladder, and urodynamic studies to assess urinary flow. Management varies depending on the cause. Lifestyle changes such as altering fluid intake or losing weight if overweight can help in some cases. Pelvic floor muscle exercises may help stress incontinence; bladder training may help urge incontinence. Antimuscarinic drugs such as oxybutynin can help urgency and urge incontinence; duloxetine (an inhibitor of serotonin and noradrenaline reuptake) can be used in stress incontinence. Surgery is considered only if conservative measures have failed.

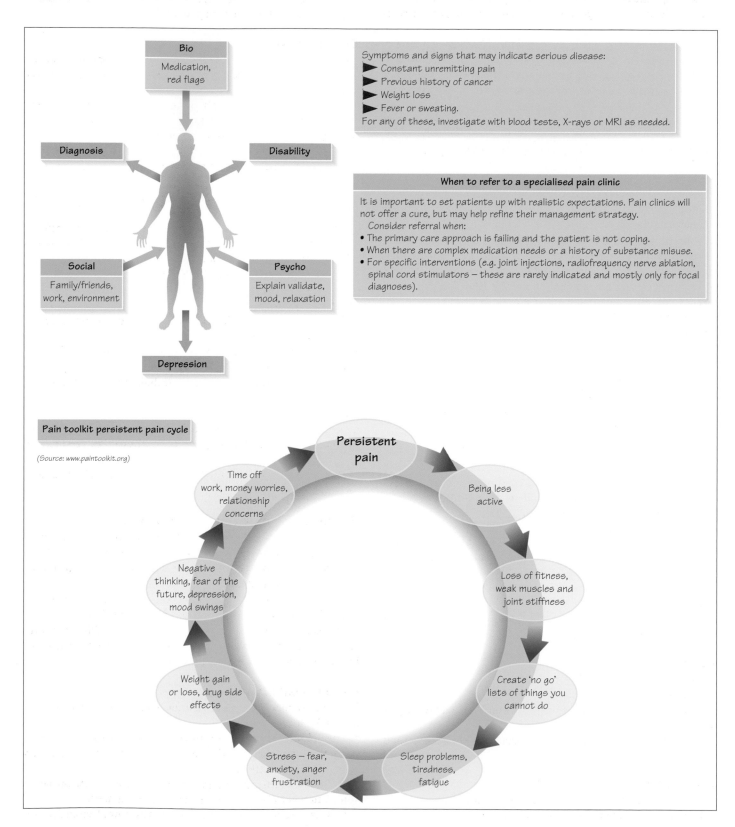

Bio

Medication, red flags

Diagnosis

Disability

Social

Family/friends, work, environment

Psycho

Explain validate, mood, relaxation

Depression

Symptoms and signs that may indicate serious disease:
▶ Constant unremitting pain
▶ Previous history of cancer
▶ Weight loss
▶ Fever or sweating.
For any of these, investigate with blood tests, X-rays or MRI as needed.

When to refer to a specialised pain clinic

It is important to set patients up with realistic expectations. Pain clinics will not offer a cure, but may help refine their management strategy.
  Consider referral when:
• The primary care approach is failing and the patient is not coping.
• When there are complex medication needs or a history of substance misuse.
• For specific interventions (e.g. joint injections, radiofrequency nerve ablation, spinal cord stimulators – these are rarely indicated and mostly only for focal diagnoses).

Pain toolkit persistent pain cycle

(Source: www.paintoolkit.org)

Persistent pain

Being less active

Loss of fitness, weak muscles and joint stiffness

Create 'no go' lists of things you cannot do

Sleep problems, tiredness, fatigue

Stress – fear, anxiety, anger frustration

Weight gain or loss, drug side effects

Negative thinking, fear of the future, depression, mood swings

Time off work, money worries, relationship concerns

General Practice at a Glance, First Edition. Paul Booton, Carol Cooper, Graham Easton, and Margaret Harper.

Chronic pain is defined as pain persisting beyond the normal healing time of tissues (usually taken to be 3 months, but may be longer in specific conditions). The majority of chronic pain is dealt with in primary care, so good management is a core general practice skill.

Chronic pain is not simply acute pain that has gone on longer. Changes occur in the neuronal pathways of the spinal cord and brain (termed 'central sensitisation'), and in the behaviour, emotions and overall function of the individual sufferer. It becomes a long-term 'biopsychosocial' condition.

The prevalence of chronic pain is around 15% of the population. More relevant to primary care is a 7% prevalence of 'significant' chronic pain that requires ongoing regular medical input.

Causes
The most common (70%) are musculoskeletal causes especially:
- Chronic low back pain
- Osteoarthritis
- Myofascial pain syndromes.

In myofascial conditions (e.g. fibromyalgia), pain originates in muscle groups or in connective tissue associated with muscles. This typically results in tight muscles and stiff joints. The pain often spreads into surrounding muscles in a domino effect.

Other causes:
- Chronic pelvic pain
- Chronic abdominal pain
- Neuropathic pain (e.g. diabetic or post-herpetic)
- Chronic headaches
- Postoperative wound pain
- Complex regional pain syndrome (sympathetic nerves start to produce pain signals).

However, any body system can produce chronic pain.

Diagnosis
Prompt diagnosis of chronic pain allows appropriate management. However, making the diagnosis is often difficult as many patients continue to worry that a serious diagnosis like cancer or infection has been missed; these need to be excluded. However, failure to recognise chronic pain for what it is can result in years of multiple unsatisfactory specialist appointments in search of a cure.

Management
Break the problem down into manageable consultations based around assessment and treatment.

Assessment
- Rule out 'red flags' (see Figure 67).
- Consider alternative diagnoses.
- Explore the duration, nature of the pain and any aggravating or relieving factors.
- Evaluate the impact of pain – especially depression and disability.

Treatment
- Rehabilitative approach aims to maximise function
- Biopsychosocial management approach
- Raise realistic expectations – a cure is unlikely.

The biopsychosocial approach
As the experience of chronic pain is influenced by biological, emotional and behavioural factors, it is important to consider a holistic approach to treatment covering all of these areas.

Biological therapy
Analgesics help, but only around one-third of patients gain up to 50% reduction in pain, so **medications are only part of the strategy.**

Consider increasing strength of analgesic medications or medication combinations: paracetamol/NSAIDs → weak opiates → medium potency opiates → strong opiates.

Tips for medication:
- Agree with patient that aim of medication is improved function, not necessarily pain relief.
- Prescribe long-acting medications to avoid an on–off analgesic effect.
- Regular review is essential. Consider benefits and side effects, and co-prescribe or stop medication as needed. Avoid escalation of dose. Once there is some functional benefit, stick with that dose.
- Is there neuropathic pain? See NICE guidance.

Psychological therapy
- Explain the nature of chronic pain. Help your patient to accept the diagnosis and move on.
- Acknowledge and validate your patient's limitations.
- Treat depression.
- Encourage relaxation, and formal techniques to assist this.

Social therapy
Consider family or work place factors that may contribute to sustained unhelpful behaviour (e.g. ongoing disputes, relationship issues).

Aim to maximise functional ability – occupational, social and physical.

'Boom and bust' versus 'base and pace'
'Boom and bust' behaviour is very common in chronic pain patients (see Figure 67). Persistent frustration → overactivity → flare of pain → prolonged reactive immobility → a downward spiral of functional ability.

A better alternative is 'base and pace'. The patient establishes a level of any activity that he or she can comfortably achieve for a manageable period of time (baseline) and then practises this level regularly. He or she gradually increases the baseline to achieve an improved functional capacity over time.

Management of flare-ups
These are an inevitable part of chronic pain, so it is useful to have a plan for flare-ups:
- Save additional medication to use only on especially bad days (i.e. do not use maximum dose of all medication all the time, step down after flare settled).
- Use non-drug treatments (e.g. transcutaneous electrical nerve stimulation [TENS], heat-ice, relaxation techniques).

It is also useful to explore the reason 'why now'. Search for new sources of stress.

Further reading and resources

General

British National Formulary Updated in print every 6 months. Pharmaceutical Press [Up-to-date, practical guidance on prescribing, dispensing and administering medicines. Useful overviews of the drug management of common conditions.]

GP Notebook. www.gpnotebook.co.uk [A concise synopsis of the entire field of clinical medicine focused on the needs of the GP.]

Healthtalkonline. www.healthtalkonline.org [Healthtalkonline and its sister website, Youthhealthtalk, let you share in more than 2000 people's experiences of over 60 health-related conditions and illnesses. You can watch video or listen to audio clips of the interviews, read about people's experiences if you prefer and find reliable information about specific conditions, treatment choices and support.]

Hopcroft, K. & Forte V. (2010) *Symptom Sorter*, 4th edition. Radcliffe Publishing Ltd.

Moulton, L. (2007) *The Naked Consultation*. Radcliffe Publishing. [A practical guide to consultation skills for any health professional working in primary care.]

Neighbour, R. (2004) *The Inner Consultation: How to Develop an Effective and Intuitive Consulting Style*, 2nd edition. Radcliffe Publishing. [An influential guide to consulting style, with everyday clinical examples.]

Patient UK. www.patient.co.uk [Evidence based information leaflets on a wide range of medical and health topics. The PatientPlus section is likely to be of particular interest to health professionals.]

Simon, C., Everitt, H. & van Dorp, F. (2009) *Oxford Handbook of General Practice*, 3rd edition. OUP, Oxford. [Comprehensive handbook of general practice, with hands-on advice and information.]

Essence of general practice
Continuity of care
General Medical Council. Good Medical Practice: Working in teams: http://www.gmc-uk.org/guidance/good_medical_practice/working_with_colleagues_working_in_teams.asp

Health Development Agency, NICE. (2003) *Teamworking guide for primary healthcare*. http://www.nice.org.uk/nicemedia/documents/teamworking_guide.pdf

Why do patients consult?
British Thoracic Society (2006) Recommendations for the management of cough in adults. *Thorax* 61 (suppl): i1–i24.

Greenhalgh, T., Helman, C. & Chowdhury, M. (1998) Health beliefs and folk models of diabetes in British Bangladeshis: a qualitative study. *BMJ* 316 (7136): 978–83.

Hannay, D.R. (1978) Symptom prevalence in the community. *J R Coll Gen Pract* 28 (193): 492–9.

Pendleton, D. (1984) *The Consultation: an approach to learning and teaching*. Oxford Medical Publications, Oxford: pp.30–44.

Saracci, R. (1997) The World Health Organization needs to reconsider its definition of health. *BMJ* 314 (7091): 1409–10.

Scambler, G. (2008) *Sociology as Applied to Medicine*, 6th edition. Saunders Ltd.

Preventive medicine
Healthtalkonline: cervical screening. http://www.healthtalkonline.org/cancer/Cervical_Screening

UK National Screening Committee. www.screening.nhs.uk

Wilson, J.M.G. & Jungner, G. (1968) *Principles and Practice of Screening for Disease*. Public Health Paper No 34. WHO, Geneva.

Significant event analysis, audit and research
http://www.patient.co.uk/doctor/Significant-Event-Audit-(SEA).htm

Pringle, M. et al. (1995) *Significant Event Auditing*. Occasional Paper 70. RCGP, London.

Communication between primary and secondary care
Scottish Intercollegiate Guidelines Network (SIGN). (1998) Report on a recommended referral document. SIGN publication no. 31. http://www.sign.ac.uk/guidelines/fulltext/31/index.html [Accessed November 2011]

Scottish Intercollegiate Guidelines Network (SIGN). (2003) The Immediate Discharge Document. SIGN publication no. 65. http://www.sign.ac.uk/guidelines/fulltext/65/index.html [Accessed November 2011]

Stephenson, A. (2011) *A Textbook of General Practice*, 3rd edition. Hodder Arnold, London.

Domestic abuse
HSC 200/007: No secrets: guidance on developing multi-agency policies and procedures to protect vulnerable adults from abuse. Available at: http://www.dh.gov.uk/en/Publicationsandstatistics/Publications/PublicationsPolicyAndGuidance/DH_4008486

The Children's Act 2004. www.legislation.gov.uk

Working Together to Safeguard Children: a guide to inter-agency working to safeguard and promote the welfare of children. (2010) www.education.gov.uk/publications

Child health
Atkinson, M. & Hollis, C. (2010) NICE guideline: attention deficit hyperactivity disorder. *Arch Dis Child Educ Pract Ed* 95 (1): 24–7.

Baumer J.H. (2009) Guideline review: management of invasive meningococcal disease, SIGN. *Arch Dis Child Educ Pract Ed* 94 (2): 46–9.

BNF for Children (BMJ Group). http://www.medicinescomplete.com/mc/bnfc/current/

British Thoracic Society and Scottish Intercollegiate Guidelines Network (SIGN). (2011) British guidelines on the management of asthma: 2008 Review.

Department of Health (2009) Healthy child programme: pregnancy and the first five years of life. http://www.dh.gov.

General Practice at a Glance, First Edition. Paul Booton, Carol Cooper, Graham Easton, and Margaret Harper.

uk/en/Publicationsandstatistics/Publications/
PublicationsPolicyAndGuidance/DH_107563

Foster, H.E., Boyd, D. & Jandial, S. (2008) Growing pains: a practical guide for primary care. *Rep Rheum Dis* (1): 1–6.

Foster, H.E. & Jandial, S. (2008) pGALs: a screening examination of the musculo-skeletal system in school-aged children. *Rep Rheum Dis* 5:7–78.

Halpin, L.J., Anderson, C.L. & Corriette, N. (2010) Stridor in children. *BMJ* 340: 1091–146.

Horridge, K.A. (2011) Assessment and investigation of the child with disordered development. *Arch Dis Child Educ Pract Ed* 96: 9–20.

Katona, C. & Robertson, M. (2009) *Psychiatry at a Glance*, 2nd edition. Blackwell.

Lissauer, T. & Clayton, G. (2007) *Illustrated Textbook of Paediatrics*, 3rd edition. Mosby.

Miall, L., Rudolf, M. & Levene, M. (2007) *Paediatrics at a Glance*, 2nd edition. Wiley-Blackwell.

National Institute for Health and Clinical Excellence (NICE). (2007) Feverish illness in children: Assessment and initial management in children younger than 5 years. www.nice.org.uk/guideline/CG47

National Institute for Health and Clinical Excellence (NICE). (2007) Urinary tract infection in children; www.nice.org.uk/guideline/CG54

National Institute for Health and Clinical Excellence (NICE). (2010) Constipation in children and young people. www.nice.org.uk/CG99

Pearce, S.H.S. & Cheetham, T.D. (2010) Diagnosis and management of vitamin D deficiency. *BMJ* 340: 142–7.

Polnay, L., Hampshire, M. & Lakhanpaul, M. (2007) *Manual of Paediatrics*. Churchill Livingstone.

Salisbury, D., Ramsay, M. & Noakes, K. (eds) (2006) *Immunization Against Infectious Disease*, 3rd edition. Department of Health. Available at: http://www.dh.gov.uk/en/Publicationsandstatistics/Publications/PublicationsPolicyAndGuidance/DH_079917

Yanney, M. & Vyas, H. (2008) The treatment of bronchiolitis. *Arch Dis Child* 93: 793–8.

Sexual health

British Association of Sexual Health. www.bashh.org/guidelines

National Institute for Health and Clinical Excellence (NICE). (2004) *CG11 Fertility: assessment and treatment for people with fertility problems.* NICE, London. www.nice.org.uk/CG011

NHS Choices: Sexual Health. http://www.nhs.uk/Livewell/Sexualhealthtopics/Pages/Sexual-health-hub.aspx

Patient.co.uk. Subfertility Investigations and Management. http://www.patient.co.uk/doctor/Subfertility-Investigations-and-Management.htm

Patient UK Information Leaflet on Erectile Dysfunction. http://www.patient.co.uk/health/Erectile-Dysfunction-%28Impotence%29.htm

Women's health

Azziz, R. (2006) Diagnosis of polycystic ovarian syndrome: The Rotterdam Criteria are premature. *J Clin Endocrinol Metab* 91 (3): 781–5.

Breast Cancer Care. www.breastcancercare.org.uk

Centre for Maternal and Child Enquiries (CMACE)/Royal College of Obstetricians and Gynaecologists (RCOG) Joint Guideline (2010) Management of women with obesity in pregnancy. http://www.nepho.org.uk/uploads/doc/vid_6151_CMACE-RCOG%20guideline%20of%20mgmt%20of%20obesity%20in%20pregnancy.pdf *or* http://www.rcog.org.uk/files/rcog-corp/CMACERCOGJointGuidelineManagementWomenObesityPregnancya.pdf

Ellis, H., Calne, R. & Watson, C. (2011) *Lecture Notes: General Surgery*, 12th edition. Wiley-Blackwell, Oxford.

Holder, A. Dysmenorrhea in emergency medicine: treatment and management. http://emedicine.medscape.com/article/795677-treatment

Hughes' Syndrome Foundation. www.hughes-syndrome.org

National Institute for Health and Clinical Excellence (NICE). (2008) *Diabetes in pregnancy. Clinical guidelines.* NICE, London. www.nice.org.uk/CG63

National Institute for Health and Clinical Excellence (NICE). (2008) *Routine care for the healthy pregnant woman. Clinical guidelines.* NICE, London. www.nice.org.uk/CG62

National Institute for Health and Clinical Excellence (NICE). (2010) *The management of hypertensive disorders during pregnancy. Clinical guidelines.* NICE, London. www.nice.org.uk/guidance/CG107

Norwitz, E.R. & Schorge, J.O. (2010) *Obstetrics and Gynaecology at a Glance*, 3rd edition. Wiley-Blackwell.

Royal College of Obstetricians and Gynaecologists. Women's health. http://www.rcog.org.uk/womens-health

Care of the elderly

Alzheimer's Society. www.alzheimersresearchuk.org

National Institute for Health and Clinical Excellence (NICE). (2006, amended March 2011) Dementia. www.nice.org.uk/CG42

Cardiovascular problems

Healthtalkonline. http://www.healthtalkonline.org/heart_disease/Heart_Attack/Topic/1981/

Healthtalkonline. www.healthtalkonline.org/Nerves_and_brain/Stroke [People who have had a stroke tell of their experiences.]

Hopcroft, K. & Forte V. (2007) *Symptom Sorter*, 3rd edition. Radcliffe Publishing.

National Institute for Health and Clinical Excellence (NICE) (2008) *Lipid modification: cardiovascular risk assessment and the modification of blood lipids for the primary and secondary prevention of cardiovascular disease.* London. NICE. http://www.nice.org.uk/CG67

National Institute for Health and Clinical Excellence (NICE) (2008) *Diagnosis and initial management of acute stroke and transient ischaemic attack (TIA).* NICE, London. http://www.nice.org.uk/CG68

National Institute for Health and Clinical Excellence (2011) *Hypertension: clinical management of primary hypertension in adults*, London. NICE. http://guidance.nice.org.uk/CG127

Patient UK: Abdominal aortic aneurysm [patient information leaflet]. http://www.patient.co.uk/health/Aortic-Aneurysm-%28Abdominal%29.htm

Patient UK: Peripheral vascular disease. http://www.patient.co.uk/showdoc/40024580

Schroeder, K. (2008) Assessment of chest pain in primary care. *InnovAiT* 1(1): 8–14.

Stroke Association. www.stroke.org.uk/

Respiratory problems

Zwar, N., Richmond, R., Borland, R., Peters, M., Litt, J., Bell, J., Caldwell, B. & Ferretter, I. (2011) *Supporting smoking cessation: a guide for health professionals*. Melbourne, The Royal Australian College of General Practitioners.

Gastrointestinal problems

Delaney, B. (2001) 10-minute consultation: dyspepsia. *BMJ* 322: 776.

Health Protection Agency: Gastrointestinal disease. http://www.hpa.org.uk/Topics/InfectiousDiseases/InfectionsAZ/GastrointestinalDisease/

Healthtalkonline: colorectal cancer. http://www.healthtalkonline.org/Cancer/Colorectal_Cancer [People who have had colorectal cancer tell of their experiences.]

Jones, R. & Rubin, G. (2009) Diagnosis in general practice : acute diarrhoea in adults. *BMJ* 338.

National Institute for Health and Clinical Excellence (NICE) (2004) *Dyspepsia: managing dyspepsia in adults in primary care*. NICE, London. http://www.nice.org.uk/CG017

National Institute for Health and Clinical Excellence (NICE) (2005) *Referral for suspected cancer*. NICE, London. http://www.nice.org.uk/CG27

NHS Choices: Diarrhoea. http://www.nhs.uk/conditions/diarrhoea/Pages/Introduction.aspx

NHS Choices: Gastroenteritis. http://www.nhs.uk/conditions/gastroenteritis/Pages/Introduction.aspx

NHS National Prescribing Centre (2006) Management of dyspepsia in primary care. MeRec briefing issue No 32. http://www.npc.nhs.uk/merec/therap/dysp/resources/merec_briefing_no32.pdf

Patient UK: Gallstones and cholecystitis. http://www.patient.co.uk/doctor/Gallstones-and-Cholecystitis.htm

Patient UK: Information leaflets on IBS, IBD, colorectal cancer, coeliac disease.

Musculoskeletal problems

National Institute for Health and Clinical Excellence (NICE) (2009) *Low back pain*. NICE, London. http://guidance.nice.org.uk/CG88

Mallen, C.D. & Porcheret, M. (2007) 10 minute consultation: chronic knee pain. *BMJ* 335, 303.

Ottawa rules for X-rays of ankle, foot and knee. http://www.gp-training.net/rheum/ottawa.htm

Pearce, S.H.S. & Cheetham, T.D. (2010) Diagnosis and management of vitamin D deficiency. *BMJ* 340: 142–7.

Eyes and ENT

British National Formulary. Section on antibacterial drugs

Centor, R.M., Witherspoon, J.M., Dalton, H.P., Brody, C.E. & Link, K. (1981) The diagnosis of strep throat in adults in the emergency room. *Med Decis Making* 1 (3): 239–46.

Clinical Knowledge Summaries (2009) Acute otitis media. http://www.cks.nhs.uk/otitis_media_acute/management/scenario_acute_otitis_media_initial_presentation

Khaw, P.T., Shaw, P. & Elkington, A.R. (2004) *ABC of Eyes*, 4th edition. Wiley-Blackwell.

Lous, J., Burton, M.J., Felding, J.U., Oveson, T., Rovers, M.M. & Williamson, I. (2005) Grommets (ventilation tunbes) for hearing loss associated with otitis media with effusion in children. *Cochrane Database Syst Rev* 25 (1): CD001801.

McDonald, S., Langton Hewer, C.D. & Nunez D.A. (2008) Grommets (ventilation tubes) for recurrent acute otitis media in children. *Cochrane Database Syst Rev* 8 (4): CD004741.

National Institute for Health and Clinical Excellence (NICE). (2008) *Self-limiting respiratory tract infections in adults and children in primary care*. NICE, London. http://www.nice.org.uk/CG69

Olver, J. & Cassidy, L. (2005) *Ophthalmology at a Glance*. Wiley-Blackwell.

Patient UK: Acute otitis media. http://www.patient.co.uk/doctor/Acute-Otitis-Media.htm

Patient UK: Common cold. http://www.patient.co.uk/health/Common-Cold.htm

Patient UK: Otitis media with effusion. http://www.patient.co.uk/doctor/Fluid-in-the-Middle-Ear-and-Glue-Ear.htm

Patient UK: Sore throat. http://www.patient.co.uk/health/Sore-Throat.htm

Mental health

Babor, T.F., Higgins-Biddle, J.C. & Saunders, J.B. *The Alcohol Use Disorders Identification Test: guidelines for use in primary care*, 2nd edition. World Health Organization, Department of Mental Health and Substance Dependence. http://whqlibdoc.who.int/hq/2001/who_msd_msb_01.6a.pdf

Healthtalkonline: depression. http://www.healthtalkonline.org/mental_health/Depression

Hodgson, R., Alwyn, T., John, B., Thom, B. & Smith, A. (2002) The FAST Alcohol Screening Test. *Alcohol Alcohol* 37 (1): 61–6.

Institute of Health & Society. (2006) *Screening Tools for Alcohol Related Risk*. Newcastle University. http://www.ncl.ac.uk/ihs/engagement/documents/screeningtools.pdf

Morgan, J.F., Reid, F. & Lacy, J.H. (1999) The Scoff Questionnaire: Assessment of a new screening tool for eating disorders. *BMJ* 319: 1467–8.

Morris, J. & Twaddle, S. (2007) Anorexia nervosa. *BMJ* 334: 894–8.

National Institute for Health and Clinical Excellence (NICE) (2004) *Eating Disorders*. NICE, London. http://www.nice.org.uk/CG009NICEguideline

National Institute for Health and Clinical Excellence (NICE) (2009) *Depression: the treatment and management of depression in adults (update)*. NICE, London. http://www.nice.org.uk/CG90

Simon, C., Everitt, H. & Kendrick, T. (2005) *Oxford Handbook of General Practice*, 2nd edition. Oxford University Press.

Treasure, J. (2009) *A Guide to the Medical Assessment of Eating Disorders*. Kings College. London.

Other common conditions

Falloon, K., Arroll, B., Elley, C.R. & Fernando, A. (2011) Clinical Review: the assessment and management of insomnia in primary care. *BMJ* 342: d2899.

GP Notebook: insomnia. http://www.gpnotebook.co.uk/simplepage.cfm?ID=1483407369

Moore, P. (2012) *The Pain Toolkit [Podcast/video]*, http://www.piperhub.com/2012/06/the-pain-toolkit-pete-moore/

Example of a sleep diary
http://www.nhs.uk/Livewell/insomnia/Documents/sleepdiary.pdf

Food intolerance and food allergy
Food intolerance and allergy. http://www.patient.co.uk/doctor/Food-Intolerance-and-Food-Allergy.htm

Antihistamines. http://www.patient.co.uk/doctor/Antihistamines.htm

Insect stings and bites. http://www.patient.co.uk/health/Insect-Stings-and-Bites.htm

Urinary problems
International Prostate Symptom Score (IPSS)

Barry, M.J., Fowler, F.J. Jr, O'Leary, M.P., et al. (1992) The American Urological Association symptom index for benign prostatic hyperplasia. The Measurement Committee of the American Urological Association. *J Urol* 148 (5): 1549–57; discussion 1564. [abstract]

Free web link for International Prostate Symptom Score (IPSS). http://www.prostate-cancer.co.uk/ipss.htm

NHS Prostate Cancer Risk Management Programme. Patient Information Leaflet. http://www.cancerscreening.nhs.uk/prostate/prostate-patient-info-sheet.pdf

Chronic pain
Guidance on strong opiate prescribing. http://www.britishpainsociety.org/book_opioid_main.pdf

National Institute for Health and Clinical Excellence (NICE) (2010) *Neuropathic pain: pharmacological management*. NICE, London. http://www.nice.org.uk/CG96

Excellent sources of patient information and self-help at www.paintoolkit.org, or www.paininfo.org.uk

Chronic obstructive pulmonary disease
National Institute for Health and Clinical Excellence (NICE) (2010) *Management of chronic obstructive pulmonary disease in adults in primary and secondary care (partial update)*. NICE, London. http://guidance.nice.org.uk/CG101/QuickRefGuide/pdf/English

Index

General Practice at a Glance, First Edition. Paul Booton, Carol Cooper, Graham Easton, and Margaret Harper.
© 2013 Paul Booton, Carol Cooper, Graham Easton, and Margaret Harper. Published 2013 by Blackwell Publishing Ltd.

Keep up with critical fields

Would you like to receive up-to-date information on our books, journals and databases in the areas that interest you, direct to your mailbox?

Join the **Wiley e-mail service** - a convenient way to receive updates and exclusive discount offers on products from us.

Simply visit www.wiley.com/email and register online

We won't bombard you with emails and we'll only email you with information that's relevant to you. We will ALWAYS respect your e-mail privacy and NEVER sell, rent, or exchange your e-mail address to any outside company. Full details on our privacy policy can be found online.

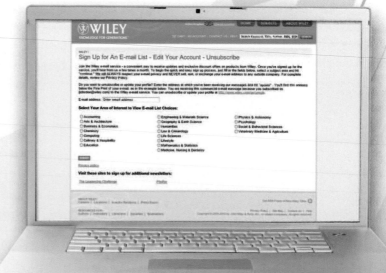

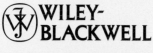

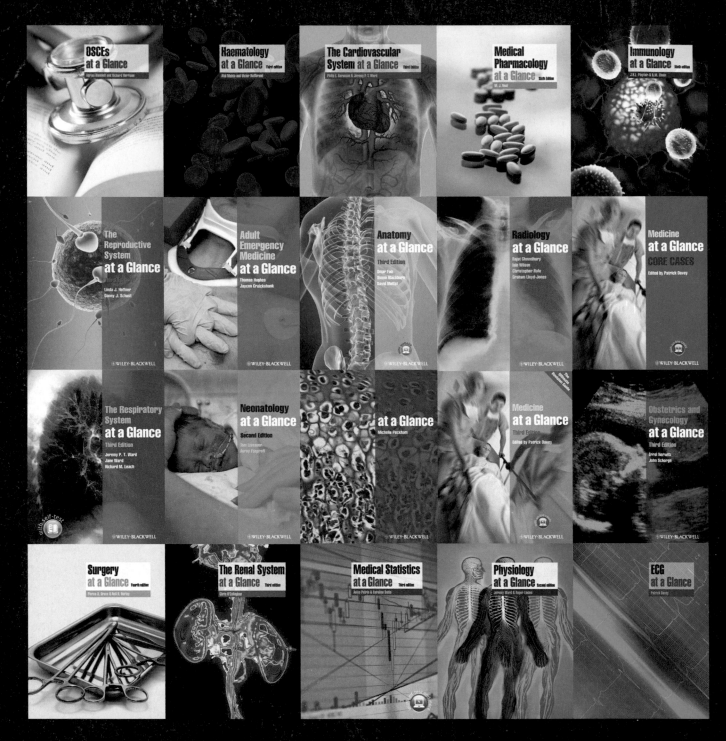
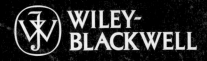